The Library, Ed & Trg Centre   KTW
Tunbridge Wells Hospital
Tonbridge Rd, PEMBURY
Kent TN2 4QJ
01892 635884 and 635489

The Library, Ed & Trg Centre KTW
Tunbridge Wells Hospital
Tonbridge Rd, PEMBURY
Kent TN2 4QJ
01892 635884 and 635489

Current Topics in Otolaryngology—Head and Neck Surgery

Lasers in Otorhinolaryngology

Editor

Karl-Bernd Huettenbrink, M.D.
Professor and Director
Department of Otorhinolaryngology
University Hospital Cologne
Cologne, Germany

With contributions by
Petra Ambrosch, Wolfgang Bergler, H.-P. Berlien, Hans E. Eckel, Ingrid Hackert, Sergije Jovanovic, Burkard M. Lippert, Christian Offergeld, Carsten M. Philipp, Thomas Zahnert

233 illustrations
 12 tables

Thieme
Stuttgart · New York

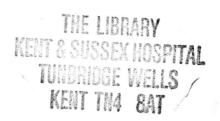

Library of Congress Cataloging-in-Publication Data
is available from the publisher

This book is an authorized translation of the German edi-
tion published and copyrighted 2003 by Georg Thieme
Verlag, Stuttgart, Germany. Title of the German edition:
Referateband 74. Jahresversammlung der Deutschen Ge-
sellschaft für Hals-Nasen-Ohren-Heilkunde, Kopf- und
Hals-Chirurgie. Herausgeber Karl-Bernd Hüttenbrink

Translator: Terry C. Telger, Fort Worth, TX, USA

Important note: Medicine is an ever-changing science undergoing continual development. Research and clinical experience are continually expanding our knowledge, in particular our knowledge of proper treatment and drug therapy. Insofar as this book mentions any dosage or application, readers may rest assured that the authors, editors, and
publishers have made every effort to ensure that such references are in accordance with **the state of knowledge at
the time of production of the book.**

Nevertheless, this does not involve, imply, or express any
guarantee or responsibility on the part of the publishers in
respect to any dosage instructions and forms of applications stated in the book. **Every user is requested to examine carefully** the manufacturers' leaflets accompanying
each drug and to check, if necessary in consultation with a
physician or specialist, whether the dosage schedules mentioned therein or the contraindications stated by the manufacturers differ from the statements made in the present
book. Such examination is particularly important with
drugs that are either rarely used or have been newly released on the market. Every dosage schedule or every form
of application used is entirely at the user's own risk and
responsibility. The authors and publishers request every
user to report to the publishers any discrepancies or inac-
curacies noticed. If errors in this work are found after publication, errata will be posted at www.thieme.com on the
product description page.

Some of the product names, patents, and registered designs referred to in this book are in fact registered trade-
marks or proprietary names even though specific reference
to this fact is not always made in the text. Therefore, the
appearance of a name without designation as proprietary
is not to be construed as a representation by the publisher
that it is in the public domain.

© 2005 Georg Thieme Verlag,
Rüdigerstrasse 14, 70469 Stuttgart, Germany
http://www.thieme.de
Thieme New York, 333 Seventh Avenue,
New York, NY 10001 USA
http://www.thieme.com

Typesetting by Satzpunkt Ewert GmbH, Bayreuth
Printed in Germany by Grammlich, Pliezhausen

ISBN 3-13-140251-2 (GTV)
ISBN 1-58890-330-3 (TNY)   1 2 3 4 5

Preface

Since lasers were first used more than 40 years ago and introduced into head and neck surgery soon after during the 1970s, this new technology has found applications in virtually all areas of the ear, nose, and throat specialty. In endolaryngeal surgery of the larynx, the use of lasers has sparked the development of new treatment options that have overcome initial resistance and gained worldwide acceptance. Also, reports are being published daily on other potential applications of lasers in otorhinolaryngology. This has led to the emergence of new therapeutic concepts, some of which appear more feasible than others.

Thus time has come to publish a comprehensive review, drawn from the proceedings of the German Society of Otorhinolaryngology, of the possible applications of lasers in our specialty. Prominent experts have contributed to the chapters in this book, sharing their wealth of experience of laser applications in the head and neck region.

The first chapter provides a detailed review of the physical principles of laser and the advantages and disadvantages of different types of laser energy. Special attention has been given to issues of laser safety and the practical precautions that must be taken during laser use.

Lasers in otology have gone beyond the experimental stage and have become an established clinical tool. This is illustrated in Chapter 2 with examples dealing with stapes surgery and the tympanic membrane. Rhinology promises to become a new, successful field for laser application. Particularly good results are being achieved in turbinate reductions and polyp surgery as discussed in Chapter 3. Lasers are also finding new applications in the oropharynx, including the treatment of snoring disorders and tonsillar hyperplasia and these are covered in Chapter 4.

Lasers have been most widely used in the larynx, trachea, and hypopharynx, providing a "bloodless" cutting instrument that not only is a welcome aid in the transoral surgery of benign disorders but has also revolutionized the treatment strategies for malignant lesions. Chapter 5 offers a comprehensive account of this successful laser application. The results from the Göttingen school in Chapter 6 offer compelling proof that, owing to the use of laser techniques, the endolaryngeal organ-conserving surgery advocated by Steiner has gained an established role in the treatment of laryngeal and hypopharyngeal cancers in appropriately selected cases.

In both otolaryngology and dermatology the laser is being used for a variety of skin diseases in the head and neck region. As illustrated in Chapter 7, the treatment of hemangiomas with interstitial laser therapy at some centers is providing a particularly impressive example of successful interdisciplinary cooperation.

In addition to using lasers as cutting instruments, the coherent waves emitted by lasers enable researchers to measure extremely tiny movements and vibrations at very low, athermal levels of intensity. This property has opened up new horizons in otologic research, for which laser vibrometry has become the standard measuring tool that may soon provide a new technique for examining patients. Chapter 8 describes the principal laser measuring technologies in use today.

This book thus provides an inventory of the many current therapeutic and diagnostic applications of lasers in otorhinolaryngology. Owing to its unique properties, the laser is certain to find many other uses, and this volume also offers a critical appraisal of these novel applications.

Cologne, 2004   K.-B. Hüttenbrink, M.D., Ph.D.

Contributors

Petra Ambrosch, M.D., Ph.D.
Department of Otorhinolaryngology
Schleswig-Holstein University Hospital
Kiel, Germany

Wolfgang Bergler, M.D., Ph.D.
Department of Otorhinolaryngology
Mannheim University Hospital
Mannheim, Germany

H.-P. Berlien, M.D., Ph.D.
Neukölln Medical Center
Berlin, Germany

Hans E. Eckel, M.D., Ph.D.
Klagenfurt Regional Hospital
Klagenfurt, Austria

Ingrid Hackert, M.D.
Department of Dermatology
Dresden University Hospital
Dresden, Germany

Sergije Jovanovic, M.D., Ph.D.
Department of Otorhinolaryngology
Benjamin Franklin Medical Center
Berlin

Burkard M. Lippert, M.D., Ph.D.
Department of Otorhinolaryngology
Marburg University Hospital
Marburg, Germany

Christian Offergeld, M.D.
Department of Otorhinolaryngology
Dresden University Hospital
Dresden, Germany

Carsten M. Philipp, M.D.
Neukölln Medical Center
Berlin, Germany

Thomas Zahnert, M.D.
Department of Otorhinolaryngology
Dresden University Hospital
Dresden, Germany

Contents

1 Basic Principles of Medical Laser Technology

C. M. Philipp, H.-P. Berlien

■ Contents

■ Abstract

The characteristics of laser light are derived from its properties as part of the electromagnetic spectrum. This chapter systematically explains the tissue effects of laser light as a function of its power and energy density. Standard medical lasers and their delivery systems are described along with typical applications. Laser safety issues are also addressed.

■ Introduction

In many types of laser application, the tissue response can be directly monitored and controlled, while in other types the effects are much more indirect. Thus, it is necessary to know not just the "how" and "where" but, in particular, the "why" to understand medical lasers and use them safely.

We begin, therefore, by reviewing some basic principles of laser physics and the optical properties of tissues. A basic understanding of physical and chemical processes is the foundation for comprehending, critically evaluating, and directing future developments, because "everything depends on the electron."

■ Physical Principles

Laser is light, the term being an acronym for *light amplification by stimulated emission of radiation*. Light occupies one region of the electromagnetic spectrum. Because of the dual nature of light it can behave both as an electromagnetic wave and as a type of particle radiation (photons). Light is classified as a wave or a particle depending on the specific context.

The Electromagnetic Spectrum

Light is a part of the electromagnetic spectrum (Fig. 1.1). The longer its wavelength, the lower its frequency and the lower the energy of the individual photons, since $E = h \times v$.

As the wavelength increases, the waves become less numerous. Thus the terms photon energy, frequency, wave number, wavelength, and color are synonyms for the same property described from different perspectives. The single-photon energy in long waves is so low, it can barely produce any effect on its own. In this case the character of the waves becomes more important, and light is usually described in terms of its wavelength (measured in km, m, cm, mm, μm, or nm). As we approach the range of the wavelengths in visible light region and especially in the ultraviolet (UV) and x-ray regions of the spectrum, the single-photon energy becomes more important. Energy beyond the UV-C range is classified as high-energy ionizing radiation. While it is customary to describe visible light, despite its relatively high single-photon energy, in terms of wavelength (usually in nanometers), radiation in the x-ray part of the spectrum is described almost exclusively in terms of its energy in electron volts (eV).

Energy and Power

On adding together all the single-photon energies in a laser beam, we obtain the total energy of the laser beam in joules. The joule (J) is widely used because it permits comparison of different forms of energy, including the conversion of radiant energy to heat. The joule energy of lasers is frequently measured by aiming the laser beam at an absorber that converts the light energy into thermal energy. But the term "laser beam" also refers to spatial and temporal propagation and velocity (the velocity of light). Thus, the distribution of laser energy within a laser beam can be equated with the corresponding photon density.

When we calculate the energy delivered by a laser beam to a particular spot in 1 second, we obtain the power, $P = J/s$, in watts (W). The laser beam and focal point must be considered as occupying a specific area. From this the concepts of power density (W/m^2) and energy density (J/m^2) are derived when considering the total duration of laser exposure or a single energy pulse.

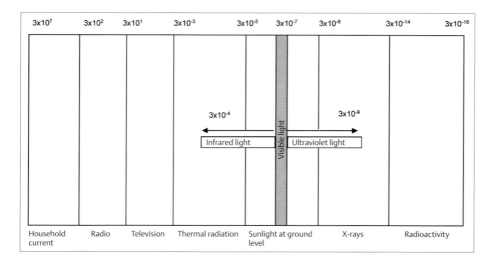

| 3×10^7 | 3×10^2 | 3×10^1 | 3×10^{-3} | 3×10^{-5} | 3×10^{-7} | 3×10^{-8} | 3×10^{-14} | 3×10^{-16} |

3×10^{-4} — Infrared light — Visible light — Ultraviolet light — 3×10^{-9}

| Household current | Radio | Television | Thermal radiation | Sunlight at ground level | X-rays | Radioactivity |

Fig. 1.1 The electromagnetic spectrum.

In medicine, it is customary to depart from the strict International System of Units (SI) when considering the power or energy delivered per cm² or mm² of tissue area, as this makes the numbers easier to handle. Thus pulsed laser beams are measured in joules or millijoules of energy. Beams from continuous-wave (CW) lasers are measured in watts of power, and the output of a CW laser operated in bursts of seconds' to milliseconds' duration is also measured in watts. Intermediate between the pulsed and CW modes are lasers that emit pulses at a very high repetition frequency but a low single-pulse energy ("free-running" mode). The output of these lasers is usually measured as the average power calculated by multiplying the single-pulse energy by the frequency in seconds (1 joule/pulse, 20 Hz = J × 20 pulses/s = 20 watts). Note that 20 watts emitted by a free-running laser may produce an entirely different effect from that produced by 20 watts emitted by a CW laser. Free-running lasers can also emit a salvo of very short bursts, treated as a single-pulse train. The temporal and spatial profiles of energy distribution across the laser beam (mode structure, etc.) and pulse durations will not be discussed here, but detailed information can be found in textbooks of laser physics [1]. The typical operating characteristics of medical lasers are summarized in Table 1.1.

Table 1.1 Units of power and of energy parameters of medical lasers

Term	CW laser	Pulsed laser
Wavelength (λ)	nanometers (nm)	
Power	watts (W), milliwatts (mW)	
Single-pulse energy		joules (J), millijoules (mJ)
Peak pulse power		watts, kilowatts (kW), megawatts
Frequency		hertz (Hz)
Average power		watts, milliwatts
Burst length		picoseconds (ps), femtoseconds (fs), nanoseconds (ns), microseconds (μs)
Spot diameter	mm², cm², m²	
Power density	W/mm², W/cm²	(W/mm², W/cm²)
Energy density	(J/mm², J/cm²)	J/mm², J/cm²
Scanning speed	mm, cm/sec	
Scan duration		μs, ms, s

For pulsed lasers the joule output is a fixed technical specification (Table 1.1) while for CW lasers it depends on the treatment technique. Thus, a statement of energy output in the context of treatment protocols is meaningful only if the power output, exposure time, and exposure area are also stated.

■ Tissue Effects of Lasers

Since light is part of the electromagnetic spectrum, laser light obeys the optical laws of reflection, transmission, scattering, and absorption (Fig. 1.2).

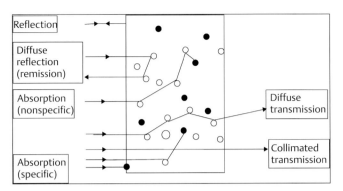

Fig. 1.2 Path taken by photons in tissue. Photons can be reflected from the tissue surface, remitted (diffusely reflected) from deeper levels, or may undergo diffuse or collimated transmission (through thin layers). The effects on the tissue occur with specific or nonspecific absorption.

Optical Properties of Tissues

To understand the interaction of a laser beam with tissue, it should be noted that when a laser beam encounters tissue, usually it is initially scattered and then finally absorbed. Only absorbed radiation can be transformed into other kinds of energy. If laser radiation were only absorbed by tissue, the spatial propagation of the beam could have been described by an exponential function. The Lambert–Beer law, however, applies only in nonscattering media. Since most tissues are optically opaque media, the phenomenon of scattering has to be taken into account. The optical properties of tissues are determined by the scattering at interfaces such as cell membranes, cell nuclei, etc. and also by absorption by tissue chromophores such as melanin, hemoglobin, water, etc. These properties can vary considerably with the wavelength of the radiation due to the different chromophores present in tissues. At UV wavelengths shorter than 300 nm, the laser radiation is chiefly absorbed by cellular proteins and nucleic acids. Visible light radiation and near-infrared (NIR) wavelengths (400–1200 nm) are absorbed mainly by chromophores such as hemoglobin, flavin, cytochromes, and carotinoids. In the far-infrared range (>1200 nm) water is the most efficient absorber. Scattering, too, varies with the wavelength. It is greatest at shorter wavelengths and steadily decreases with increasing wavelength. With the neodymium:yttrium aluminum garnet (Nd:YAG) laser, which emits in the NIR range of the spectrum (1064 nm), scattering predominates over absorption (Fig. 1.3). It is possible for one photon to return to a given tissue site several times, increasing the local light intensity and the likelihood that absorption will occur at that site (or in the affected tissue layers).

The scattering coefficient (μ_s) is the probability that a photon will undergo a scattering event while traveling over a certain path length. The absorption coefficient (μ_a) is the probability that a photon will be absorbed over a certain path length. Both are stated in units of reciprocal length (cm^{-1} or mm^{-1}). The albedo (a) is calculated by dividing the

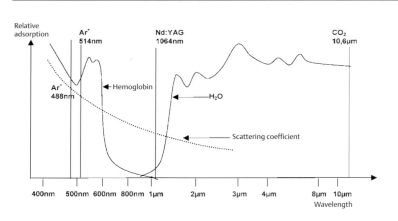

scattering coefficient by the sum of the scattering and absorption coefficients:

$a = \mu_s/(\mu_s + \mu_a)$.

With an albedo of 0 (i.e., $\mu_s = 0$), all the radiation is absorbed by the medium and is not scattered. A completely transparent medium does not scatter or absorb, while an albedo of 1 (i.e., $\mu_a = 0$) means that all the radiation is scattered and none is absorbed. The albedo expresses the proportion of the radiation that is scattered before reaching an optical depth of 1. It is a dimensionless quantity. The optical depth τ is defined as the distance from the tissue surface (z) multiplied by the sum of the absorption and scattering coefficients ($\tau = (\mu_s + \mu_a)\,z$). It, too, is a dimensionless quantity. With a value of 1, z is equal to the mean free path. This is the average distance that a photon can travel before it is scattered or absorbed by interacting with the tissue.

The probability that a photon will be scattered at the angle θ may be equal for all angles (isotropic scattering) or may favor a particular scattering axis (anisotropic scattering). The degree of anisotropy is expressed by the anisotropic factor g. When g = 1, scattering occurs almost exclusively in a forward direction. When g = 0, scattering is isotropic—that is, the photons are scattered with equal probability in all directions. (Mathematically, g is defined as the cosine of the scattering angle X averaged over all possible angles; Fig. 1.4). When considering the phenomenon of scattering, we should bear in mind that tissues favor a particular scattering direction: scattering tends to occur in continuity with the axis of the incident scattering photon. The g value for tissues in vitro is between 0.7 and 0.99, and g increases with the wavelength of the light.

Knowledge of the optical properties of tissues can be helpful in predicting the actual tissue effects of lasers. It is not always possible to distinguish between the scattering and absorption components, in particular, of lasers that are not selectively absorbed (Nd:YAG lasers, diode lasers). Nor is this necessary, since the decisive factor is the total amount of scattering and absorption occurring over the penetration depth of the laser energy. The penetration depth is defined as the tissue depth at which the original laser power has been diminished by the factor $1/e$. Even the Nd:YAG laser does not penetrate deeply into blood. This is not because of strong absorption by hemoglobin but because of heavy scattering by the cellular constituents of blood. In ordinary tissues, however, the Nd:YAG laser has the highest specific penetration depth of any medical laser system—ranging from 3 mm to 10 mm, depending on the tissue [2].

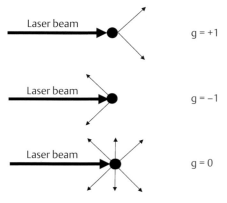

Fig. 1.4   The anisotropic factor g.

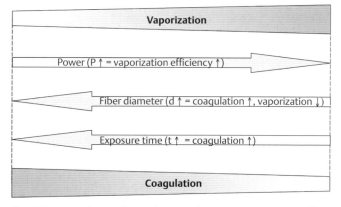

Fig. 1.5   Dependence of coagulation and vaporization on power, fiber diameter, and exposure time.

Tissue Reactions

The possible tissue effects depend on the wavelength of the laser light, the power and duration of a single pulse, the repetition rate, and the spot diameter (Fig. 1.5). Besides these properties of emission, specific tissue reactions and perifocal reactions are critical determinants of the penetration depth and effect.

With low power and energy densities, the tissue effects are determined chiefly by photochemical processes. Light absorption causes little or no initial heating of the tissue (e. g., a CW dye laser). Clinical applications of photochemical reactions include photodynamic therapy and fluorescent diagnosis. At higher power and energy densities, photothermal effects begin to occur (Fig. 1.6).

For laser light to produce a thermal effect, the energy contained in the light must be converted into heat. Propagation of heat in the tissue depends both on the wavelength of the light and on the exposure time. With exposures in the microsecond range, heating is confined largely to the absorbing structure. With a longer exposure time (longer than the thermal relaxation time of the medium) or with continuous exposure, heat diffusion assumes major importance. Heat conduction from the absorbing tissue into the environment causes damage to the surrounding tissues. The extent of this damage depends on the magnitude and duration of the temperature increase. This can already be seen at exposure times greater than 500 µs. If the exposure time is long enough, the thermal effect may even spread beyond the range of the optical penetration depth. This distance, called the active depth, may be as much as 20 mm for certain lasers and tissues. Beyond the optical penetration depth, thermal effects are determined entirely by the thermal properties of the tissue such as heat conduction, heat capacity, and heat dissipation due to blood flow. The latter process will have little impact if the perfusion rate is low or if vessels are occluded due to clotting. But in tissues with a high rate of perfusion, heat is efficiently removed by transport along the vessels. This can reduce the local

thermal effect, but it can dissipate the effect of the (moderated) temperature increase over a greater volume of tissue.

Photothermal Tissue Reactions

Tissue temperatures between 40 °C and 60 °C, which occur at the margins of areas that have been directly coagulated, cause a disturbance of cellular metabolism which Katalinic calls a "thermodynamic reaction" (e. g., argon laser, Nd:YAG laser) [3]. The therapeutic principle of this reaction involves a thermally induced vasculitis and perivasculitis, resulting in apoptosis and regressive structural changes.

When tissue is heated to a temperature above 60–100 °C, it undergoes coagulation (protein precipitation). Definitive coagulation with stasis of blood flow may be achieved. The local effect of coagulation is tissue destruction, the extent of which depends on the maximum temperature reached and the time course of the heating effect. A temperature of 51 °C must be maintained for at least 1 second to cause irreversible cell damage. This process takes 100 seconds at 57 °C, but only 1 ms at 68 °C. Also, the reactions at the cellular level are not uniform: endothelial cells, for example, show less thermal stress tolerance and undergo denaturation before other cells are devitalized. When tissue is heated to a temperature above 100 °C, the tissue water vaporizes and desiccation occurs. Carbonization (charring) occurs at approximately 150 °C and tissue vaporization (burning) begins at 300 °C (e. g., Nd:YAG laser, CO_2 laser).

Besides wavelength, the extent of coagulation also depends on the spot diameter, power density, and exposure time. Wavelength is important in the sense that a wavelength with high specific absorption—resulting in shallower penetration—cannot produce volume coagulation and the width of the coagulated area is limited by thermal conduction. With a strongly penetrating wavelength, such as of the Nd:YAG laser (1064 nm), the active depth is dependent on the factors mentioned above. The spot diameter, and thus the exposed volume, defines the interfacial area with sur-

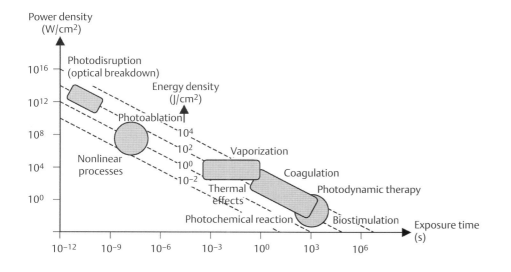

Fig. 1.6 Various tissue effects in relation to the power density and pulse duration.

rounding tissues. As this area increases, greater numbers of photons scatter in the surroundings and a larger area is available for heat conduction from the irradiated tissue. Thermal conduction is also affected by the duration of exposure. Heat transfer takes time. With short exposure times, the pulse is already over before the thermal front can reach the surrounding tissues. In this case coagulation occurs only from stored heat, which is very little when the spot diameter is small. With longer exposure times, however, heat builds up and produces coagulation zones extending well beyond the penetration depth of the wavelength [4].

Photomechanical Tissue Reactions

If the pulse duration is much shorter than the thermal relaxation time and heat conductivity of the medium, few if any collateral thermal effects occur in the surrounding tissues. When the laser beam is focused on the surface, it causes an explosive tissue ablation with no significant thermal effects on adjacent tissues (e. g., erbium laser, photoablation).

When pulsed lasers with very high energy densities are used, a nonlinear interaction known as optical breakdown occurs. This generates a plasma that is no longer transparent to the radiation and acts as an absorber of the additional energy delivered to the site. The explosive expansion of the plasma induces a shockwave that can cause tissue cavitation and fragmentation, depending on the elasticity of the tissue (e. g., pulsed dye laser, frequency-doubled Nd:YAG laser, lithotripsy). Tissue ablation and destruction may occur on the surface of a tissue with high absorption and low optical transparency or may be shifted to deeper levels in transparent tissue [5].

Lasers also produce secondary mechanical effects. A very rapid energy influx into vessels can cause violent heating of the vascular contents with secondary endothelial damage and the rupture of small vessels (flashlamp-pumped dye laser). The expansion caused by the water vapor and gas formation results in tears in the vessel wall and the extravasation of thermally altered blood at the center of the laser pulse. With short laser pulses, only a negligible amount of heat is transferred to areas directly adjacent to the vessel. As a result of this, the coagulating effect is limited to capillary-size blood vessels. In larger vessels, the side of the vessel facing away from the laser is protected by a "shielding effect" due to strong absorption in the upper part of the vessel lumen. The heating effect of a single laser application is limited and the increase in pressure caused by outgassing can dissipate into the vascular system via the mobile blood phase.

Photochemical Tissue Effects

Although photoablation with lasers operating in the UV-C range is included among the photomechanical tissue effects occurring at the high end of the power density scale, it can also be classified as a photochemical effect since the high single-photon energy can break chemical bonds directly without prior conversion to heat. Ordinarily, however, photochemical reactions are interpreted as tissue effects occurring at the lower end of the power density scale. These reactions have two main clinical applications:

- Photodynamic therapy with the formation of cytotoxic oxygen radicals
- Fluorescent diagnosis

For photochemical effects to occur, molecules with ligands, central atoms, etc. must be present. These can be excited to a higher energy state by photons of a certain energy (= light at a certain wavelength). There are two ways in which the excited molecules return to the ground state. First, if the difference between the higher-energy state and ground state is exactly equal to a certain quantum, an "allowed transition" can occur. In this case the transition between levels occurs immediately and spontaneously, accompanied by the emission of a photon along with a certain amount of heat (fluorescence). Thus, fluorescence refers to the immediate emission of light following excitation. Second, if the two levels are not separated by an exact quantum difference, only a "forbidden transition" can occur. Despite the term "forbidden," the transition is not impossible but simply occurs more slowly and by a circuitous route. If light is emitted in the process, this phenomenon is called phosphorescence (once used in luminous clock dials). Both phenomena are collectively referred to as luminescence [6].

If the processes take place slowly, another phenomenon can occur: chemical reactions take time, and in this case sufficient time is available. There is time for the stored energy to be transferred to other molecules. The excited state of one such molecule can react with ground state triplet oxygen, energizing it into an excited singlet state called a radical. The formation of radicals is the basic principle of photodynamic therapy. Two radical-forming mechanisms can be distinguished: type I and type II. Type I is a chemical reaction in which the substrate is consumed and superoxide and hydroxy (OH) radicals are produced. This type of reaction occurs in alkylating chemotherapy and in radiotherapy with high photon energy. Type II is a pure energy transfer from one excited molecule to another molecule, producing a radical. Owing to the special configuration of oxygen in nature, this involves the formation of singlet oxygen radicals [7]. Oxygen radicals can destroy cell membranes, mitochondria, nuclear membranes, and other cell organelles but they cannot disrupt the DNA double helix. This distinguishes them particularly from type I radicals, which have this capability. However, both types of radical induce a biological process which, unlike thermal coagulation or mechanical disruption, falls short of the immediate, definitive destruction of cells (necrosis) and results in necrobiosis or apoptosis. First recognized during the 1920s and 1960s, this process has attracted growing interest in recent years, owing in part to its role in photodynamic therapy.

Photosensitizers

While many endogenous substances, particularly respiratory-chain enzymes and endoporphyrins, can fluoresce, only exogenous agents can induce the formation of singlet

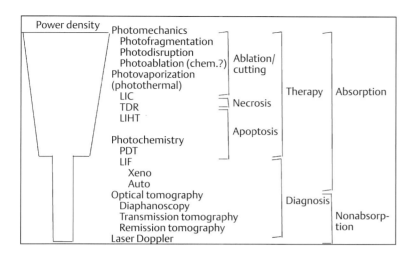

oxygen radicals. Protoporphyrin (PP) IX occupies an intermediate position. It is a potent oxygen-radical former, but even in tumor cells its concentration is normally so low that it is detectable only by high-resolution detection systems. However, when its precursor, 5-aminolevulinic acid (ALA), is applied, PP IX accumulates in dysplastic cells, making it possible to stimulate fluorescence and even carry out photodynamic therapy with a simple light source. Otherwise, however, an exogenous photosensitizing compound must be administered [8].

Another principle of photodynamic diagnosis or therapy is based on the accumulation of the sensitizer in the target tissue. This accumulation can occur through an active process such as special membrane affinity, increased membrane permeability due to a decrease in pH, or an increase in metabolism. It can also occur passively based on a decrease in substrate clearance or a decreased breakdown of the metabolites of active photosensitizers, as in the case of ALA-induced PP IX photodynamic therapy. While fluorescent diagnosis requires only the presence of an adequate excitatory wavelength, therapy requires the additional presence of oxygen. It is not the excited photosensitizer but the oxygen activated by it that is pharmacologically active. Without oxygen, there can be no photodynamic therapy.

Optical Diagnosis

Absorption is crucial for photodynamic therapy and for fluorescent diagnosis. Without absorption, there can be no energy transfer. But reflected, remitted, and transmitted photons are by no means wasted. They are used for diagnostic imaging. It should be recalled that the use of light in diagnosis predated the invention of the laser. Transmission microscopy employs the selective transmission of light through stained specimens for diagnosis, while in clinical examination secondary remissions from the examiner's light source are used. In the pre-ultrasound era, transillumination was an established tool in neonatology, urology, and otolaryngology. Due to the pronounced scattering with polychromatic, noncoherent light sources, these methods of examination have been completely superseded by ultra-

sonography. But with the development of NIR diode lasers, which provide maximum tissue transmission due to a lack of selective absorption and low scatter, plus the development of highly sensitive NIR cameras with image analysis systems, optical diagnosis is again assuming importance. Another technique of remitted light imaging is laser Doppler, in which emitted and remitted laser light is used to detect the Doppler effect (red shift) caused by moving red blood cells [9] (Fig. 1.**7**).

■ Principle of Laser Generation

The laser is a type of feedback amplifier. Several conditions must be met to initiate the lasing process. An atom or molecule normally returns to the ground state after its electrons have been excited, immediately emitting the absorbed energy in the form of a photon. Laser emission can take place only in a medium in which this process occurs in steps proceeding at different rates. This can be illustrated with the four-level laser as an example. The lasing medium is "pumped" by adding energy (e. g., in the form of light, electric current, chemical energy, etc.), thereby raising the electron to a higher energy level. The first step occurs very rapidly as a "radiation-free transition," usually involving the production of heat. Initially the electron stays at this first intermediate level. When more than 50% of the electrons in the medium reach this level, a population inversion is said to have occurred and is a necessary prelude to initiating the laser process. When an electron in this excited state is struck by a photon whose energy is equal to the energy that would be released on transition to the next lower level, their interaction stimulates the emission of a photon. The excited photon does not lose any energy in this process and is preserved. Both photons now continue this process by interacting with other electrons, resulting in the formation of an exponentially expanding photon cloud. This process is perpetuated by initiating it within a mirror-enclosed space (the resonant cavity). One of the mirrors is partially silvered to allow some of the light to escape from the resonant cavity (Fig. 1.**8**).

Because of the multiple back-and-forth reflections between the mirrors, the photons taking part in the lasing

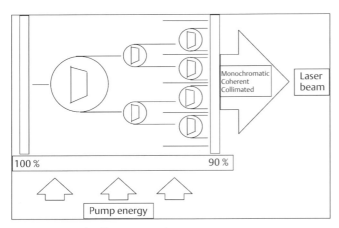

Fig. 1.8 Principle of laser generation.

process are only those moving precisely along the mirror axis. As a result, the laser beam is collimated (parallel). Since all the photons have the same energy, the laser beam is monochromatic. In addition because a standing wave is generated within the cavity, the laser beam is also coherent. An ordinary light source can have any one of these properties, but only a laser can produce a beam with all three properties and a sufficiently high total power output. The laser process may be pulsed (pulse durations <1000 µs) or continuous (continuous wave, CW), depending on the type of excitation used and the electron structure and levels of the lasing medium. A population inversion is easy to produce in a CW laser, i. e., the electrons are pumped to a higher energy level faster and more efficiently than their spontaneous return to the lower energy level or ground state with the emission of photons. In a four-level laser, the transition from the lowest energy level to the ground state is very rapid and efficient, allowing for continuous laser operation in which a steady beam can be produced by pumping the laser with an arc lamp, or a pulsed beam can be generated by using a flashlamp. In a three-level laser,

the laser transition takes place between the first laser level and the ground state. A new laser transition cannot occur until the ground state has been drained through population inversion. As a result three-level lasers can operate only in a pulsed mode. In the Q-switched laser, the pulse energy produced in the laser is stored until it exceeds a threshold value, at which point it is released in a sudden burst by an optical shutter. These lasers usually operate in the nanosecond range and produce photomechanical effects [1].

■ Laser Systems

Various laser media are available: gases, dye solutions, crystals, glasses, fibers, and semiconductors. Most lasing media have several possible energy transitions with various energy differences, i. e., several wavelengths. Generally speaking, however, medical laser systems are optimized to one wavelength. (Exceptions with several standard wavelengths are argon lasers, diode lasers, dye lasers, Nd:YAG lasers, and titanium-sapphire lasers; when these devices are used, the wavelength should be specified in the written documentation.) Tables 1.2–1.5 summarize the features of the major current medical laser systems, grouped according to their typical tissue effects [11].

■ Application Systems

Aside from "biostimulation" and low-level laser therapy (LLLT), which are based on laser pointers, medical laser light cannot be applied directly to the patient from the laser device. Laser application systems consist of delivery systems as well as accessories that are sometimes needed to direct or modify the output of the delivery system.

Table 1.2 Laser systems producing a photoablative tissue effect

Laser	Wavelength (nm)	Pulse duration	Typical pulse energy/cm^2	Repetition frequency	Property of emitted radiation	Indications	Applicators, delivery systems, accessories
Excimer	193	10 ms	180 mJ	20 Hz	Ionization, absorption by water	Corneal surgery	Direct, slit lamp
Excimer	308	100–250 ms	5–200 mJ	1–200 Hz	Absorption by water	Ophthalmology, angioplasty	Fiber/ multifiber catheter
Nd:YAG pulsed	1064	100–200 µs	100–200 mJ	15–30 Hz	Nonspecific absorption	Oral medicine	Fiber, handpiece
Ho:YAG	2100	1–2 ms	0.8–4.5 J	2–20 Hz	Absorption by water	Surgery, orthopedic surgery, urology	Fiber/bare fiber contact, side-fire, handpiece
Er:YAG	2900	0.1–1 ms	200 mJ–1.5 J	1–20 Hz	Absorption by water	Surgery, dental surgery, plastic surgery	Articulated arm, hollow waveguide, sapphire fiber
CO_2 pulsed	106 000	<950 µs	1–500 mJ	1–10 Hz	Absorption by water	Plastic surgery	Articulated arm, hollow waveguide, scanner

Table 1.**3** Laser systems producing a photodisruptive tissue effect

Laser	Wavelength (nm)	Pulse duration	Typical pulse energy/cm²	Repetition frequency	Property of emitted radiation	Indications	Applicators, delivery systems, accessories
Flashlamp pumped dye laser (FPDL)	504	1.4–1.5 μs	80–120 mJ	1–10 Hz	Absorption by chromophores	Lithotripsy	Fiber
Flashlamp pumped dye laser (FPDL)	585	200–500–800–1500 μs	4–9 J	2 Hz	Absorption by blood vessels, hemoglobin	Plastic surgery, dermatology	Fiber, focusing handpiece
Ruby (Q-switched)	694	10–30 ns (Q-switched) 120 μs (non-Q-switched)	5–30 (–50)	1–2 Hz	Absorption by pigment	Plastic surgery, dermatology	Fiber, focusing handpiece
Alexandrite	755	300–500–700 ns	10–150 mJ	1–20 Hz	Absorption by chromophores	Lithotripsy	Fiber
Nd:YAG laser (Q-switched)	1064	20–25 ns	10–100 mJ	1–20 Hz	Photoacoustic disruption (mechanical)	Secondary cataract membrane, oral medicine	Fiber, slit lamp
Double pulse Nd:YAG laser/KTP	1064/532	1–1.2–1.4 μs	120 mJ	10 Hz	Photoacoustic disruption (mechanical)	Lithotripsy	Fiber

Table 1.**4** Laser systems producing a photothermal tissue effect

Laser	Wavelength (nm)	Temporal modality, pulse width	Exposure time	Power (W)	Property of emitted radiation	Tissue interaction	Applicators, delivery systems, accessories
Ar+	488/514	CW	0.01 s CW	0.3–5 (–15)	Specific absorption by hemoglobin and melanin	Specific coagulation	Fiber, focusing handpiece
Kr+	350–800	CW	0.1 s CW	2–5	Specific absorption by xenogenic chromophores	Specific coagulation, photodynamic therapy	Fiber, focusing handpiece
KTP	532	CW	0.01 s CW	1–30	Specific absorption	Specific coagulation, vaporization	Fiber/bare fiber contact, side-fire, diffuser tip, focusing handpiece
Diode	780–980	CW	0.1 s CW	1–60	Nonspecific volume absorption	Nonspecific coagulation, vaporization	Fiber/bare fiber contact, side-fire, diffuser tip, focusing handpiece
Nd:YAG	1064 1032	CW	0.01 s CW	1–120 1–40	Nonspecific volume absorption	Nonspecific coagulation, vaporization	Fiber/bare fiber contact, side-fire, diffuser tip, focusing handpiece
CO₂	10 600	CW	0.05 s CW	0.03–80	High absorption by water	Vaporization, coagulation	Articulated arm, micro-manipulator, hollow waveguide, scanner, focusing handpiece

Table 1.**5** Laser systems for photodynamic therapy

Laser	Wavelength (nm)	Temporal modality, pulse width	Exposure time	Power (W)	Property of emitted radiation	Tissue interaction	Applicators, delivery systems, accessories
KTP/Ar+ Dye	532/488 633 (–650)	CW	0.02 s CW	0.2–7	Specific absorption by natural and synthetic chromophores (photosensitizers)	Photodynamic therapy	Fiber, side-fire, microlens, spherical or cylindrical diffuser tip
Diode	633 650–750	CW	0.01 s CW	3–5–25	Specific absorption by xenogenic chromophores (photosensitizers)	Photodynamic therapy	

Delivery Systems

Articulated Arms

When laser light is delivered to the target tissue through an articulated arm, all the properties of the laser beam are preserved, including its collimation and coherence. The articulated arm can also transmit all wavelengths from the far UV-C of the excimer laser to the mid-infrared of the CO_2 laser. Moreover, there are virtually no limits on pulse energy or power output, so that even lasers with a short pulse durations can deliver peak outputs in the gigawatt range. These features make the articulated arm a universal delivery system for all lasers. However, it has a number of disadvantages. First, if one of the (usually) seven mirrors in the articulated arm is out of alignment, the transmitted light will be off-center, causing the beam to deviate from the cross-sectional axis of the tube. This also occurs when one of the tubes in the articulated arm is twisted or bent. Consequently, the articulated arm must meet very stringent requirements in terms of mechanical stability, making the device very expensive as well as heavy and cumbersome to use—the second disadvantage of the articulated arm system. Third, although seven-mirror systems provide a high degree of mobility, their flexibility is greatly limited. Articulated arms cannot be used in small endoscopes or in flexible endoscopes.

Hollow waveguides, composed of thin ceramic tubes, represent an attempt to solve this problem. But these still have an outer diameter of approximately 3–5 mm and the flexibility of only a thin rod. They are also limited in their ability to transmit laser power, since the walls of the waveguide absorb a significant portion of the laser radiation. In any case, the output beam of a waveguide lacks the coherence and collimation necessary for focusing and optical scanning. Thus, waveguides are an option only in cases where an articulated arm is too cumbersome.

Fiber Optics

Whenever fiberoptic transmission is technically feasible, it should be used. The principle of fiberoptic transmission is based on the total reflection occurring at the interface between a medium of higher optical density and a medium of lower optical density (e.g., a water spout in a lighted fountain). Most optical fibers in current medical use have a quartz core surrounded by a thin plastic sheath, or cladding, where the total reflection actually occurs. The entire fiber has an outer jacket made of plastic (plastic-coated silica) or quartz (quartz/quartz fibers). This jacket imparts mechanical stability on the one hand and high flexibility on the other. Fibers which transmit wavelengths from the ultraviolet range (308 nm) to the mid-infrared wavelengths of the holmium:YAG laser (2.1 µm) are now available for clinical use. Fibers for the erbium:YAG laser at 2.94 µm or the CO_2 laser at 10.6 µm have not yet progressed beyond the experimental stage.

Fibers can transmit pulse energies of 1 J in the VIS and NIR ranges, even in the Q-switched mode, without being de-

stroyed. Possible fiber diameters range from 50 µm for the argon laser to 800 µm or 1000 µm. It can be relatively difficult to couple laser light into a 50-µm fiber, but 800- and 1000-µm fibers are so rigid, they sacrifice flexibility, which is the major advantage of fiberoptic cables. As a result, these thick fibers should be used only in cases where the laser energy cannot be delivered through thinner fibers (e.g., a high-power NIR diode laser). The fiber diameters that are most often used clinically are 400 µm and 600 µm. For laser light to be coupled into the fiber, the beam must be focused to the diameter of the fiber core with a fairly high degree of precision. If the focal spot is too large, some of the laser energy will be absorbed by the connector, damaging the input surface. If the focus is too small, it may create a hot spot that destroys the input end of the fiber, or a "downspout" phenomenon may occur within the fiber, analogous to water spiraling down the wall of a rain gutter rather than being evenly distributed over its cross-section. This results in a very uneven power distribution over the cross-section of the beam at the output end of the fiber.

Since the cross-section of the beam leaving the laser cavity is always larger than the diameter of the fiber core (except in "fiber lasers"), the laser beam must be focused (given the cross-sections involved, this is possible with no other light source than a laser). However, focusing the laser beam at the input end means that the beam will leave the output end of the fiber at the same divergent angle. A laser transmitted by an optical fiber loses one of its properties, collimation. Additionally, the light emitted from the fiber is no longer coherent (except in highly specialized fibers). This can be problematic in diagnosis, but it is often advantageous in laser therapy since the modal structures tend to offset the original nonhomogeneities of power distribution in the laser beam. Looping the fiber into several coils with a relatively small radius of curvature can further homogenize the output beam [10].

Lens systems can be used to refocus the divergent beam at the end of the fiber. The smallest possible focus at this stage is limited only by the fiber cross-section, since focusing replicates an image of the fiber core diameter. Thus, the smallest focus and highest power density can be achieved by using a very small fiber diameter and lenses with short focal lengths. These lenses again create a large divergence past the focus, however, resulting in a short beam waist with a very limited focal depth. This is neither good nor bad, simply a fact. An advantage is that the desired high power density is achieved only in tissues within the beam waist, while deeper tissues are protected since the power density falls off rapidly with increasing depth. The disadvantage is that precise focusing is needed; otherwise the desired effect is not obtained.

Application Accessories

Focusing Handpiece

A focusing handpiece can be connected to an articulated arm or to an optical fiber. The collimated emission from the articulated arm can then be focused on a very small spot size (subject to theoretical wavelength limits) using lenses with a short focal length; longer focal lengths can be used to obtain a larger spot size with a long beam waist and a correspondingly large depth of focus. Additionally, zoom focusing systems are available for adjusting the desired spot size at a specified distance from the handpiece. In cases where it is critical to maintain a particular spot size, it is helpful to use a spacer in conjunction with a zoom system. Of course, the focal spot can also be adjusted simply by varying the distance from the handpiece to the tissue surface. The more sophisticated the lens system, the better the optical precision and the better the quality of the spot. Since losses due to reflection and absorption occur at every interface, even with coated optics, multilens systems of this kind are sensitive and require gas cooling, especially when an infrared laser is used. Also, even the smallest amount of dust or other impurities on the lens surface can absorb the laser light, severely damaging the lenses. Because glass is not transparent to mid-infrared wavelengths, CO_2 lasers should be used with lenses made of zinc-selenite, which themselves are very susceptible to mechanical and chemical damage.

Micromanipulators for Operating Microscope, Colposcope, or Slit Lamp

The micromanipulator is another type of focusing system. After the laser light has been coupled into the operating microscope, the beam is redirected with a mirror in the visual field of the scope using a joystick to control the mirror position. This is a very precise method of aiming the laser beam in the operative field. The focal length, and thus the position of the focal spot, is matched to the focal length of the operating microscope so the surgeon can work accurately and consistently within the focal plane. The long beam waist makes it possible to work through narrow openings (e.g., laryngoscope or colposcope), even in the noncontact mode.

Endoscopic Delivery

In cases where the laser beam cannot be delivered through optical fibers, an alternative is to couple the laser light into a rigid endoscope. Endoscopic delivery systems are derived from micromanipulators, i.e., the laser beam is coupled into the visual field of the endoscope by a mirror, and its movements within the visual field are precisely controlled with a micro-joystick. The focal length is defined, of course, by the length of the endoscope. Endoscopic delivery systems have little practical importance today because they are very cumbersome and imprecise, and their indications have been almost entirely superseded by lasers that can be transmitted through fiberoptic carriers such as the Nd:YAG laser, holmium laser, and diode laser.

Scanner Systems

In a scanner system, the laser beam is not aimed manually with a joystick but is directed automatically by means of electrically controlled mirror systems.

Scanners have two main applications:
- accurate placement of individual laser shots at a specified distance from one another (Hexascan); and
- sweeping a beam over a surface at a predetermined speed (Swiftlase, line scanners).

The first involves the use of gated or short-pulse lasers. It was originally developed in the early 1980s as an automated scanning unit (Hexascan) for the treatment of port-wine stains with an argon laser. The individual shots are patterned so that two shots are never placed directly adjacent to each other; this avoids treating the same spot twice due to overlapping thermal conduction. Today this principle is applied in the potassium-titanyl-phosphate (KTP) laser and derivative scanner systems for tissue ablation using a short-pulse CO_2 or erbium laser. In these systems the individual shots are spaced at designated intervals or in an overlapping pattern to achieve uniform ablation. The depth of ablation is controlled by the power density, while the width of the coagulation zone is controlled by the exposure time. Since the laser operates with an expanded, round beam, two problems arise. The operator can avoid overlapping the individual shots, leaving untreated areas between the circles, or allow the individual exposures to overlap. With lasers that have a gaussian beam profile, an overlapping pattern can just compensate for the power fade toward the edges. With a rectangular beam profile, an overlapping pattern may produce collateral thermal damage or may cause the overlapping areas to be ablated twice.

The second method—scanning continuously with a focused beam—is free from these hazards. The laser passes consist of fine, closely-spaced adjacent lines permitting uniform ablation of the tissue surface. The passes may be in the form of a single or double spiral, a figure-of-eight pattern, or a meandering pattern. A critical issue in continuous scanning is the reversal point, where there is a risk of double-irradiation or training the beam on one spot for too long. The depth of ablation for a given scan diameter is determined by the laser power and scanning speed, and the depth of coagulation is determined by speed. Data stated in millijoules or the like in these systems are calculated values that cannot be directly compared with the values for short-pulse single-step scanners.

Both scanning methods can produce a variety of patterns such as lines, rectangles, squares, hexagons, octagons, and circles. The hexagon has proved effective for surface ablation over large areas, as it permits the figures to be placed in an interlocking ("bugeye") pattern. Also, if a second pass is necessary, the scanner can be rotated 90° to avoid pattern structures and achieve a uniform surface.

Noncontact Laser Accessories

Unlike the Nd:YAG laser, for example, the CO_2 laser requires the use of metallic mirrors to redirect the laser beam. Also, endoscopic CO_2 lasers are typically used with backstops designed to protect tissues located behind the target structure. Contact lenses are used chiefly in ophthalmology to navigate the laser beam.

Fiber Tips

While the accessories described above can be used with articulated arms and fiberoptic carriers, the following applicators are used exclusively with laser fibers. They are necessary and helpful whenever the laser output of the fiber is not directly suitable for producing the desired effect. Sapphire contact tips are the oldest fiber applicators. Fiber tips have two main functions:
• increasing the power density while improving mechanical and thermal stability for contact cutting, and
• focusing the laser beam beneath the tissue surface.

Sapphire contact tips consist of synthetic sapphires that are screwed onto the end of the fiber with a metal connector. Since the transmission of laser light from the fiber to the sapphire was very inefficient, the metal connectors underwent significant heating, requiring continuous gas cooling. Also, only a small fraction of the laser power was actually available for cutting, and the tips tended to break easily, making them tedious to use. Today, sapphire contact tips for laser cutting have been completely superseded by bare-fiber contact surgery. Nevertheless, they did provide an important impetus in the early 1980s for the further refinement of contact techniques. They have not proved suitable for modifying (focusing or diverting) the output beam due to significant coupling losses. However, they did prompt much discussion in this area, culminating in the two different fiber applicator systems available today:
• Focusing and diverting systems
• Diffusers

Focusing and Diverting Systems

The spot diameter from an endoscopic laser fiber is controlled strictly by altering the fiber–tissue distance, but in many cases endoscopy does not allow sufficient room for this maneuver. With microlens fibers, in which a tiny lens is glued to the end of the fiber, it is possible to emit a focused beam with a greater or lesser degree of divergence. Special cylindrical lenses can provide homogeneous illumination of the treated area, even in the far field. This is particularly helpful for achieving uniform dosimetry in photodynamic therapy.

The beam can also be modified by diverting it with a 70° or 90° prism mounted onto or ground into the end of the fiber. This creates a side-firing fiber, also with defined beam parameters, that is particularly useful in narrow or sharply angled body cavities. Glued surfaces are very susceptible to mechanical damage, however, and cannot handle arbitrarily high power outputs. Prisms require a protective glass dome and must therefore be handled carefully.

Diffusers

Scattering applicators are used in interstitial therapy and photodynamic therapy. Where a clean, freshly cleaved bare fiber cannot be used for interstitial coagulation, two applicator designs have become established commercially: the ring-mode applicator and the isotropic diffuser. The ring-mode applicator has a forward-directed, ring-shaped emission pattern. The distribution of photons is homogenized as a result of multiple photon scattering in the tissue. This applicator requires extra tissue contact for scattering, and so far it has been widely used only for prostatic coagulation.

The light from an isotropic diffuser is already emitted in a scattered form. The applicator may consist of cauterized fiber ends (which also require a glass dome) or of flexible, variable-length plastic fibers doped with scattering materials and glued to the actual end of the fiber. Mirrors (gold film) can be used to contain the emission within a particular spatial angle. Plastic fibers are used chiefly in photodynamic therapy for homogeneous light application in body cavities.

Adjuvant Accessories

The clinical effects of lasers are determined not only by the application accessories described above but also by the additional measures in use. The two basic principles of primary importance are:
• augmenting the laser effect, and
• preventing or reducing collateral effects.

The latter mainly involves compression and cooling methods, which can also augment the effect in the target area by permitting the use of higher wattages.

Augmenting the Laser Effect

Laser effects on and in tissues can be augmented for a given power and energy density in two ways:
• Conditioning the tissue to increase its absorption of laser energy. This is done mainly with photosensitizers. Laser power that is too low even to produce a clinically significant temperature rise, let alone a thermal effect, may be sufficient to trigger photochemical reactions as in photodynamic therapy. Tissues can also be conditioned with fluorescent dyes, which can increase absorption in cases where tissue-specific absorption is inadequate. Through the complete utilization of photons for energy conversion, even lasers with low power and energy densities can produce thermal or photomechanical effects in tissues that would otherwise be almost transparent to the applied wavelengths. An example of this principle is the use of UV absorbers for corneal surgery or angioplasty.
• The laser effect can be enhanced not only by better photon utilization but also by a more effective photon distribution. As described in the application techniques above, using a laser in contact or interstitially can prevent losses due to reflection and remission, allowing all of the laser energy to be distributed in the tissue. Besides scattering applicators, a more uniform photon distribution can be achieved by the use of scattering solutions such as intralipid irrigants, especially in body cavities. Intravascular irrigating solutions can also be used to decrease light absorption by blood so that more photons

can penetrate into the tissue. This can also be done by applying surface pressure to reduce superficial perfusion, enabling the photons to penetrate more deeply.

Preventing or Reducing Collateral Effects

If heat conduction from the absorber into the surrounding tissue is not desired, the heat must be dissipated. Again, irrigating solutions, despite their limited heat capacity, can be used (but only physiologic solutions). Even continuous gas cooling provides only a small degree of superficial protection and serves mainly to reduce pain. Liquid spray coolants with a low evaporation point are effective for surface cooling but have a number of disadvantages. These liquids have a very low heat capacity, thus their cooling action is based entirely on evaporation. This can effectively cool only a very superficial layer—less than 1 mm thick. When applied while the laser is off, these coolants can easily cause superficial tissue freezing, as in the well known case of ethyl chloride. Therefore sophisticated controls are necessary. The liquids also desiccate the skin and can cause formation of ice crystals, with increased scattering and reflection of the laser light from the surface. Some modern lasers have built-in cooling and compression systems. The three cooling and compression methods described below can be used with all lasers emitting at visible and NIR wavelengths [12].

Glass Slab Compression

To reduce the shielding effect of laser light absorption by blood or hemoglobin, the blood must be expressed from the superficial vessels. This is quite easy to do with an ordinary microscope slide applied over a liquid immersion film of saline solution. Besides luminal compression of the vessels by the contact pressure, this has two additional effects:
• wetting of the cornified surface with saline solution prevents scattering, and
• wet keratin lamellae are more resistant to vaporization.

The added presence of materials (glass, water) with a refractive index between that of the epidermis and air provides an "index matching" similar to that produced by the optical coatings on fine lenses (between the glass and air). Just as capillaries become distinctly visible, the laser light reaches its target with much less reflection and scattering. The focal point can even be shifted beneath the epidermis, avoiding higher power densities at the surface. Use of other glass instruments (e.g., for intranasal use) is based on the same principles. In cases where index matching and simple compression are not enough to protect the surface, additional measures must be used.

Flow-Through Cooling Cuvette

The epidermis can be protected with a flow-through cooling system in the form of a cooling cuvette. The coolant consists of a 40% propylene glycol solution cooled to an initial temperature of −18 °C. An elastic latex membrane at

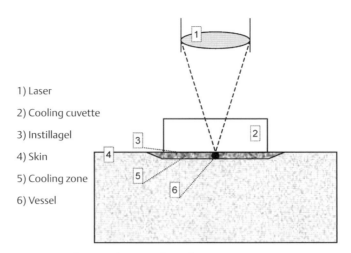

1) Laser
2) Cooling cuvette
3) Instillagel
4) Skin
5) Cooling zone
6) Vessel

Fig. 1.9   Schematic diagram of a cooling cuvette.

the base of the cuvette maintains good contact with the skin on uneven surfaces, even without pressure. A contact gel (2% lidocaine [Instillagel]) is put on the skin, which behaves as an immersion film improving heat transfer and index matching (Fig. 1.9).

The skin is compressed to reduce the thickness of the tissue and bring the undersurface of the vessel closer to the tissue surface. This provides better "illumination" of the vessel within the treated area and allows the light pulse to induce primary heating of the vessel undersurface. Reducing the outflow from the cuvette causes the membrane to bow outward, exerting pressure on the larger superficial vessels and narrowing their lumen. Conversely, reducing the inflow of coolant into the cuvette creates a slight negative pressure that bows the membrane inward. Good adhesion between the skin and membrane induces luminal expansion of the cutaneous vessels, causing the tiniest vessels to fill with blood thus increasing local absorption of the laser light. The adverse effects of increased pulse energy on the epidermis can be offset by cooling the tissue to a limiting value (cooling capacity).

Continuous Ice Cube Cooling

An interposed ice cube not only provides index matching but also exerts pressure, reducing the luminal cross-section of superficial vessels. An active penetration depth of 1 cm can be achieved in this way. Energy absorption in the superficial layers is decreased due to the diminished amount of blood in the tissue, thereby reducing thermal damage to the skin. At the same time, the heat generated in the upper skin layers is dissipated so efficiently that the temperature at skin level does not exceed 45 °C. Cooling is ineffective beyond a depth of approximately 1.5 mm due to the limited thermal conductivity of the skin. Temperatures below that level rise to more than 60 °C, causing vascular coagulation (Fig. 1.10). The advantage of ice-cube cooling lies in the high heat capacity of melting ice. Within limits, this system is self-regulating since the melting ice maintains a constant contact temperature of 0 °C.

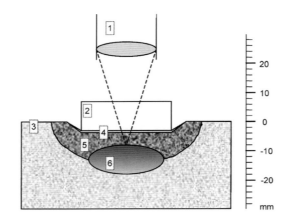

1) Nd:YAG laser

2) Ice cube

3) Skin

4) Water film (0 °C)

5) Cooling zone

6) Coagulation zone

Fig. 1.**10**   Schematic diagram of continuous ice cube cooling.

When this type of cooling is used, the ice cube should be in direct contact with the skin during the laser application and the beam should be directed only through the intact ice. The ice cube should be changed frequently and slid or rotated during treatment to maintain effective cooling. If the ice cube covers a large area, however, it may restrict perfusion so severely that there is a danger of secondary skin necrosis. For this reason, an area no larger than 5 cm^2 should be treated at one time.

■ Application Techniques

For many applications, especially in microsurgery, it is highly advantageous to laser tissues without any force and any visual obstruction, which occurs when an instrument is in contact with the tissue. On the other hand, contact laser application has resulted in many new treatment options. Both the contact and noncontact modes are equally appropriate for specific indications. Another aspect to consider is the route by which the laser light is delivered to the target area [13] (Fig. 1.**11**).

Noncontact Mode

Holding the fiber above the target site is the most obvious mode of laser use. Unobstructed vision and lack of contact pressure are particular advantages in microsurgical operations and when operating in a narrow field. Moreover, working with fewer instruments improves safety by reducing iatrogenic tissue damage and the transmission of infectious organisms. Various focusing accessories (handpiece, micromanipulator) can be used to achieve different tissue effects. By varying the distance from the tip to the tissue, the surgeon can adjust the spot size from a focal point to a divergent spot with low power density, easily changing from vaporization (focal point on the tissue surface) to coagulation (postfocal, divergent) without altering the laser parameters. In lasers with high penetration depth, the focal point can be moved beneath the tissue surface for applications such as tattoo removal. If the overlying medium is completely transparent to the laser light and is nonscattering, a plasma can be ignited at the focal point, even without specific absorbers, to produce a photodisruptive effect (postcataract membrane).

The properties of the surface tissue do not necessarily match those of the underlying target tissue, such as water content and heat-conducting properties as well as scattering, remission, reflection, and specific absorption. With

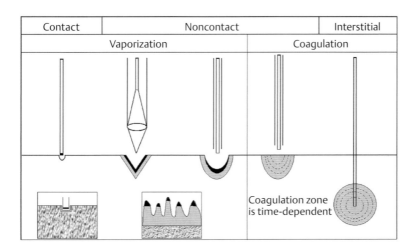

Fig. 1.**11**   Possible modes of laser application.

strongly reflective or scattering surfaces or larger tissue layers, contact or interstitial laser application may be better for delivering the laser energy to deeper tissues.

Contact Mode

A laser can be used in the contact mode in two ways:
• touching the fiber to the tissue surface; and
• interstitial application.

Two techniques can be used for tissue-surface contact. When interfacial absorption is high (with a precharred fiber tip), the laser light is absorbed at the contact surface. The surface tissue is vaporized at once, and perifocal coagulation is limited to thermal conduction. Short pulse durations (neodymium:YAG laser, diode laser) can provide a vaporizing and cutting effect otherwise available only with a CO_2 laser. If carbonization is avoided by using a freshly cleaved fiber and a lower power setting or short pulse durations, the coagulation zone can be localized to a point equal to the diameter of the fiber core.

If limiting the volume or depth reaction is a primary goal in the techniques described above, contact application can also be used to expand the treated volume while protecting the surface. When the laser power is reduced further with long exposure times, the light will spread in an almost spherical pattern beneath the surface where the fiber is applied. Pressing on the fiber can shift this treatment volume to a deeper subsurface level. This technique marks the threshold to interstitial laser application.

As with surface contact, various tissue effects can be achieved with an interstitial laser fiber. In all cases the target tissue is punctured with a needle, and the fiber is placed in a way that avoids irradiating adjacent areas and especially the underlying tissue. In lasers with a high basic absorption such as the holmium:YAG and neodymium:YAG, vaporization begins immediately after the fiber end is charred. With short pulse durations or low repetition rates, the target tissue can be ablated with little thermal damage to the surrounding areas. When lasers with high penetration depth are operated at long exposure times and low power density that prevents charring of the fiber end, a large volume of tissue can be treated. The use of scattering applicators can further enhance this effect; this can be used in PDT. With thermal lasers, the interstitial coagulation zone can be extended beyond the depth of penetration of the beam by heat conduction. If irrigating fluid is also applied through the puncture needle, the thermal stress at the fiber–tissue interface can be reduced and a higher power setting can be used without charring or destroying the fiber. When used intravascularly, irrigation may permit intraluminal laser application without thrombus formation or charring. Strictly speaking, however, this is no longer considered contact application.

Interstitial and Intraluminal Application

Any part or region of the body accessible to needle insertion can be treated with interstitial laser therapy [14].

Since little or no direct visual control is possible, imaging procedures are usually necessary for the puncture itself and for process control. Image intensifier control can be used in musculoskeletal procedures such as intervertebral disk surgery and in vascular angiographic procedures. The indications for color duplex sonography both overlap and complement the indications for radiographic imaging. The main advantages of color duplex scanning are that it involves no exposure to radiation and does not require contrast media for vascular imaging. If the puncture site is obscured due to acoustic shadowing or poor ultrasound contrast, computed tomography (CT) guidance can also be used. CT is not suitable for process control, however, and may have to be followed by magnetic resonance imaging (MRI). Similar to ultrasound, an open MRI system is useful both for monitoring needle insertion and for process control [14, 16].

The puncture instruments vary with the type of delivery system used. An indwelling Teflon venous catheter is suitable for a bare laser fiber, or a steel puncture needle (Turner) can be used for deeper sites. These instruments are available with an ultrasound contrast tip, making it somewhat easier to check needle placement. For laser application, care should be taken that the fiber tip projects an adequate distance from the needle. With the exception of ring-mode applicators for interstitial coagulation of the prostate, which are inserted directly into the prostate under endoscopic control, diffuse scattering applicators require the use of special puncture sets. First the needle is advanced into the target tissue using the Seldinger technique. Next a guidewire is placed, the tract is dilated, and a tubular sheath is introduced for placement of the actual scattering applicator. The advantage of the sheath is that its diameter effectively increases the radius of treatment so that higher powers can be applied with a constant power density. The sheath also protects the applicator from mechanical damage and prevents direct contact with tissue and blood. Unlike the needle used with a bare fiber, these more elaborate puncture sets are very difficult to reposition once placed, and so larger tumors require an afterloading technique involving the placement of multiple treatment sheaths.

Interstitial Bare-Fiber Technique

The steel needle is removed leaving the Teflon catheter in place, and a quartz fiber is introduced. The catheter is then withdrawn about 5 mm, leaving the tip of the bare fiber in direct contact with the tissue. The fiber should protrude at least 5 mm, preferably 8 mm, to prevent charring of the Teflon cannula or heating of the steel needle due to thermal conduction and backscattering. At the same time, the fiber should not be advanced more than 10–15 mm beyond the end of the needle, as it would be unstable in this situation and could break off.

With the room darkened, the position of the fiber end can be identified with the aid of the aiming beam to a depth of about 2 cm. Two different application techniques can be used in interstitial therapy:
• leaving the fiber in place, with an end-point determination and limited application time; and

- withdrawing the system at 1 mm/s while constantly applying laser energy.

The first technique is generally preferred, as it permits a more precise application and the extent of coagulation can be controlled by varying the application time. Power of 5 W and exposure time up to 180 s are recommended, depending on the desired coagulation diameter. Longer exposure times can lead to unwanted charring of the tissue and fiber.

Interstitial lasing produces a spherical coagulation zone distributed around the end of the fiber and centered on the fiber tip. The coagulation zone spreads along the fiber in a retrograde fashion. The diameter of the zone can be controlled by varying the application time. Heat retention and decreasing perfusion facilitate expansion of the zone.

For larger lesions, the fiber is repositioned and a new area is treated using the same parameters. After the fiber has been repositioned, an application time of 120 s is sufficient to produce a coagulation zone 15 mm in diameter. With steel needles, compared with Teflon, the increased heat conduction can lead to unwanted coagulation of the puncture tract. Steel needles should therefore be used only in special cases (e. g., positioning problems) and with the needle retracted somewhat further from the fiber tip.

In the technique where the system is withdrawn with constant laser application, the bare fiber should not be drawn back into the catheter or needle to avoid damaging the catheter and leaving debris in the tissue or vessel. To avoid coagulation necrosis of the overlying skin, the spread of heat can be monitored by superficial digital (fingertip) palpation over the area being treated. The finger should not exert pressure on the tissue, as this might press the skin against the fiber end and cause burns. The needle tract should not be lased more than once to avoid uncontrolled coagulation of the skin at the puncture site [17].

Intraluminal Bare-Fiber Technique

The same procedures are used for needle insertion and temperature control of the overlying skin as in interstitial application. The intraluminal fiber end should be irrigated continuously to avoid direct coagulation of blood at the fiber tip. A physiologically neutral medium such as 0.9 % saline solution is a suitable irrigant. The end of the fiber should protrude no more than 5 mm to maintain constant tip irrigation and ensure a steady flow and no less than 3 mm to avoid damaging the catheter. A 600-μm fiber diameter should be used at a power setting of 88–12 W. Whenever possible, the puncture site should be located at least 1 cm from the target vessel to obtain a tract of sufficient length. The vessel may be punctured again if post-treatment bleeding occurs.

■ Lasers and Safety

Laser safety has become a matter of considerable public interest, due in part to controversies regarding the safety and appropriate classification (see below) of laser pointers. To view this sometimes very emotional debate in more objective terms, the general hazards of laser use in medicine will be explored in this section, which then concludes with some practical guidelines on the prevention of laser accidents [18–20].

Classes of Laser

Lasers are generally divided into four classes based on their potential hazards. Class 1 lasers pose no safety hazard because their emissions are completely shielded by a housing (e. g., a CD player), even though the device may contain a relatively powerful laser. Class 2 lasers emit only wavelengths in the visible range of the spectrum and are not hazardous even when shined directly into the eye, since the blink reflex permits only a very brief exposure. This class includes helium-neon laser pointers. Class 3a lasers are hazardous to the eye if, for example, the cross-section of the beam is narrowed by the convergent optics of an endoscope and there is direct intrabeam exposure to the eye. With a class 3b laser, looking directly into the beam close to its emergence from the applicator can injure the eye regardless of the lens systems used. Class 4 lasers are hazardous to the eye from the direct beam and from reflected laser light. Medical lasers are in classes 3b and 4.

Laser Control Area

Laser radiation is light, and all tissue effects are photobiological effects. Unlike x-rays, therefore, diffuse stray laser radiation does not pose a biological hazard. In contrast with industrial lasers, the laser systems used in medicine are subject to stringent supervision and control. For an accident to occur, two mishaps would have to occur simultaneously. First, the operator would have to direct the laser beam away from the patient toward a bystander. Second, the bystander would have to be looking directly into the beam at that precise moment because eye injuries are the only relevant hazard with medical lasers. For safety purposes, it is sufficient to have protective eyewear available just outside the area in which direct or reflected laser exposure can occur. Anyone wanting access to the laser area must put on the protective glasses before entering.

Laser glasses are designed to withstand exposure to a direct laser beam for a prolonged period of time. A divergent reflection from a steel door, wall tile, or window pane never poses a greater risk than the direct beam itself. Since the operating room is designated as the laser control area during open laser use, and everyone present in the room must wear safety glasses that protect against direct exposure, this eyewear will naturally protect against reflected laser light as well. As a result, operating rooms in which lasers are used do not require any special structural modifications, except for exterior warning lights that come on when the laser sockets are activated. This alerts those outside the room that they should wear protective glasses before entering. It is also a good idea for warning signs to indicate the type of laser being used, since the eyewear needs to be appropriate for the particular laser in use. In contrast with open laser use, protective glasses need not be worn for endoscopic or interstitial laser procedures since the laser control area is contained within the patient's body. The laser may then be considered a class 1 device (like a CD player) such as when the treatment fiber of an operational laser is placed inside the patient's body. The fiber used in these procedures must be protected from kinking, as this could rupture the fiber and allow laser light to escape from the side. An aiming beam visible outside the endoscope indicates a defective fiber, which should be replaced right away.

Finally, video endoscopy is mandatory in the setting of endoscopic operations. Laser light cannot be transmitted back through the fiberoptic bundles of the endoscope and injure the eye. The real danger is that mishandling may cause a laser fiber to break at the instrument valve near the eyepiece. If video endoscopy is not available, laser glasses should be worn. There is no point in using an eyepiece safety filter. If the operator's unprotected eye is within a few millimeters of an accidental fiber break, the escaping laser light, though divergent, can still cause injury since it is very close to the eye.

Eye and Skin Injuries

Due to the high power density of medical lasers and the fact that the optical media of the eye focus light onto a small area of the retina, injuries to the unprotected eye can occur during open laser use. Lasers that are strongly absorbed by water (e. g., CO_2) tend to damage the anterior portions of the eye (especially the cornea and lens), while wavelengths in the visible and NIR range (e. g., argon and Nd:YAG lasers) pass through the optical media of the eye and damage the retina. To prevent these eye injuries, everyone in the laser control area should wear protective glasses during the open use of medical lasers. Care should be taken that the wavelength(s) emitted by the laser match the wavelength(s) for which the protective eyewear is designed. The only time it is not necessary to wear laser glasses is when the laser control area is within the patient's body during an endoscopic or interstitial procedure, or when the laser has been put in standby mode. It is good practice to cover the patient's eyes with an adhesive cotton compress, which can also be moistened when a CO_2 or erbium beam is used. The closed eyelids provide the best possible eye protection; if necessary, metal spatulas can be placed over the eyelids or may be actively held and positioned under the eyelids. In this case the spatula should lift the lid away from the eye without touching the cornea or conjunctiva to avoid thermal conduction injury.

Inadvertent skin injuries from laser light are very rare. If the laser beam accidentally strikes an area of the skin, a painful recoil response by the person usually quickly moves the affected part away from the beam, often resulting in no injury or at most a mild, low-grade burn. Moreover, the high temperatures developed during laser treatment kill any bacteria or viruses that are present, so even a skin injury from a direct-contact fiber poses very little risk of infection. A skin injury from a scalpel is far more hazardous, as the lesion usually extends to deeper skin layers with a higher risk of infection, e. g., human immunodeficiency virus (HIV) infection.

Fire and Explosion Hazards

In principle, a risk of fire or explosion is present whenever energy is transmitted in an environment where flammable materials may be present. This risk is not laser-specific and also exists in electrosurgical procedures and when endoscopic light cables are used [21–23]. Flammable materials consist of surgical drapes, adhesive films, compresses, pledgets, and most plastic items (especially tracheal tubes, cuffs, and catheters). This group also includes organic and disinfectant solutions. Most solutions will not burst into flame when struck by a laser beam, but they can reach combustible temperatures more quickly when they have been spread over the skin in a thin film. Gases such as oxygen, nitric oxide, and halothane can potentiate the combustive effect.

An endotracheal tube fire is definitely the greatest hazard associated with oral, laryngeal, and tracheal laser use—although lasers are not the only source of combustion. It can also occur in electrosurgery. The best safeguard against a tube fire is to keep the endotracheal tube at a safe distance from the operative field. For this reason, nasal intubation should be used for intraoral procedures whenever possible, while jet ventilation is preferred for laryngeal procedures if the operation and patient's condition will allow it. A rigid bronchoscope offers the greatest protection during tracheoscopy, but often a flexible tube must be passed down the endoscope for recanalizing a malignant stricture. This illustrates the general nature of the problem: a "laser-resistant" tube is designed to protect against external laser radiation, but an actual tube fire is caused by the combustion of laser gases inside the tube, which acts like a flamethrower. In other situations as well, an endotracheal tube does not burn on the outside; a fire occurs when the laser beam pierces the tube wall and ignites the inside of the tube. As a result, a "laser-resistant" tube offers no protection during a bronchoscopic operation, but if the tube is located within the operative field, a "laser-resistant" tube should still be used. Tubes are made laser safe in two ways by using:
- noncombustible or fire-resistant materials such as a metal spiral tube; or
- compressed foam (Merocel Laser-Guard), which is made laser resistant by moistening.

Metal spiral tubes reflect laser light diffusely, posing only a theoretical risk to surrounding tissues. With prolonged exposure, the metal tube can become heated through radiation absorption, causing the cuff hoses, for example, to melt to the inside of the tube. Other disadvantages of metal tubes are that they are very rigid and have an unfavorable lumen:outer diameter ratio. The foam tubes designed for infrared lasers are considerably more flexible than metal tubes and can also be used for nasal intubation. However, they have several disadvantages.
- The foam is not laser-resistant in itself but only through its high water-binding capacity. The foam must be dripping wet or it is liable to catch fire.

- The foam covering does not extend all the way to the end of the tube. All portions of the tube not covered by foam may be instantaneously ignited by a laser beam.
- Since the foam binds water, the vocal cords abutting the tube may become adherent to the foam surface, resulting in mucosal injury when the tube is withdrawn.

So when metal and foam tubes are described as "laser-resistant," it means that they do offer some protection from accidental laser exposure but are not designed to withstand continuous laser irradiation.

An even more common situation is one in which it would be desirable to use a laser-resistant endotracheal tube, but this cannot be done due to anatomical constraints, intubation problems, or other factors. The best solution in these cases is to keep the laser beam from striking the tube. This means that the surgeon must be able to locate and identify the tube throughout the operation. This can be difficult if the tube is hidden beneath drapes, sponges, or other materials. Wrapping the tube with aluminum foil is not advised, since the laser beam can perforate the foil in an instant. In situations where a laser-resistant tube cannot be used, an alternative is a transparent polyvinyl chloride (PVC) tube, which is transparent to scattered radiation from the Nd:YAG laser and undergoes only slight surface melting by scattered emissions from the CO_2 laser. Near the surgical site, it is best to cover the tube surface with moist neurosurgical cotton so that the tube can be easily identified in the operative field and an accidental laser beam strike will not cause instant perforation and combustion.

Neuroleptic analgesia and room air ventilation can enhance laser safety, but the usual indication for an endobronchial procedure is respiratory insufficiency due to stenosis, and these patients require high oxygen concentration just to maintain adequate saturation. In any case, lowering the oxygen concentration is not an effective safety measure in itself. The difference between room air (20 % O_2) and 100 % O_2 is entirely in the combustion time, and once a fire has been ignited, the anesthetic gas, tube, and flexible endoscope will continue to burn even in room air. Similarly, intermittent apnea does not protect against combustion, though it is effective for keeping laser fumes out of the lung during laser use. When a laryngeal mask (or mask ventilation) is used during laser surgery in the facial region, an explosive "pop" can occur over vaporized skin or hair due to the combustion of leaked gas, and therefore masks should be used only in conjunction with neuroleptic analgesia. The protective measures covered so far are summarized below, in order of priority:
1. An endotracheal tube should be kept out of the operating field if at all possible.
2. If this cannot be done, a laser-resistant tube should be used.
3. If a laser-resistant tube cannot be used, the surgeon should be able to identify the tube in the operative field at any time.
4. In this case the part of the tube closest to the surgical site can be protected by covering it with wet neurosurgical cotton.
5. Wrapping the tube with aluminum foil can give a false sense of security and is not advised.

6. Room air ventilation or apnea can also give a false sense of security and can do no more than slightly delay tube combustion. Oxygen should be given to patients who require it.

We also recommend that a large-bore suction catheter with an attached syringe containing 50 mL of saline be placed within the operative field in every laryngotracheal procedure. It can provide a fast and effective fire extinguisher in the event of an emergency. Wisps of smoke and the odor of burned plastic are often the initial warning signs of a tube fire. If a burned plastic smell is noted during laser treatment, it should be assumed that a tube fire has occurred until proved otherwise.

Hazards from Toxic Compounds

The toxic compounds present in some lasers are of little importance when due attention is given to maintenance, service, and dye changes. Numerous medical procedures involve the generation of smoke and fumes with mutagenic and carcinogenic properties (e. g., methylmethacrylate in bone cement, formaldehyde, acrolein and other compounds that form as pyrolytic products in tissue vaporization). Even without a smoke evacuation system, the amounts generated are well below the maximum allowable concentration (MAC). Even then good suction is essential for maintaining a clear operative field and eliminating objectionable odors during surgery. In terms of the total volume of the smoke and fumes produced, compared with high-frequency electrosurgery, most laser operations generate fewer pyrolytic products.

As a general strategy for reducing the spread of infectious materials, it is preferable to avoid pulsed lasers (e. g., erbium lasers) in situations where there is an increased risk of transmitting pathogenic organisms (human papillomavirus [HPV] lesions, infected wounds) [24]. The use of an ultrasound dissector, incidentally, can significantly increase the risk of disease transmission.

Electrical Hazards

There are no specific electrical hazards associated with the use of an appropriately operated and maintained laser device. Of course, the manufacturer's manual should be consulted for specific power supply recommendations.

Routine Clinical Laser Safety

While trade organizations have established occupational safety standards to promote employee safety, physicians bear responsibility both to their employees and also to their patients, whose well-being is a priority concern. These caregiver responsibilities will inevitably clash with prescribed safety standards. Measures to protect patients from laser radiation must always be tailored to the specific therapeutic situation and therefore should have the status of a recommendation rather being a hard and fast rule. Moreover, safety measures should be formulated only by persons who have a position of responsibility in the treatment of patients [25, 26].

Table 1.6 lists the seven "golden rules" of medical laser safety developed over years of medical laser practice. These rules have proved effective both in ensuring the safety of the personnel and in providing an optimum degree of safety and care for the patients.

Table 1.6 The seven "golden rules" of clinical laser safety

1. Keep lasers in standby mode when not in operation
2. Bystanders should remain at a safe distance
3. Wear protective glasses (the right kind) in the laser environment
4. Never use the laser as a pointer (coworkers are not a target)
5. Do not aim the beam at other instruments (reflections)
6. Do not aim the beam at flammable materials (especially the endotracheal tube)
7. Check your system (be informed)

To expand upon the final rule, be aware of the temptation to boost the power or energy setting of the laser device if the beam does not produce the desired effect on the tissue. This is a common error when using medical laser systems. Thus the laser device and especially the terminal part of the delivery system (applicator) should be checked before each use. The applicator is particularly susceptible to damage and often constitutes a weak point in the system as a whole. Since it is easy for the operator to check these components, he or she is obliged to do so.

When using a flexible fiberoptic delivery system, check:
- the fibers for visible external defects and contaminants (ethylene oxide dissolves softening agents, formaldehyde oxidizes metal);
- the fibers for optical patency (hold one end to a light source; the opposite end should appear uniformly bright);
- the light from the aiming beam should not come out of the side of the fiber;
- Check the aiming beam against a dark background (it should be round and uniform).

When a rigid delivery system is used, a trial exposure should be made (e. g., on a wooden tongue depressor) to check for perfect alignment of the aiming and treatment beams.

Medical lasers are highly complex systems whose effect depends on various properties such as wavelength, pulse duration, power, etc. Safe and specific laser application requires not only theoretical knowledge of optical physics but also hands-on training. For insurance purposes as well, it is strongly recommended that laser practitioners enroll in qualified training courses. Additional practical knowledge can be gained from instructional visits to colleges and other institutions with experience of medical lasers. Often it is the "little" tips and tricks that are of greatest help in facilitating practical laser use and avoiding potential hazards. Reading the manufacturer's instructions (manual) is no substitute for this kind of training and information.

The seven "golden rules" mentioned above do not mean that established safety standards are irrelevant. All laws, regulations, standards, etc. are based on the concept of using lasers safely and correctly. Tailoring these to a concrete situation requires sound knowledge of laser physics, the safety standards derived from laser physics, and of typical treatment situations. For this reason, in every department where laser surgery is regularly undertaken, a responsible physician (e. g., a senior staff member) should be designated as the local laser safety officer responsible for setting up safety protocols based on the local circumstances and specific requirements of that department. It is also good practice, especially at larger hospitals, to appoint a laser technician as a coordinating safety officer whose duties include maintaining equipment standards, providing regular instruction, and issuing reports.

Occupational safety standards cover a broad spectrum of possible safety measures, all of which do not necessarily have to be implemented. The overriding goal is safety: occupational safety standards should apply in any given situation only if the goal of safety cannot be achieved through other means, such as placing the laser in standby mode. It is helpful to recall one of the oldest mottos in workplace safety: a danger recognized is a danger averted.

■ References

1 Berlien H-P, Müller G. Angewandte Lasermedizin, Handbuch für Praxis und Klinik. Landsberg: Ecomed, 2000; 3. Auflage
2 Müller G, Berlien H-P. Fortschritte in der Lasermedizin. In: Roggan A (Hrsg). Dosimetrie thermischer Laseranwendungen in der Medizin. Landsberg: Ecomed, 1997; Bd. 16
3 Katalinic D. pers. Mitteilung. Sion, CH: ISLMS, 1984
4 Müller G, Roggan A. Laser-Induced Interstitial Thermotherapy. In: Roggan A, Dörschel K, Minet O, Wolff, D, Müller G (Hrsg). The Optical Properties of Biological Tissue in the Near Infrared Wavelength Range – Review and Measurements. Bellingham: SPIE-Press, 1995
5 Fujimoto JG, Lin WZ, Ippen EP, Puliafito CA, Steinert RF. Time Resolved Studies of Nd:YAG Laser Induced Breakdown, Plasma Formation, Acoustic Wave Generation and Cavitation. Invest Ophthalmol Vis Sci 1986; 26: 1771–1777
6 Förster T. Fluoreszenz organischer Verbindungen. Göttingen: Vandenhoek und Ruprecht, 1951
7 Nelson JS, Liav LH, Orenstein A, Roberts WG, Berns MV. Mechanism of tumor destruction following photodynamic therapy with hematoporphyrin derivative, chlorin and phthalocyanine. J Natl Cancer Inst 1988; 80: 1599–1605
8 Jori G. Photosensitizing Compounds: Their Chemistry, Biology and Clinical Use. Chicester, UK: Wiley, 1989: pp. 78–86
9 Goldman L. The Biomedical Laser: Technology and Clinical Applications. In: Riva C, Feke G (eds). Laser Doppler Velocimetry in the Measurement of Retinal Blood Flow. New York: Springer Verlag, 1981: 135–181
10 Naht G, Gorisch W, Kiefhaber P. First laser endoscopy via a fiber optic transmission system. Endoscopy 1973; 5: 208
11 Berlien HP, Müller G. Applied Lasermedicine. New York: Springer, 2002
12 Philipp CM, Algermissen B, Quint C, Poetke M, Urban P, Müller U, Berlien H-P. Surface cooling during laser treatment, cooling and compression – twofold action of contact cooling. Laser Physics 2003; 13: 1–8
13 Philipp CM, Rhode E, Berlien HP. Nd: YAG laser procedures in tumor treatment. Sem Surg Oncol 1995; 11: 290–298

14 Bown SG. Phototherapy of tumors World. J Surg 1983; 7: 700–709
15 Philipp C, Bollow M, Krasicka-Rohde E, Fobbe F, Berlien HP. Color-coded duplex sonography as a new method for monitoring of laser-induced thermotherapy. SPIE Proceedings 1994; 2132: 287–294
16 Vogl TJ, Weinhold N, Muller P, Mack M, Scholz W, Philipp C, Roggan A, Felix R. MR-controlled laser-induced thermotherapy (LITT) of liver metastases: clinical evaluation. Roentgenpraxis 1996; 49: 161–168
17 Poetke M, Philipp CM, Urban P, Berlien HP. Interstitial laser treatment of venous malformations. Med Laser Appl 2001; 16: 111–119
18 Unfallverhütungsvorschriften der Berufsgenossenschaften, BG V2 (Laser), (ehem. UVV VBG 93)
19 Medizinproduktegesetz (MPG)
20 Medizinprodukteanwendergesetz (MPAG)

21 Altomare DF, Memeo V. Colonic explosion during diathermy colotomy. Dis Colon Rectum 1993; 3: 291–292
22 Axelrod EH, Kusnetz AB, Rosenberg MK. Operating room fires initiated by hot wire cautery. Anesthesiology 1993; 5: 1123–1126
23 Bailey MK, Bromley H, Allison JG, Conroy JM, Krzyzaniak W. Electro-cautery-induced airway fire during traceostomy. Anesth Analg 1990; 71: 702–704
24 Capizzi PJ, Clay RP, Battey MJ. Microbiologic activity in laser resurfacing plume an debris. Lasers Surg Med 1998; 23: 172–174
25 Philipp C, Albrecht H, Hug B, Berlien H-P, Müller G. Significance of Laser Safety. Lasers in Gynecology. Berlin, Heidelberg: Springer-Verlag, 1992: 435–446
26 Rockwell RJ. Laser Accidents: Reviewing thirty years of incidents: What are the concerns – old and new. J Laser Application 1994; 6: 203–211

2 Lasers in Otology

S. Jovanovic

■ Contents

■ Abstract

Ongoing efforts to refine surgical techniques in otology are based on the desire to minimize the critical aspects of these procedures, especially the hazards to the inner ear. One approach is to optimize conventional operative techniques through the precise and controlled use of lasers. This chapter deals with the various indications for noncontact laser use in the external auditory canal, on the tympanic membrane, and in the middle and inner ear and reviews the surgical techniques involved in the use of various laser wavelengths, placing special emphasis on the techniques that are best for specific indications. For example, today it is hard to conceive of stapes surgery without lasers, both in primary operations and revision surgery. Other indications for laser use are chronic hyperplastic mucosal suppuration, cholesteatoma, tympanosclerosis, malleus fixation, adhesive processes, external auditory canal exostoses near the tympanic membrane, and vascular lesions of the middle ear. Particularly in revision surgery, the laser often provides a surgical treatment option that would not be available with conventional instruments. Lasers applied to the tympanic membrane in the operative treatment of middle ear ventilation problems, transtympanic endoscopy, and the treatment of perforations are additional procedures that can be carried out on an ambulatory basis. With regard to the inner ear, the use of lasers in the treatment of peripheral vestibular disorders as well as tinnitus and sensorineural hearing loss is discussed. The chapter concludes with a description of laser use in the surgical treatment of acoustic neuroma.

■ Introduction

In otology, surgical techniques using conventional instruments are widely practiced and have been established for many years. All manual instrument techniques involve the manipulation of tissues (external auditory canal, tympanic membrane, middle ear mucosa, ossicular chain, etc.) to produce and transmit mechanical energy. Some of the instruments, such as drills, cause additional energy transmission through vibrations. In the past, various types of energy have been used to eliminate these unwanted effects during the surgical alteration of tissues. For a review see the article "The Argon Laser in Otology" by DiBartolomeo and Ellis [1]. Clarke, for example, used electrocautery needles in 1973 to remove exostoses from the external auditory canal [2]. Mülwert and Voss used ultrasound in 1928 for the treatment of otosclerosis [3]. Krejci, in 1952, was the first to surgically expose the mastoid and selectively ablate the vestibular apparatus with ultrasound as a treatment for Ménière's disease [4]. Sjöberg and Stahle optimized the ultrasound therapy for Ménière's disease in 1965, but this treatment was not widely accepted due to lack of precision in selective ablation [5]. Similarly, the selective cryosurgical destruction of anatomic structures has failed to offer significant advantages [6].

In the continuing search for a precise and "noncontact" form of tissue alteration, the application of laser beams appeared to be the ideal approach. Stahle and Högberg [7], in 1965, were among the first to investigate the potential of lasers in otologic surgery, initially using a ruby laser to carry out inner ear surgery in pigeons. Later the same group of authors used the argon laser on the organ of Corti in guinea pigs to produce surface changes in the stria vascularis without damaging the bony cochlea [8]. Sataloff [9], in 1967, was the first to experimentally vaporize isolated human footplates with a neodymium:glass laser. Kelemen et al. [10] were able to induce bleeding in the inner ear of mice with pulsed ruby and neodymium:yttrium aluminum garnet (Nd:YAG) lasers. Wilpizeski et al. [11] produced selective vestibular ablation in monkeys by irradiating the semicircular canals with an argon laser. However, the conflicting experimental data prevented clinical application. Escudero et al. [12] used an argon laser in human tympanoplasties to spot-weld a temporalis fascia graft to the margin of the perforated eardrum. DiBartolomeo and Ellis [1] reported on the clinical application of argon laser surgery of the external auditory canal and middle ear for the treatment of various soft-tissue abnormalities (adhesions, granulations, persistent stapedial artery, etc.), the ossicular chain, and bony lesions of the external auditory canal (exostoses, osteomas). Finally, Perkins [13] introduced the argon laser in clinical stapes surgery in 1980. Silverstein et al. [14] first used the potassium-titanyl-phosphate (KTP)-532 laser in stapes surgery in 1989 and Lesinski [15] the carbon dioxide (CO_2) laser also in 1989. Among the pulsed laser systems, the erbium (Er):YAG laser was first used clinically for otologic surgery in 1992 [16]. Recently, an experimental study was published on the use of fiberoptically transmitted near-infrared diode lasers in otologic surgery [17]. To date, their clinical use has been limited to a few cases. More recently, otosurgical applications of the argon, KTP-532, CO_2 and Er:YAG lasers have been described in various publications, with some degree of controversy [1, 13–15, 19–71, 73–94].

Many otosurgical procedures involve removing large amounts of bone and soft tissue with conventional instruments. In contrast, the application of laser energy using a noncontact technique allows for vibration-free tissue removal and enables surgeons to carry out some procedures with greater precision, leading to better results and fewer complications. The transmission of potentially harmful energy to the surrounding tissues can be limited in a very precise way by selecting the optimal laser parameters for removing particular types of tissue.

For the present, lasers are still not widely used in otologic surgery. Using a laser means leaving behind traditional, established surgical techniques with conventional instruments. The safe and effective use of lasers in otology requires knowledge of the basic principles of laser–tissue interactions and the possible applications of laser use in otologic surgery. However, theoretical knowledge is no guarantee for achieving good surgical results, which depend more upon clinical experience acquired in a supervised setting.

In this chapter first the general principles of laser use in otologic surgery are reviewed. Then the following sections deal with clinical laser application in selected otologic disorders.

■ Role of Various Lasers in Otology

Laser–tissue interactions have already been dealt with in some detail in Chapter 1. Here we consider the specific features of these lasers as they apply to otologic surgery.

Suitability of Different Wavelengths

Not infrequently, the selection of a laser for otosurgical procedures is dictated by the availability of a wavelength intended for use in other ENT regions. The tissue effects of lasers and the extent of the thermal damage zone in the surrounding tissues can vary considerably among lasers with different wavelengths. The ability to transmit the beam through fiberoptic cables is another factor that has an important bearing on laser applications. Finally, the individual enthusiasm for a new technology can also be the decisive factor in choosing a particular laser.

Three types of continuous-wave (CW) thermal laser are currently used in otologic surgery: the argon laser (which emits at wavelengths of 488 nm and 514 nm), the KTP laser (532 nm), and the CO_2 laser (10,600 nm). The Er:YAG laser (2940 nm) is a pulsed laser that produces an oligothermal tissue effect.

Argon and KTP Lasers

The argon and KTP lasers are discussed together because of their similar laser–tissue interactions. They emit energy in the visible range of the electromagnetic spectrum.

In some circumstances, a low-intensity argon laser beam can pass through bone tissue without altering it. At high energies, the argon beam vaporizes bone and is used for laser fenestration of the stapes footplate in otosclerosis. The suitability of the argon laser for stapedotomy is doubtful, however, due to the low absorption coefficient of its radiation in the stapes footplate. Its effectiveness depends strongly on the degree of pigmentation of the treated tissue, resulting in poor reproducibility of its ablative (perforative) effect [56, 62, 63]. Moreover, the light from visible-wavelength lasers passes through the perilymph with almost no interaction. Because it is strongly absorbed by the perfused tissue and pigmented cells, it can pose a threat to inner ear structures. Clinical experience with these lasers to date, however, has not confirmed this potential theoretical hazard. The most likely explanation for this is that the beam delivered by an optical fiber diverges immediately after leaving the fiber. The power density falls off so rapidly that the laser radiation still being absorbed in the tissue causes no thermal damage to the inner ear structures because of its low power density.

Argon and KTP laser light is strongly absorbed by hemoglobin, making it an excellent tool for hemostasis. Well-vascularized or inflamed tissues can be effectively treated with very little bleeding by coagulating the tissue before cutting or vaporizing it. These lasers can also be used to destroy cholesteatoma cells within the middle ear and mastoid [83, 95, 96].

CO_2 Laser

The continuous beam of the CO_2 laser is effective for removing soft tissue, and it can vaporize thin bony structures when focused to a small spot [56, 62, 63]. The CO_2 laser beam is more strongly absorbed by bone than the argon laser, with the result that the CO_2 laser is more effective, can create a more reproducible stapedotomy opening, and causes less collateral thermal damage.

One of the main advantages of the far-infrared emission of the CO_2 laser is its strong absorption by water, resulting in a shallow penetration depth of only 0.01 nm from the irradiated surface. This property of CO_2 laser light is particularly useful in stapes surgery. During a stapedotomy, the perilymph completely absorbs the CO_2 laser energy and thus protects the inner ear structures from direct injury.

The hemostatic effect of CO_2 laser is poorer than that of the argon and KTP lasers. It can be enhanced, however, by deliberately defocusing the laser beam with the micromanipulator or by using a microprocessor-controlled scanner (see Delivery Systems below). As a result, this laser is generally satisfactory for all surgical procedures in the middle ear. The CO_2 laser is also applied in cholesteatoma surgery [69, 97].

Er:YAG Laser

The effect of the pulsed Er:YAG laser differs from that of the CW CO_2 laser. By emitting short bursts of high power density in the microsecond range, the Er:YAG laser induces "nonlinear" processes, known also as "photoablation." The exposure times, and thus the duration of the temperature rise in the tissue, are so short that heat conduction is virtually eliminated. Thus, the target tissue is ablated with no significant heating of the surrounding structures. However, due to the explosion-like nature of photoablation, pulsed lasers produce acoustic phenomena (pressure and shock waves) which can damage the inner ear. The wavelength of the Er:YAG laser has a higher absorption coefficient in bone (stapes footplate) than that of the CO_2 laser. Scholz and Grothues-Spork [98] note that Er:YAG laser radiation is absorbed mainly by water and collagen, whereas CO_2 laser waves are absorbed by inorganic salts.

The Er:YAG laser offers the greatest advantages when used on bony structures [57, 63, 65, 99–103]. The tissue-ablating effects of the pulsed Er:YAG laser permit the precise and controlled treatment of middle ear structures with low, reproducible ablation rates. Thermal side effects are less extensive than with CW lasers.

Given the strong absorption of Er:YAG laser radiation by water, the beam has a low penetration depth in perilymph when used for stapedotomy. However, the pressure waves generated by the pulsed beam in the perilymph are higher than with CW lasers and can cause inner ear injuries [63, 71, 78, 85, 102]. Clinical studies have shown that transient or permanent high-frequency hearing loss and tinnitus can result from Er:YAG laser use ([85, 104] and personal experience). These safety concerns have reduced the frequency of clinical use of the erbium laser [85, 86, 88–90, 101, 103].

Today, the Er:YAG laser is considered less safe than the CO_2 laser and can be hazardous when used in stapes surgery. In addition, the Er:YAG laser is not effective for hemostasis. When bleeding occurs, the Er:YAG laser beam is completely absorbed by the extravasated blood and no longer reaches the target tissue. This is a particular disadvantage in revision surgery.

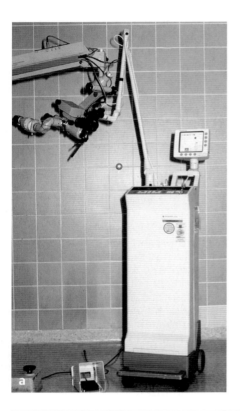

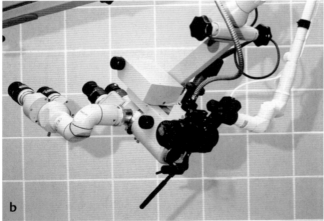

Fig. 2.1 **a** CO_2 laser with an articulated arm and micromanipulator (Lumenis model 40C). **b** Precision micromanipulator with a variable focal distance f = 200–400 mm (Lumenis Acuspot 712).

Nd:YAG and Diode Lasers

The Nd:YAG laser (1064 nm) and the new diode lasers (810 nm, 830 nm, and 940 nm) emit at near-infrared wavelengths and can be transmitted through fiberoptic cables. To date they have been used only sporadically in otologic surgery due to their high penetration depth in tissue.

The hemostatic effect of the Nd:YAG laser and various diode lasers is very good despite their nonspecific absorption by blood owing to the greater penetration and scatter of their radiation.

Delivery Systems

Micromanipulators

CO_2 and Er:YAG laser energy cannot be transmitted efficiently through optical fibers without significant losses. The output of the CO_2 laser is delivered to the operative site through an articulated arm and a micromanipulator coupled to an operating microscope (Fig. 2.**1 a, b**). A joystick is used to move the laser beam within the operative field. The micromanipulator and the attached articulated arm of the laser can limit the mobility of the operating microscope. The new generation of micromanipulators, with their lower weight (approximately 500 g) and size and shape better adapted to otologic surgical requirements, make the microscope easier to handle and allow the comfortable use of additional surgical instruments (Fig. 2.**2**).

The CO_2 laser can be used with micromanipulators allowing a spot size of 0.18–0.2 mm at a working distance of 250 mm. With a good beam profile and perfect alignment of the helium neon (HeNe) aiming beam with the CO_2 treatment beam, extremely fine microsurgical work can be carried out on middle ear structures. Newer systems also offer a variable working distance of 200–400 mm, which can be changed simply by turning a knob on the micromanipulator, eliminating the need for cumbersome lens changes. This is particularly advantageous when the CO_2

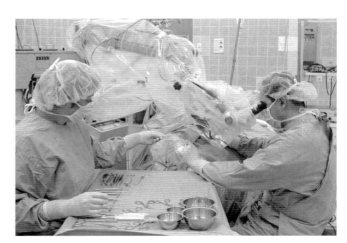

Fig. 2.**2** Intraoperative setup for middle ear surgery with the CO_2 laser.

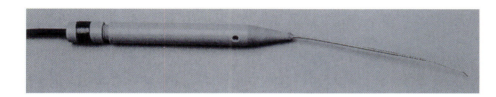

Fig. 2.**3** Hand-held applicator designed by Gherini-Causse (Endo-Otoprobe).

laser is used for other indications requiring a different focal distance.

The Er:YAG laser currently available for clinical use has been designed exclusively for otologic surgery and has an integrated microscope (TwinEr, Carl Zeiss). It is equipped with a micromanipulator with a working distance of 300 mm, which some ear surgeons consider to be too large. The spot size at the focal point is approximately 0.4 mm.

Delivery systems can differ greatly in their ability to transmit laser power. With the CO_2 laser, the delivered output ranges between 70% and 90% of the primary output, depending on the laser system and micromanipulator. The surgeon must be knowledgeable about the amount of power loss and use a correspondingly higher power setting on the laser device to correct for it and achieve the desired effect on middle ear structures.

The main advantage of the micromanipulator delivery system compared with fiberoptic carriers is the unobstructed view of the treatment site. The laser beam remains focused at a predefined working distance, thus maintaining its power density when focused onto the selected site.

Fibers

The output from lasers that emit at visible and near-infrared wavelengths is delivered through an optical fiber mounted in a handpiece that is controlled separately from the microscope (Fig. 2.**3**). This can increase the flexibility of the delivery device and is helpful in treating hard-to-reach sites (e.g., cholesteatomas, the anterior crus of the stapes, etc.).

Because the power density of fiberoptically delivered lasers is maximal only at the output end of the fiber, the fiber tip must be held close to the target site to achieve the desired effect. As a result, the fiber and fiber-bearing applicator can partially obscure the operative field and the structure being treated.

Scanner Systems

When a CO_2 laser beam is directed with microprocessor-controlled rotating mirrors known as scanner systems (SurgiTouch, Lumenis), the beam is automatically tracked in a spiral-shaped pattern within a designated pulse duration (Fig. 2.**4 a, b**). In this way the CO_2 laser can deliver high power densities even over a relatively large treatment area with minimal collateral effects. At a working distance of 250 mm, the size of the treated area can be freely selected in accordance with the local anatomic configuration and the desired size of the perforation. In middle ear surgery, the treated areas will range from 0.3 mm to 0.8 mm in diameter. Areas of 1–3 mm are used in tympanic membrane procedures. Thus, an opening of a specified diameter can generally be made in the stapes footplate or tympanic membrane when the correct laser parameters are used.

At present, no scanner systems are available for the Er:YAG laser used in otologic surgery.

Laser Otoscope

Designed for laser myringotomy, the CO_2 laser otoscope is a special delivery system (OtoScan, Lumenis) consisting of a mirror system with a built-in video camera (Fig. 2.**5**). Ear specula of assorted lengths and diameters are available for

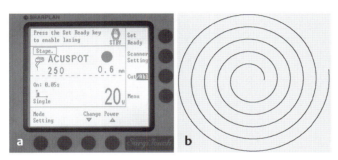

Fig. 2.**4** Microprocessor-controlled scanner for the rotary application of laser energy. **a** SurgiTouch scanner (Lumenis). **b** Spiral lasing pattern applied within 0.03–0.05 seconds.

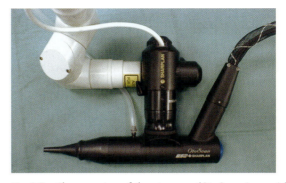

Fig. 2.**5** Close-up view of the otoscope (OtoScan, Lumenis). The otoscope consists of a mirror system (center), a video camera (right), and ear speculum attachments of varying sizes (left). Mounted on the otoscope is a computer-controlled scanner system, to which the articulated mirror arm is connected.

both children and adult patients. The diameter of the focused laser beam is approximately 400 µm. The otoscope is used in conjunction with a computer-controlled scanner system.

Thermal and Acoustic Effects of Laser Radiation

Tissue removal with a laser beam is based on the physical principles of laser energy absorption in tissue and its conversion into other forms of energy, initiating thermal and acoustic processes. The possible hazards posed by thermal and acoustic phenomena must be recognized and understood in quantitative terms.

When lasers are used in otologic surgery, the structures that are most susceptible to injury are the cochlea and the labyrinth. Prior to clinical laser use it is necessary to investigate the physical processes and assess the potential for harm. Since losses occur whenever energy is transported, laser light does not pose a critical threat to structures more distant from the inner ear. On the other hand, laser application in direct proximity to the oval window niche (e. g., laser stapedotomy) is particularly hazardous to inner ear structures. Similarly, prolonged laser application without sufficient pauses can produce a critical summation of tissue effects. The phenomena associated with laser stapedotomy have been rigorously investigated and the results have been applied to other laser procedures in otology. To illustrate the problem, a summary of the results of studies by the present author on the suitability of various lasers for stapes surgery is given below [41, 42, 50, 53, 55, 60, 61, 63, 68, 70, 71, 78].

When laser energy is applied to middle ear structures, the results are a surface- and wavelength-dependent absorption of the radiation and its conversion to thermal energy. This heat then spreads from the target site to adjacent areas, including the inner ear. In a laser stapedotomy, local absorption-dependent heating of the perilymph occurs at the application site. Heat is also transferred into the cochlea directly behind the perforation, potentially causing thermal injury to more deeply situated cochlear structures. Focal energy delivery into the fluid leads to varying degrees of local, energy-dependent vaporization followed by rapid, intense, radiation- and flow-related heat exchange processes. Temperature increases depend on the laser energy needed to produce an adequate stapedotomy opening and the resulting convection currents. Thermal conduction is of only minor importance in fluids briefly exposed to a laser beam.

Temperature Measurements

Based on the present author's measurements of a calorically approximated cochlear model, the time course of local temperature changes in the cochlea in response to laser application shows a rapid, transient, convection-induced temperature rise that becomes maximal at about the end of the laser pulse and then shows a gradual cooling that lasts for several seconds. The duration of the strong, transient heating effect approximates the duration of the laser pulse, which was only 0.05 s or 0.1 s. Longer application times would lead to higher, more prolonged temperature peaks due to the greater energy delivery. The potential of laser radiation to cause thermal injury to biological structures depends both on the maximum temperature reached and on the length of time the tissue is exposed to the elevated temperature.

In all systems, increasing the power and energy density of the laser beam leads to an increase in the temperature increments. With a CO_2 laser operating in the CW and superpulse modes, the maximum temperature rise at a distance of 2 mm past the stapes fenestra in the effective power density range needed for multiple applications averages 8.8 °C and 4.6 °C, respectively, at a power of 8 W and a pulse duration of 0.05 s. For a single-shot application with the SurgiTouch Scanner in the CW mode, the average temperature rise is 4.4 °C at a power setting of 20 W and a pulse duration of 0.05 s. Given the short exposure time, these temperature increases do not appear to be harmful for the inner ear (Fig. 2.6).

Laser light acting directly on the perilymph after perforating the stapes footplate does not pose an increased risk to inner ear structures with the CO_2 lasers tested in our study. When multiple applications are used to make a sufficiently large opening in the footplate, a slight rise occurs in the basal fluid temperature. But when the laser pulses are applied at a low repetition rate (≤1 Hz), there is no evidence that the additive effect of the temperature increments has a deleterious effect on inner ear structures. In contrast, the temperature increases following argon laser treatment show almost no site-dependent variations and exhibit a large scatter (from 5.5 °C to 13 °C). Given the low absorption of argon laser light by the perilymph, the temperature increases are due to the absorption of scattered radiation by the thermoprobe itself.

The pulsed lasers we investigated were found to cause smaller temperature increases. In the pulsed systems as

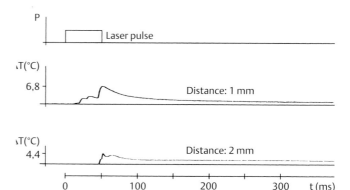

Fig. 2.**6** Time course ΔT (°C) of fluid heating in the cochlear model at a perpendicular distance of 1 mm and 2 mm behind the fenestra for a continuous-wave CO_2 laser used with a scanner (power output 20 W, pulse duration 0.05 seconds, power density 80,000 W/cm², scan diameter 0.6 mm).

well, increasing the energy density and the number of pulses (= more total energy) results in higher measured temperatures. The Er:YSGG laser (<5 °C) and the Er:YAG laser (5.5 °C) produced the lowest temperature peaks at a distance of 2 mm past the stapes fenestra in the effective energy density range and necessary number of pulse applications.

These results indicate that a stapedotomy opening made with a CO_2 laser in the CW and superpulse modes over a relatively broad range of power densities will not cause thermal damage to the inner ear. We recommend working with low energies by selecting a small beam diameter and short pulse duration (≤0.05 s). Among the pulsed laser systems, the erbium lasers appear to be most suitable for stapedotomy from a thermal standpoint.

Acoustic Measurements

Besides thermal stresses, acoustic phenomena (pressure and shock waves) also result from laser application and can cause additional damage to the inner ear. Hence they are another important criterion in the selection of suitable laser types and modes of delivery.

The acoustic effects associated with laser surgery are based on two different physical mechanisms. In the first, the photoablative effect of pulsed laser systems generates pressure waves in the lased tissue. These waves can disrupt the tissue and, when the laser is applied to the auditory ossicles, can create a vibratory stimulus in the ossicular chain similar to that caused by impulse noise. The physiologic transmission of the vibrations across the auditory ossicles to the inner ear can result in "noise trauma."

In the second mechanism, which occurs in laser stapedotomy, the energy from any laser system can cause local, transient heating and vaporization of the perilymph during and especially after perforation of the stapes footplate. This creates turbulent convection currents and causes the formation of gas and steam bubbles, which implode on cooling (cavitation) and trigger a stochastic train of pressure impulses in the cochlea. These impulses also stimulate the physiologic vibratory structures of the inner ear (basilar membrane and organ of Corti), producing a type of impulse–noise trauma in the inner ear similar to that caused by sound transmitted via the tympanic membrane and middle ear.

When the CO_2 laser is used in the CW mode, the cavitation-induced, stochastic pressure impulses in the fluid produce a noise-like signal pattern with spectral amplitude peaks in the range of 2–7 kHz. The thermally induced signal generation begins a moment after the start of the laser pulse and lasts longer than the pulse itself because of delayed cooling. The duration of the "noise" exposure corresponds roughly to the duration of laser application. When the CO_2 laser is used in the superpulse mode, the pressure variations reflect the temporal profile of the laser device (series of short laser pulses with a constant peak pulse power) and display higher pressure amplitudes compared with the CW mode. Because the mean power setting is controlled by the

pulse frequency, the temporal profile at higher power settings shows a higher frequency of the generated pressure impulses with no change in the amplitudes.

In the CW mode, increasing the power density (and thus the laser energy) leads to greater fluid heating with increased bubble formation and implosion, resulting in higher signal amplitudes. The measured signal patterns, which were converted to a comparable sound pressure transmitted through the external auditory canal, showed that tripling the power density led to a 10-dB increase in the peak sound pressure level (from approximately 120 dB-SPL to 130 dB-SPL). We found a maximum peak pressure level of approximately 135 dB-SPL. Lasing in the superpulse mode with a peak pulse power of approximately 300 W and a small beam diameter (180 µm) generates higher peak sound pressure levels of approximately 145 dB-SPL, which are independent of the mean power setting and pulse frequency.

Laser application through an existing stapes fenestra does not increase the peak sound pressure level in either operating mode compared with initial laser fenestration. Increasing the pulse duration from 0.05 s to 0.1 s does not cause higher amplitudes in either mode, but it does double the exposure time and also the noise dose.

These results show that laser energy is the only parameter to critically affect the induction of pressure waves in the ear.

With the argon laser, the only frequency components measured were low-frequency signals. This means that cavitation did not occur in the fluid at the laser settings used. We can attribute this to the low absorption of the argon wavelength, which leads to almost complete transmission of the argon beam in the model, causing very little rise in the local fluid temperature.

The pressure–time curve for pulsed laser systems shows a single, short pressure impulse whose effective duration is approximately equal to the laser pulse duration (Er:YSGG laser approximately 600 µs, Er:YAG laser approximately 250 µs) based on the "10-dB down duration" used for impulse noise. We did not find measured peak sound pressure level to be dependent on energy density with the Er:YSGG laser. With the Er:YAG laser, however, the levels did rise slightly with the energy setting. The comparable peak sound pressure levels were higher with pulsed lasers than with CO_2 lasers in the CW and superpulse modes. The highest levels, at 175 dB-SPL, occurred with the Er:YAG laser.

When interpreting the results, we drew upon studies of impulse–noise effects (which show similar signal patterns) as documented in tolerance level diagrams. The sound pressure level (SPL)–exposure time diagram is used to determine the risk of hearing loss based on the critical noise dose defined by Pfander [105]. When exposure exceeds this tolerance limit, it is reasonable to expect that permanent noise-induced hearing loss will occur. (The values in the diagram represent an extrapolation of the tolerance limits from occupational medicine with an equivalent sustained noise level of 85 dB-A over an 8-hour work day.) The

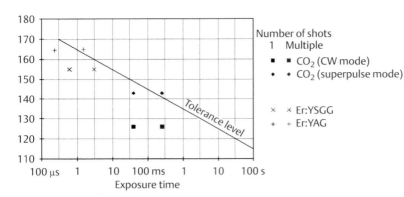

Fig. 2.**7** Sound pressure level–time diagram for determining the risk of hearing loss (tolerance limit defined by Pfander, 1975 [105]).

diagram shows that with a single application of laser energy from any of the systems tested, the dose of the noise does not reach the critical level that can cause hearing impairment (Fig. 2.**7**). On the other hand, multiple applications like those sometimes needed to produce an adequate fenestra in the stapes footplate can exceed the critical limit for noise-induced hearing loss due to the cumulative exposure time. According to the diagram, five shots from the CO_2 laser in the CW mode are not hazardous and provide good operational safety. In the superpulse mode, however, five pulses are sufficient to enter the critical range. The high peak levels of the Er:YAG laser exceed the tolerance limit despite the short exposure time. The Er:YSGG laser, which is not yet available for clinical use, remains below the critical range with its longer pulse duration of 500 µs, but it does not equal the operational safety of the CO_2 laser in the CW mode.

Experimental Animal Studies

Experiments have been done in guinea pigs to determine whether the lasers tested could damage the inner ear when used at the settings necessary for stapedotomy, and to identify lasers that could produce these effects. The basal turn of the guinea pig cochlea was selected as the laser target because its thickness is similar to that of the human stapes footplate. Auditory evoked potentials (AEPs) yielded information on inner ear function.

Perforation of the basal turn of the cochlea and laser applications into the open cochlea using effective laser parameters (high power densities with a small beam diameter of 180 µm) caused no measurable AEP changes with the CO_2 laser operated in the CW mode. Even the application of power densities approximately 10 and 20 times higher than those necessary for stapedotomy did not produce AEP changes. Since injury would occur only at power and energy settings much higher than those used clinically, the CO_2 laser in the CW mode is considered to provide high operational safety in laser stapedotomies. In the superpulse mode, however, the CO_2 laser caused significant and sometimes irreversible AEP changes in approximately 40% of animals when used at effective settings. This suggests that a stapedotomy with the CO_2 laser in the superpulse mode, which generates peak powers of approximately 300 W, would be hazardous to the inner ear. On light and scanning

electron microscopy, the sensory and supporting cells of the organ of Corti were identified as the damaged sites. CO_2 laser application in the superpulse mode damaged the inner and outer hair cells in more than 40% of guinea pigs. The pathologic changes included torsion and collapse of the stereocilia and the fusion and partial clumping of stereocilia with the formation of giant cilia [63, 80]. On the other hand, CO_2 lasing in the CW mode did not damage the organ of Corti even up to energies of 2 J (Fig. 2.**8 a, b**).

The pulsed Er:YSGG laser, which is not yet available clinically, has a relatively long pulse duration of 500 µs. When it was fired at the cochlea at the settings necessary to create an opening of 0.5–0.6 mm in the footplate, it did not cause AEP changes in any of the animals tested. Only when the total energy required to fenestrate the footplate was increased 10-fold by increasing the number of pulses did the laser cause irreversible changes in the AEPs. These results demonstrate the high operational safety of the Er:YSGG laser. The present author has not tested the effects of the Er:YAG laser in experimental animals.

Light and scanning electron microscopy following use of the Er:YSGG laser in up to 25 applications showed no adverse effects on the organ of Corti in the guinea pig cochlea. When the number of firings was increased to 50 and 75, however, pathologic changes were found ranging from a

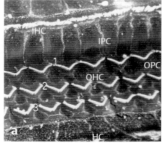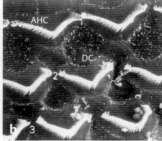

Fig. 2.**8** Normal-appearing organ of Corti with a regular arrangement of the outer and inner hair cells in the basal turn. (IHC, inner hair cells; IPC, inner pillar cells; OPC, outer pillar cells [Deiter cells, DC]; OHC 1, 2, 3, outer hair cells; HC, Hensen cells.)
a magnification ×2000. **b** Magnification ×5000. (CO_2 continuous-wave laser, single application, power 8 W, pulse duration 0.05 seconds, 1-day-old animal.)

localized loss of outer hair cells to the loss of all hair cells in all the turns. These histomorphologic findings show good agreement with the results of electrophysiologic measurements [71].

It should be emphasized that the results presented here are valid only for the laser systems investigated. They cannot be applied to other pulsed laser systems, especially those with shorter pulse half-widths and higher peak pulse powers.

Of the laser systems tested, the infrared-emitting CO_2 laser in the CW mode was found to be the safest and most effective instrument for carrying out a stapedotomy.

■ Laser Use in the External Auditory Canal

Vascular Lesions

Parkin [106] reported on the treatment of hemangiomas and telangiectasias of the external auditory canal with argon laser light delivered through a handpiece. The laser was operated at 2 W in the CW or single-pulse mode. The laser coagulation of superficial hemangiomas and telangiectasias of the external auditory canal yielded very good results, although the meatal skin after healing was thinner and more friable than normal skin.

Larger vascular lesions require a combined treatment strategy that includes embolization and/or interstitial laser therapy followed by surgical removal and plastic repair of the defect. The Nd:YAG laser is particularly suited for this purpose owing to its greater penetration depth in tissue.

Polyps and Granulations

Conventional techniques of removal of granulations and polyps from the external auditory canal generally cause bleeding. Laser removal is an almost bloodless procedure that affords an unobstructed view of the underlying tympanic membrane defect and any accompanying cholesteatoma [106].

This type of surgery can be carried out with fiberoptically delivered lasers emitting at visible wavelengths (argon, KTP lasers) and near-infrared wavelengths (diode lasers) as well as lasers that emit in the far-infrared range (CO_2 lasers). The necessary power settings for fiberoptically transmitted lasers range from 2 W to 6 W for a pulse duration of 0.5 s and 10–18 W for a pulse duration of 0.1 s. For CO_2 lasers, the settings without a scanner range from 1.5 W to 3 W (pulse duration 0.05 s). With a scanner, the power should be set at 4–8 W (pulse duration 0.03 s and 0.05 s), depending on the selected scan diameter.

Exostoses

It should be stipulated that no laser system at the present time is more effective for removing exostoses of the exter-

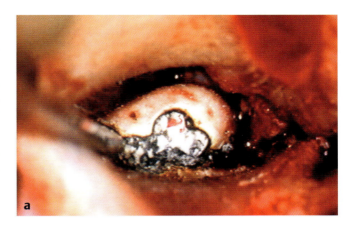

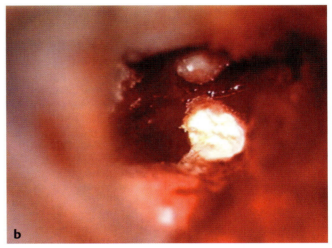

Fig. 2.**9**   Noncontact laser removal of an exostosis near the tympanic membrane. **a** Removed with the CO_2 laser and SurgiTouch scanner (20 W, pulse duration 0.04 s, scan diameter 0.6 mm). **b** Removal with the Er:YAG laser (40 mJ).

nal auditory canal than a conventional drill. Nevertheless, the use of a laser for this indication may be appropriate in selected cases. Removing auditory canal exostoses close to the tympanic membrane with a drill carries a risk of inner ear trauma from the direct transmission of vibrations across the tympanic membrane. When certain precautions are taken, such as covering the tympanic membrane with moistened gelatin sponge and applying single pulses separated by intervals of at least 1 s, exostoses bordering on the tympanic membrane can be removed atraumatically with the laser.

Both the CO_2 laser (Fig. 2.9 a) and pulsed Er:YAG laser (Fig. 2.9 b) are suitable for this application. The Er:YAG laser provides slightly better bone removal with no significant thermal effects, but its photoablative effect induces high-pressure waves that can potentially damage the inner ear. The CW CO_2 laser is slightly less effective for removing bone, but it appears to be the better choice owing to its high operational safety.

Laser bone ablation generates considerable amounts of thermal products such as char and crystalline debris. Because crystalline debris tends to reflect the CO_2 laser energy and decrease its ablative effect, it should be removed with a suitable instrument so that the ablation process can be continued more efficiently.

The CO_2 laser parameters for stapes surgery are similar to those used for bone work (see Otosclerosis below). Energy of 25–50 mJ is effective when the Er:YAG laser is used.

Stenoses

Membranous stenoses of the external auditory canal can be easily excised with the CO_2 laser [106]. When the laser is used to vaporize fibrotic stenoses caused by scar tissue, it may be necessary to graft the resulting defect with split-thickness skin. Bony atresias of the external auditory canal cannot be effectively vaporized with the laser due to their dense, ivory-like structure.

Kumar et al. [107] used the KTP-532 laser in eight patients to treat hyperplastic stenoses of the external auditory canal caused by chronic otitis externa. All of the patients were diagnosed as having severe stenosis (>66 % occlusion of the external meatus). The laser was operated at 2 W in the continuous mode, and the authors used a 0.2-mm fiber to obtain a small spot size for precision work. The stenosis was vaporized on a broad front in the anteroposterior direction without creating deep, narrow channels to prevent inadvertent laser beam entry into the middle ear. During the vaporization, an attempt was made to identify the tympanic membrane anteriorly to avoid possible damage to the ossicles. Skin grafting was generally not required, as the defect reepithelialized from the surrounding meatal skin. The laser procedure was quick, with an average operating time of 10 minutes. Two patients had a tympanic membrane perforation; one healed during the initial week, the other after 12 months. None of the patients had restenosis of preoperative proportions (>66 % occlusion), but two developed mild restenosis (<33 %) and one had moderate restenosis (33–66 %). The author uses the CO_2 laser with an automated scanner for this indication, using the same parameters as for soft-tissue work in stapes surgery (see Otosclerosis below).

To date the author has had experience in 18 patients treated for varying degrees of stenosis. As the degree of the stenosis increased, so did the necessity of skin grafting, which was done in 12 cases in the author's series. In the remaining six patients, it was sufficient to splint the ear canal with silicone strips and pack it with small gelatin sponges. The ear canal was packed for several weeks postoperatively to prevent any tendency toward restenosis. Up to 2 years' follow-up confirmed a good, stable postoperative result in 16 patients. The remaining two patients had complete restenosis requiring revision surgery with the CO_2 laser and skin grafting in the same sitting. The revision was successful in both cases. The CO_2 laser facilitates the surgery of membranous stenoses of the external auditory canal owing to the noncontact technique and good hemostatic effect, while minimizing the risk of damage to the ossicular chain and inner ear.

Debulking Inoperable Tumors

Large, inoperable carcinomas of the external auditory canal causing bleeding and recurrent otorrhea can be debulked with the CO_2 laser or with fiberoptically transmitted lasers emitting at visible wavelengths [106]. Fiberoptically transmitted lasers in the near-infrared region (Nd:YAG and diode lasers) are also suitable for this indication.

■ Laser Use on the Tympanic Membrane

Laser myringotomy is a tested procedure that is increasingly used in the clinical setting. The ventilation time of the middle ear depends mainly on the diameter of the myringotomy opening and to a lesser degree on the thermal effects of the laser on the tympanic membrane [108–113].

A myringotomy opening of the desired size should be made with a single laser application to the topically anesthetized tympanic membrane. CO_2 laser myringotomies generally heal without scarring [113, 114]. Alternative procedures such as thermoparacentesis (burn perforation) and mono- or bipolar electrothermoparacentesis do not offer the same precision and operational safety as laser myringotomy, and the duration of the procedure may too long for topical anesthesia to be effective [115, 116].

On the basis of the effects of their emissions, the CO_2 and Er:YAG lasers are suitable instruments for laser myringotomy [52, 108, 117–119]. The CO_2 laser offers several advantages over the Er:YAG laser: Computer-based scanner systems (SurgiTouch, Lumenis) can be programmed to treat an area of predetermined size and shape. Also available are high-precision micromanipulators (e. g., Acuspot 712, Lumenis) and otoscopes (OtoScan, Lumenis), which can be combined with the scanner systems (see Fig. 2.**5**).

A laser myringotomy of adequate size can be created with these systems using one or just a few laser applications. The CO_2 laser also produces an adequate hemostatic effect so that when the laser is reapplied to the same site, its energy is not absorbed by the extravasated blood. Moreover, the high operational safety of the CO_2 laser permits the use of high power settings in cases with greatly thickened tympanic membrane and middle ear effusion.

To create a sufficiently large myringotomy with the Er:YAG laser, it is necessary to apply several focused pulses in a closely spaced pattern. The weak hemostatic effect of this laser makes repeated applications difficult due to bleeding at the edge of the opening [120]. The single-pulse energy should not exceed 100 mJ due to the risk of acoustic trauma to the inner ear. At present there are no scanner systems available that could be used to enlarge the treated area on the tympanic membrane.

Other lasers used in clinical medicine such as the argon laser or Nd:YAG laser cannot be safely used on the tympanic membrane due to their greater penetration depth, tissue effects, and lack of absorption by blood-free fluids.

The CO_2 laser is considered the laser of first choice for performing a myringotomy.

Secretory Otitis Media

Secretory otitis media (SOM), which is caused by deficient ventilation of the middle ear, is one of the most common disorders in otolaryngology/head and neck surgery. The treatment of choice after an unsuccessful trial of medical therapy is surgical ventilation of the tympanic cavity by paracentesis, with or without the placement of a myringotomy tube [121, 122]. The majority of patients are children, in whom the incidence of SOM secondary to eustachian tube dysfunction is approximately 5% [123].

A conventional myringotomy incision heals in a day or two, which is usually too short to be of therapeutic benefit. On the other hand, the average ventilation tube is left in place for approximately 4–6 months, which is too long. Three weeks of transtympanic middle ear ventilation is generally considered to be sufficient [121]. Perforating the eardrum with a laser to ventilate the middle ear space can provide a solution to this clinically important problem when the laser system, delivery mode, and laser parameters are properly selected [59, 124, 125]. This method can also avoid rare adverse side effects of middle ear intubation such as chronic otorrhea, persistent perforation, atrophic scarring of the tympanic membrane, and the development of tympanosclerosis or cholesteatoma [126–128].

Laser myringotomy in children is usually carried out under general endotracheal anesthesia so that the frequently enlarged adenoids can be removed in the same sitting. If the adenoids are not enlarged, the myringotomy can be done under topical anesthesia. An opening of at least 2 mm should be created with the CO_2 laser, otherwise the therapeutic patency time will be too short (Figs. 2.**10 a, b,** 2.**11**). Myringotomy openings of this size will generally close in an average of 17 days and heal without scarring (Fig. 2.**12 a, b**). Based on experience to date, this provides adequate ventilation time in most cases [110, 111]. In a series of 85 patients (159 ears), approximately 15% of patients developed recurrent effusion over a follow-up period of 6 months. This

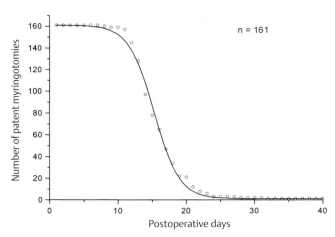

Fig. 2.**11**   Graphic representation of the healing of laser myringotomies (power 12 W, pulse duration 0.18 s, scan diameter 2.2 mm, myringotomy size approximately 2 mm) in 84 patients (161 ears). The average ventilation time was 17 days (range 8–32).

recurrence rate is no higher than in conventional procedures for transtympanic middle ear ventilation, especially when a tube has been inserted [129].

At our center, the primary treatment for children with SOM and nasal airway obstruction is adenotomy combined with a CO_2 laser myringotomy. If there is an initial recurrence in the absence of further nasal airway obstruction, a CO_2 laser myringotomy is carried out under topical anesthesia. If the adenoids reappear, a second adenotomy is done under general anesthesia and the CO_2 laser myringotomy is repeated. In the event of a second recurrence, a ventilation tube is inserted.

Operative Technique

The myringotomy can be done with the otoscope or micromanipulator. Prior to laser application, the external auditory canal is cleaned and the tympanic membrane is anesthetized with a 32% solution of tetracaine base in isopropyl alcohol applied to the tympanic membrane for 30 minutes.

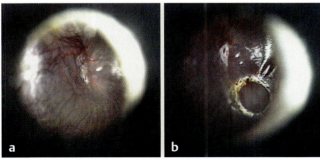

Fig. 2.**10**   **a** Secretory otitis media of the right ear before laser myringotomy. **b** Appearance after CO_2 laser myringotomy in the anteroinferior quadrant (power 12 W, pulse duration 0.18 s, scan diameter 2.2 mm, myringotomy diameter approximately 2 mm). Cautery residues are visible on the margin of the opening.

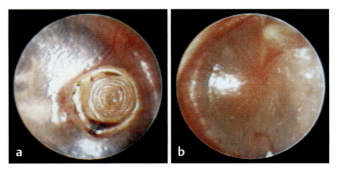

Fig. 2.**12**   **a** Healing of a CO_2 laser myringotomy. At 3 weeks postoperatively, the opening is sealed by an onionskin-like membrane of keratinized material. **b** At 4 months postoperatively, the tympanic membrane at the site of the former laser myringotomy appears normal.

The solution is dripped into the ear canal, making certain that no air bubbles come between the anesthetic and the tympanic membrane. We place a small cotton swab or thin Merocel ear wick (Pope Ear Wick, Merocel Surgical Products) on the tympanic membrane to keep the topical anesthetic from running out of the ear canal and eliminate the possible need to suction the solution before proceeding.

Whenever possible, the myringotomy opening should be placed in the anteroinferior quadrant to avoid laser damage to the annulus and malleus handle. In patients with a prominent anterior canal wall or narrow ear canal, the posteroinferior quadrant can be lased. In this case the power setting should be reduced if there is no definite evidence of middle ear effusion. The laser beam should be optimally focused, regardless of whether the otoscope or micromanipulator is used. The focal plane is adjusted by varying the distance between the target site and delivery system. The beam is optimally focused when maximum visual sharpness is noted. When a micromanipulator is used, the operating microscope should be set to the highest magnification for adjusting the focal plane. The aiming beam outlines the desired target area, the exact diameter of which depends on the indication. Generally the tympanic membrane is perforated with the first laser application by setting the parameters indicated below.

When the OtoScan CO_2 laser otoscope is used, the beam is set to 12 W and scanned to produce a spot size of 2.2 mm. The system sets a predetermined pulse duration of 180 ms. When the AcuSpot 712 micromanipulator is coupled to an operating microscope, the beam is set to 10 W and scanned over a spot size of 2.2 mm. The system provides a pulse duration of 260 ms.

In patients with a definite middle ear effusion or thickened tympanic membrane, the power setting can be increased to 15 W with the OtoScan otoscope and to 13 W with the AcuSpot 712 micromanipulator. With a scan diameter of 2.2 mm, an opening approximately 2 mm in diameter is obtained with both delivery systems. If the tympanic membrane is greatly thickened, multiple applications may be required. For a myringotomy opening, present but smaller than desired in the presence of middle ear effusion, additional pulses can be applied to the same site until an adequate opening is obtained. If the middle ear space is filled with air, the myringotomy should be enlarged by ablating the edge of the opening with the smallest scan diameter or without a scanner; this is necessary to protect the promontory from an accidental laser strike. When a scanner is used with the otoscope, the recommended parameters are 10 W with a scan diameter of 1 mm and pulse duration of 50 ms; when used with the AcuSpot 712 micromanipulator, the recommended parameters are 10 W with a 1-mm scan diameter and 60-ms pulse duration. A lower power setting of 2 W and 50-ms pulse duration are recommended when a scanner system is not used.

With the laser parameters stated above, an accidental laser strike to the promontory will not damage the vestibulocochlear organ, but it will cause pain with a topically anesthetized tympanic membrane, since the middle ear mucosa is not anesthetized. The laser plume is suctioned from the field between laser applications when the micromanipulator is used. With the OtoScan otoscope, ablation products are cleared with a built-in air jet.

It is possible in principle to undertake a CO_2 laser myringotomy without a scanner system or otoscope, using a different type of micromanipulator. The critical parameter in this case is the power density (W/cm^2) at the target site. Perforation of the normal human tympanic membrane requires an effective power density of approximately 2000 W/cm^2. The diameter of the focused laser beam is a characteristic feature of a given micromanipulator and depends on the working distance from the target. When a focused laser beam is used without a scanner system to define the pulse durations, it is best to work with a short pulse duration of 50 ms. A series of adjacent burns are made in the tympanic membrane to achieve the desired diameter of the laser myringotomy.

Defocusing the laser beam to create a larger myringotomy reduces the power density at the target in proportion to the square of the radius of the irradiated area. The power setting must be increased considerably to achieve effective power density. Defocusing the beam to a 2-mm spot size would require a power setting of approximately 60 W to achieve the effective power density indicated above. Moreover, the laser beam profile becomes imprecise when the beam is defocused, also resulting in less effective perforation.

For the reasons stated, computer-controlled scanner systems that move the focused laser beam in a programmed pattern are a better way to increase the spot size than the application of a defocused beam.

Acute Otitis Media With Vestibulocochlear Complications

Acute otitis media (AOM) is a bacterial infection that generally develops in the wake of a viral infection. Rarely, it leads to vestibulocochlear complications with impaired hair-cell function of the auditory and vestibular apparatus—presumably a toxic insult caused by bacterial products. The primary treatment is myringotomy. More serious complications such as acute inflammatory facial nerve palsy, mastoiditis, or intracranial spread of bacterial infection via the cranial sinuses or meninges require mastoidectomy or, if necessary, sigmoid sinus ligation.

Very often the inflammatory process involves the tympanic membrane, causing it to become thickened and covered by fluid-filled vesicles. This affects the response of the tympanic membrane to laser application. Whenever possible, the myringotomy is placed at the standard site in the anteroinferior quadrant (Fig. 2.**13 a, b**). The necessary ventilation time is usually shorter than in secretory otitis media, and so a spot size of 1.6 mm should be adequate. When the OtoScan otoscope is used, the beam power is set to 20 W with a pulse duration of 80 ms. When the AcuSpot micromanipulator is used, the beam should be set to 20 W with a pulse duration of 110 ms. After the anesthetized tympan-

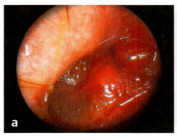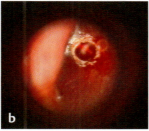

Fig. 2.**13** **a** Inflammatory redness and thickening of the tympanic membrane in acute otitis media. Small fluid-filled vesicles are seen in the anteroinferior quadrant. **b** Appearance after CO_2 laser myringotomy under topical anesthesia. Note the coagulated rim of the opening, which is approximately 1.2 mm in diameter.

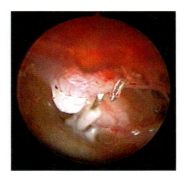

Fig 2.**14** Endoscopic appearance of a platinum–Teflon stapes prosthesis 5 years after CO_2 laser stapedotomy. The patient presented with an unexplained recurrence of conductive hearing loss. The prosthesis does not appear to be displaced.

ic membrane has been perforated with the laser, a bacteriologic smear can be taken from the alcohol-prepped ear canal under sterile conditions to determine antibiotic sensitivity. In cases of bullous myringitis with involvement of the external auditory canal, the application of an alcohol solution can be painful, and infiltration anesthesia is preferred.

Even in AOM, laser myringotomies will generally heal without scarring. Prospective randomized studies are currently underway in the U.S. and Germany to assess the role of laser myringotomy in the primary treatment of AOM to prevent persistent middle ear effusion and multiple antibiotic regimens. Definitive results are yet to be reported.

Acute Eustachian Tube Dysfunction

Acute eustachian tube dysfunction is usually caused by acute inflammatory edema of the mucosa about the tubal orifice and in the lumen of the tube. The inflammation may be caused by an acute viral infection or may have an allergic etiology. Prolonged negative pressure in the tympanic cavity causes fluid to accumulate in the middle ear. Primary surgical ventilation of the middle ear is rarely indicated and should follow a trial of medical therapy. If conservative therapy is ineffective or if rapid hearing improvement is desired, a laser myringotomy is done using the same parameters as in the treatment of SOM (see above). If effusion is not definitely present, the laser should be used at a reduced power setting.

Barotrauma

Barotrauma results from a rapid change in ambient pressure in the presence of eustachian tube dysfunction. It can occur during flying, diving, or rapid altitude changes in the mountains when acutely painful positive pressure, or rarely negative pressure, develops in the middle ear causing a bulging or retraction of the tympanic membrane. Recommended medical treatment options include decongestion of the nasal membranes and analgesia. The painful symptoms can be relieved at once by a CO_2 laser myringotomy under topical anesthesia. This requires only short-term ventilation of the middle ear. The OtoScan otoscope is used

with a 10-W power setting, 1-mm scan diameter, and 50-ms pulse duration, creating an opening approximately 0.8 mm in size. The micromanipulator is used with a 10-W power setting, 1-mm scan diameter, and 60-ms pulse duration.

Transtympanic Endoscopy

Inspection of the middle ear through a laser myringotomy under local infiltration anesthesia using a 1.7-mm rigid endoscope (0°, 30°, 70°) or special flexible micro-endoscope may be done to exclude a window rupture in patients who experience acute hearing loss. Other indications include checking the placement of a prosthesis when conductive hearing loss recurs after stapedotomy (Fig. 2.**14**) and investigate other unexplained middle ear problems. A laser myringotomy can also provide access for applying local medications to the round window. The tympanic tubal orifice and lower portions of the sound conduction apparatus can be inspected through an opening in the anteroinferior quadrant. The round window can be viewed through an opening in the posteroinferior quadrant. The OtoScan otoscope is used with a power setting of 10 W and pulse duration of 270 ms, the AcuSpot 712 micromanipulator with a power setting of 10 W and pulse duration of 360 ms. As the middle ear is dry in these indications, physiologic saline solution should be instilled into the tympanic cavity before laser use to protect the round window membrane from accidental injury. The scan diameter in both delivery systems is 2.6 mm.

Tympanic Membrane Perforations and Atrophic Scars

Lasers that emit at visible as well as invisible wavelengths help in promoting the healing of a persistent traumatic eardrum perforation or a small, residual mesotympanic defect following a myringoplasty for chronic otitis media (Fig. 2.**15 a**). The practice at our hospital, is to vaporize the mucocutaneous connection at the edge of the perforation with several CO_2 laser pulses of low wattage (1 W, pulse duration 0.05 s) delivered through an otoscope or micromanipulator (Fig. 2.**15 b, c**). Generally this can be done without using topical or infiltration anesthesia. The procedure is painless and bloodless and avoids the ossicular chain irritation that can occur with conventional treat-

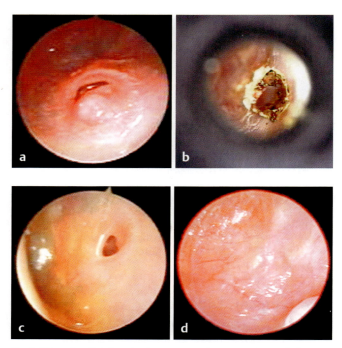

Fig. 2.**15** **a** Small defect in the posteroinferior quadrant of the tympanic membrane. **b** The margins of a tympanic membrane perforation are vaporized with the CO_2 laser (1 W, pulse duration 0.05 s). **c** Perforation on the sixth postoperative day. **d** by 6 weeks postoperatively, the tympanic membrane perforation has closed without atrophic scarring.

ments. The author has achieved a better than 80 % closure rate in selected primary and revision procedures for chronic otitis media with small central defects (Fig. 2.**15 d**). Even in cases with atrophic mesotympanic retraction pockets, CO_2 laser vaporization of the affected area appears to result in a normal configuration of the tympanic membrane with no new retraction.

Graft Fixation for Tympanic Membrane Defects

The argon [130] and KTP [131] lasers have been used clinically in myringoplasties to weld fascial grafts to the residual tympanic membrane. The middle ear is packed with physiologic saline-soaked gelatin sponges, and the graft (temporalis fascia or tragus perichondrium) is underlaid to repair the tympanic membrane defect. It is then spotwelded to the residual membrane with single 0.2–5-W laser pulses applied in the noncontact mode. The low power settings prevent thermal damage and charring of the graft and residual membrane. The perforations range from subtotal to small defects usually located anteriorly. Tissue welding was successful in 29 of 30 patients using the argon laser and in 10 of 12 patients using the KTP laser.

Epidermoid Cysts of the Tympanic Membrane

When conventional instruments such as small hooks and needles are used to remove epidermoid cysts of the tympanic membrane, bleeding often obscures vision and hampers complete cyst removal. The author uses the CO_2 laser in the CW mode to vaporize small epidermoid cysts that may form in the graft following myringoplasty or tympanoplasty. A micromanipulator is used with a power setting of 1–3 W in CW mode and a pulse duration of 0.05 s. Single shots are fired to vaporize the cyst surface layers, and the contents are aspirated to marsupialize the cyst. The procedure causes little bleeding and provides excellent healing rates. Among the author's patients, there have been no instances of tympanic membrane perforation or cyst recurrence.

■ Laser Use in the Middle Ear

Medialization of the Malleus

In some myringoplasties, medialization of the malleus handle makes it difficult to insert a fascial or perichondrial underlay graft. The malleus handle may be retracted because of adhesions tethering the handle to the promontory, even when the rest of the ossicular chain is still intact. Saeed and Jackler [132] described the use of the KTP laser for dividing scar tissue and exposing the malleus. Resecting the distal third of the malleus handle with the laser permits additional lateral advancement of the malleus handle, enabling a secure graft placement. With this technique the mechanical trauma to the ossicular chain that usually occurs with conventional procedures is avoided. The author prefers to use the CO_2 laser. The laser parameters are the same as those used for soft-tissue and stapes work in stapes surgery. When the distal malleus handle is vaporized, care should be taken to avoid any heat transfer from the malleus handle to the remaining tympanic membrane, which could damage the tympanic membrane and enlarge the membrane defect. In some cases this thermal damage goes unnoticed intraoperatively and is usually manifested after a latent period. Heat transfer can also cause wound healing problems with necrosis of the malleus handle. This can be avoided by waiting at least 1 s between laser applications.

Malleus Fixation

Sands and Napolitano [133] were the first to describe the use of the argon laser in a clinical case of malleus fixation. They used a power setting of 7.5 W and exposure time of 1 s to remove bone connecting the malleus head to the canal wall. Char was removed after each laser application. Hearing sensitivity after the procedure was normal. With conventional techniques, malleus fixation in the attic requires drilling to free the malleus head from sclerotic plaques or a special punch to transect the malleus neck and remove the malleus head. This invariably transmits gross movements to the remaining ossicular chain. Noncontact vaporization of the malleus neck or sclerotic foci around the malleus head with the laser can mobilize the chain while avoiding significant chain manipulation and trauma to the inner ear [69, 133, 134].

The author has used the CO_2 laser for this indication since 1997. After the lateral attic wall is taken down with a bur, either the malleus neck is transected with the noncontact laser beam and the malleus head extracted, or the beam is used to free the malleus head from its bony fixation in the epitympanum, restoring mobility to the intact ossicular chain. To date the author has completed this procedure in 25 patients. It remains to be seen whether the very good initial hearing results (currently up to 4.5 years follow-up) will remain stable in the long term.

Tympanosclerosis

Noncontact laser use has also proved effective for tympanosclerotic changes in the middle ear. Tympanosclerotic plaques on the tympanic membrane and on the ossicular chain and its surroundings causing fixation and obliteration of the window niches can be removed with point laser application or by scanning the beam over a larger area; it is unnecessary to manipulate the ossicular chain. Using laser technique, fixed portions of the chain can be partially remobilized or removed virtually without contact to create better conditions for surgery to improve hearing and/or insert a fascial or cartilage-perichondrial graft. Laser usage makes it possible to carry out operative procedures that are not feasible by conventional means. The CO_2 laser is the instrument of choice for this indication (Fig. 2.**16**). The Er:YAG laser, despite its excellent properties for bone work, should not be used because of potential shock-wave trauma to the inner ear.

Ossicular and Prosthetic Dislocation after Tympanoplasty

In some cases the initial hearing improvement produced by tympanoplasty with ossicular reconstruction will dete-

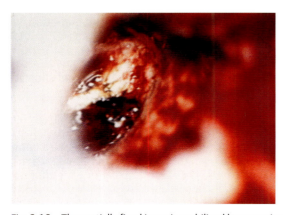

Fig. 2.**16** The partially fixed incus is mobilized by removing tympanosclerotic plaques with the CO_2 laser (4 W, pulse duration 0.05 s).

riorate after the procedure. This may result from ossicular dislocation, prosthetic migration, and/or adhesions in the middle ear space restricting the mobility of the reconstructed chain. In other cases the cause may be tympanosclerotic changes with the fixation of individual ossicular chain elements. Laser technology can assist in the treatment of these conditions in several ways.

Diagnostically, a laser myringotomy can be combined with transtympanic endoscopy using a 0° or 30° scope, as an outpatient procedure under local anesthesia. In this way the audiologic results can be correlated with preoperative visual findings to direct surgical planning.

Lasers can be used in the noncontact mode to vaporize adhesions, thereby freeing up an ossicle or prosthesis and restoring ossicular chain mobility. Since this technique causes no mechanical irritation, it does not jeopardize the integrity of the sound conduction apparatus or the function of the inner ear. Both the argon and KTP lasers and the CO_2 laser are suitable for this indication. The author prefers the CO_2 laser in the CW mode using the parameters recommended for soft-tissue and ossicular work in stapes surgery.

Park and Min [135] conducted in vitro studies to investigate another mode of laser use in ossicular reconstruction. They attempted to weld human ossicles to prosthetic implants with the CO_2, Nd:YAG and argon lasers to increase the stability of the reconstructed ossicular chain. The laser beam was not applied directly to the ossicles and prosthesis because it would damage the surface, and so it was necessary to use a solder melted by the laser at a relatively low temperature. Of the several proteinaceous solutions tested, a 40 % albumin solution and commercially available fibrin glue provided the best bonding strength and adhesion. Park and Min concluded that the denatured proteins in the solder formed bridges between the ossicular and prosthetic surfaces. At present, the advantages of "laser welding" over conventional techniques have not yet been definitely established.

Chronic Otitis Media

The pathology of chronic otitis media consists essentially of hyperplastic mucosa, granulations, and squamous epithelial structures. Anatomic landmarks are often obscured by inflammatory tissue and previous surgery. The conventional removal of these soft-tissue structures with manual instruments often causes intraoperative bleeding that further obscures the operative field. Removal of these pathologic entities with conventional instruments can dislocate auditory ossicles, accidentally mobilize the stapes, and cause damage to the inner ear. The most risky procedures are those in which the stapes and its surroundings are completely obscured by granulations or hyperplastic mucosa. When used in chronic otitis media surgery, the laser permits noncontact ossicular work and soft-tissue ablation with almost no bleeding.

To date there have been no detailed studies on laser use in chronic ear surgery. Thedinger [95] reported on the use of the KTP laser in 103 cases of chronic otitis media following tympanoplasty and mastoidectomy. The laser was used in the treatment of granulations, hyperplastic mucosa, adhesions, sclerotic foci, and cholesteatomas. Regions around the stapes, stapes footplate, round window niche, and facial nerve were of particular interest. The laser energy was delivered through a 0.4-mm optical fiber or a micromanipulator. The fiber provided tactile feedback so that the surgeon could "feel" the pathologic tissue with the fiber tip before vaporizing it, while the micromanipulator provided unrestricted beam access to the target site. According to Thedinger, both delivery devices were well suited for middle ear surgery and were occasionally combined. Typical KTP laser parameters included a power setting of 1–3 W and a pulse duration of 0.2 s in the CW mode.

The laser was used as needed to cut, vaporize, or coagulate. Because the mucosa (unlike the ossicles) contains hemoglobin that strongly absorbs KTP laser energy, the mucosa was effectively removed without transmitting mechanical trauma. In some situations it was necessary to vaporize part of the ossicle to gain or improve access to the diseased tissue. Excessive heat spread was avoided by firing the laser intermittently and irrigating the target site and its surroundings with water. Since the KTP laser energy is not well absorbed by water, a thin irrigant film was used to dissipate the laser-generated heat. The remaining energy was sufficient to be absorbed by the mucosa and effectively vaporize it. Pathologic processes near vulnerable structures were removed with single laser pulses at low power to avoid thermal damage to the inner ear or facial nerve.

This type of surgery can also be done with the CO_2 laser, aided by various scanner systems (e. g., SurgiTouch), owing to its shallow penetration and limited thermal spread (Fig. 2.**17**) [69]. This laser appears to be safer and more effective than lasers that emit at visible wavelengths. The laser parameters are the same as those used for stapes surgery. To date, the present author has had experience in more than 200 patients with various pathologic entities and has noted definite advantages over conventional techniques.

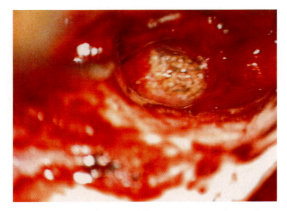

Fig. 2.**17**   Hyperplastic middle ear mucosa and granulations vaporized with the CO_2 laser and SurgiTouch scanner (4 W, pulse duration 0.05 s, scan diameter 0.6 mm).

Cholesteatoma

Currently cholesteatomas are usually removed through a retroauricular incision providing access to the middle ear space and mastoid. Generally an effort is made to preserve the posterior canal wall and spare the patient a radical cavity. This procedure is associated with a higher risk of recurrence since the surgeon cannot see into all niches and may leave residual cholesteatoma in the middle ear [136], resulting in a second operation to exclude or treat recurrent disease. Different authors describe recurrence rates of 20–50 % after primary cholesteatoma removal, with a higher overall rate in pediatric cases [137–145]. It is reasonable to conclude that laser use can lower the recurrence rates in the operative removal of cholesteatoma.

In 1989, Schindler and Lanser [97] described their concept of using the CO_2 laser and KTP laser in selected patients with small cholesteatomas and following up with a second operation and high-resolution computed tomography (CT) scans of the petrous bone. Raslan [146] tested the ability of the argon laser to vaporize cholesteatoma fragments and also investigated several dyes for staining the squamous epithelium to enhance its absorption of the argon laser energy. After in vitro staining with Janus green, a significant increase in the ablation of cholesteatoma tissue was confirmed.

Thedinger published his experience with KTP laser use in chronic ear surgery [95]. Hamilton [96], in a textbook on laser applications in otorhinolaryngology published in 2002, reported the preliminary results of an ongoing comparative, prospective clinical study of recurrence rates after cholesteatoma surgery with or without use of the KTP laser. The initial results indicated a lower recurrence rate with KTP laser use [96]. The author attributes this to the more effective removal of squamous epithelial remnants, especially in the ossicular chain region.

Lasers are particularly useful for removing cholesteatoma tissue covering a mobile stapes and spreading between the crura and oval window. The laser can be used in these cases to transect the crura at their base with no risk of footplate mobilization or dislocation, permitting the exposure and removal of all cholesteatoma tissue from the oval window niche. The CO_2 laser is particularly effective for this purpose. The parameters correspond to the safe and effective laser parameters that are used in stapes surgery (Fig. 2.**18 a, b**) [69]. For large cholesteatomas in the mastoid, some surgeons apply a defocused laser beam to various areas of the mastoid cavity to vaporize any residual foci of cholesteatoma [83].

It is the overall impression of various authors [69, 83, 95, 96] that argon, KTP, and CO_2 lasers in cholesteatoma surgery lower the recurrence rate by providing a more complete removal of cholesteatoma tissue than is possible with conventional methods. The laser applications for cholesteatoma removal published to date are nonspecific, i. e., the laser energy is aimed at the target tissue and acts on cholesteatoma cells and adjacent structures alike. Shadowed areas are not accessible to this type of laser application, and

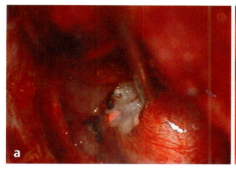
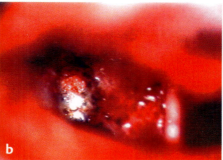

Fig. 2.**18** **a** The cholesteatoma sac has been separated from the stapes superstructure with the CO_2 laser (1.5 W, pulse duration 0.05 s). **b** Cholesteatoma matrix on the footplate has been vaporized with the CO_2 laser and SurgiTouch scanner (2 W, pulse duration 0.04 s, scan diameter 0.6 mm).

very small squamous epithelial remnants difficult to recognize as such will also be missed. A new approach would be the selective antibody-mediated staining of in situ squamous epithelial cells, which could then be devitalized with low-dose laser energy applied over a large area. The delivery system could apply the laser energy in a circular pattern, enabling the entire operative site to be treated in one pass.

Laser is a valuable adjunct to conventional methods in cholesteatoma surgery. It can reduce the incidence of residual and recurrent disease while preserving the anatomical and functional integrity of the auditory apparatus. The technique of laser-assisted surgery is safe when the user is familiar with laser–tissue interactions and knows the limits of the laser wavelengths being used.

Vascular Lesions

Glomus tympanicum tumors (paragangliomas) are richly vascularized true tumors of the middle ear that arise from paraganglia in the neural plexus of the middle ear (tympanic plexus). Laser-assisted surgical treatment starts by reducing the vascularity of the tumor by photocoagulation of the peripheral feeding vessels. The tumor is then debulked and vaporized with the laser beam. The argon and KTP lasers are excellent for this purpose owing to their high absorption in perfused tissue. The author has had some experience with the KTP-laser–assisted removal of glomus tympanicum tumors. The laser makes the operation easier by coagulating and debulking the tumor and then vaporiz-

ing it, completely clearing it from surrounding structures like the promontory and ossicular chain. Power settings of 1–5 W and single short pulses of 0.05 s duration, separated by intervals of at least 0.04 s, have proved effective. The pulses are delivered through a 0.4-mm laser fiber. The author has also had experience with the combined treatment of glomus tympanicum tumors using the CO_2 laser with a micromanipulator plus a fiberoptically delivered diode laser (940 nm). The CO_2 laser has proved to be an effective no-touch tool for dissecting the tumor from adherent structures such as the tympanic membrane, chorda tympani, auditory ossicles, etc., while the diode laser provides effective hemostasis and tumor shrinkage by coagulation and vaporization (Fig. 2.**19** **a–c**). The hemostatic effect of the diode laser (940 nm) is slightly less than that of the KTP laser. The CO_2 laser is used at the parameters described earlier for soft-tissue work in stapes surgery. The diode laser is used at 2–6 W with a pulse duration of 0.05–0.2 s to control heavy bleeding from larger vessels. The beam is delivered through a 0.6-mm fiber.

The Nd:YAG laser is also considered useful in glomus tumor surgery owing to its deep coagulating effect. Robinson et al. [147] described the case of a 60-year-old woman with a glomus tumor filling the hypotympanum inferiorly and extending to the horizontal portion of the facial nerve. The Nd:YAG laser energy was delivered through a 0.4-mm fiber held 2–3 mm above the tumor surface. The laser was first used at 1 W for 1–2 s, and then the power was gradually increased to 5–6 W. At that power level, the tumor contracted at its center and shrank. The tumor was vaporized piecemeal. Though draped over the incudostapedial joint,

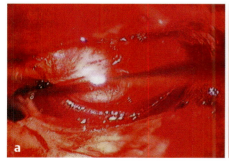
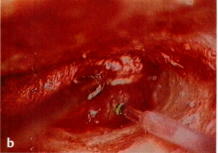
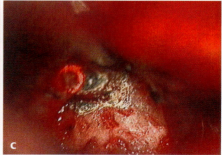

Fig. 2.**19** **a** Glomus tympanicum tumor after elevation of the tympanomeatal flap. **b** Shrinkage of the vascular tumor after diode laser treatment (6 W, pulse duration 0.1 s). **c** Tympanic cavity after complete tumor removal. The promontory has been vaporized with the CO_2 laser using the SurgiTouch scanner to prevent recurrence (4 W, pulse duration 0.04 s, scan diameter 0.6 mm).

the tumor was effectively removed by noncontact vaporization with no need to manipulate the joint. The intraoperative blood loss was 50 mL. Facial nerve function and vestibular function were normal. Postoperative hearing loss with tinnitus was attributed to the thermal damage to the hair cells resulting from energy absorption through the round window. The patient's hearing subsequently improved, returning to the preoperative level by 18 months, and the localized high-pitched tinnitus also improved.

These results demonstrate the advantages of noncontact laser use in paraganglioma surgery, which normally is a very bloody procedure which can damage the ossicular chain, the round and oval windows (with inner ear compromise), and the facial nerve. The improved hemostasis permits a better view of the lesion, allowing for greater microsurgical precision. Separation from normal tissues is simplified, resulting in better protection of adjacent anatomic structures such as the round and oval windows and facial nerve. Most tumors can be completely removed through an endaural approach with no need to disrupt the ossicular chain [69, 106, 147].

Laser use is controversial for larger glomus jugulare tumors arising from the paraganglia of the jugular bulb wall, which may invade the middle ear and petrous bone causing destruction of bone.

Otosclerosis

Given the many modifications of stapes surgical techniques that have been devised, it is evident that the ideal procedure has not yet been found. It is difficult to make a perfectly round stapedotomy opening using mechanical instruments such as drills and perforators. Hazards are also there in that these instruments may accidentally mobilize a partially fixed footplate (floating footplate), for example, or cause a thin footplate to become fractured. Using a drill to perforate a thick footplate obliterating the oval window niche (as in obliterative otosclerosis) can cause harmful vibrations to be transmitted to the inner ear.

The goal of laser stapedotomy is to create a precise opening while protecting the inner ear and avoiding damage to the remaining middle ear structures. Advocates of the laser

technique agree that noncontact vaporization of the bone covering the vestibule with the laser beam is less traumatizing to the inner ear than manual instrument extraction or perforation of the stapes footplate. It is also true, however, that the absorption of laser energy and the generation of heat during the stapedotomy pose a potential hazard to the membranous structures of the inner ear.

Owing in part to experimental and clinical studies by the present author on the suitability of the CO_2 laser, with its far-infrared emissions, as a stapedotomy tool [43–72], the laser has become more widely accepted and used as an otosurgical instrument in recent years. In primary operations and especially in revision stapedotomies, clinical studies document significantly better hearing results with the CO_2 laser than with conventional methods [15–32, 58, 64, 72, 79, 84, 87, 91, 93, 148]. Advocates of the visible-wavelength argon and KTP lasers point to the advantages of fiberoptic transmission over laser delivery through a microscope-mounted micromanipulator in both primary and revision procedures [13, 29, 38, 80–82, 149]. The fiberoptic microhandpiece (Endo-Otoprobe) is advantageous in that increasing the distance from the fiber tip to the tissue reduces the power density by creating a divergent beam (14–15°) [38, 40, 150]. This minimizes the risk of damage to the inner ear from excessive beam penetration at these wavelengths and/or heating of the perilymph. Also, a fiberoptic microhandpiece makes it easier to vaporize the anterior crus and avoids the use of conventional instruments that can transmit damaging mechanical forces [86].

Numerous experimental and clinical studies have also been done on the suitability of pulsed laser systems (excimer, holmium:YAG, Er:YSGG, Er:YAG) in stapes surgery [16, 41–43, 46, 54, 57, 61, 63, 65, 68, 71, 78, 85, 86, 88, 90, 102, 103, 151–160]. Of these, only the Er:YAG laser has been used clinically owing to its suitability for bone work [85, 86, 88, 90, 103, 159, 161]. Its photoablative effect, however, generates pressure waves in the perilymph that can cause transient or permanent inner ear damage with tinnitus (see Delivery Systems and Thermal and Acoustic Effects of Laser Radiation above). This danger has discouraged the more widespread use of the Er:YAG laser in stapes surgery ([85, 86], personal experience).

Table 2.1 Effective laser energy parameters for CO_2 laser stapedotomy (1030, 1041, 20c, 30c, and 40c CO_2 lasers, Lumenis)*

Anatomic structure	Actual power (W)	Power density (W/cm²)	Pulse duration (s)	Mode	Spot size (mm)	Number of pulses	Diameter of fenestra (mm)
Stapedial tendon	2	8000	0.05	CW	0.18	2–3	
Incudostapedial joint	6	24 000	0.05	CW	0.18	8–14	
Stapes crus	6	24 000	0.05	CW	0.18	4–8	
Stapes footplate	6	24 000	0.05	CW	0.18	6–12	0.5–0.7
or	20–22†	80 000–88 000	0.03–0.05	CW	ca. 0.5, 0.6, or 0.7	1	0.5–0.7

* The wattage data represent the actual power levels at the output of the delivery system. When the SurgiTouch scanner system (Lumenis) is used on the stapes footplate, additional single applications without the scanner (6 W, pulse duration 0.05 s) may be necessary to enlarge the opening (focal distance f = 250 mm, focal spot size = 0.18 mm [Acuspot 712]).
† Laser energy delivered with rotating mirrors (SurgiTouch).

Table 2.**2**   Effective laser energy parameters for revision stapedotomy (1030, 1041, 20c, 30c, and 40c CO_2 lasers, Lumenis)*

Anatomic structure	Actual power (W)	Power density (W/cm²)	Pulse duration (s)	Mode	Spot size (mm)	Number of pulses	Diameter of fenestra (mm)
Soft tissue	1–2	4000–8000	0.05	CW	0.18		
Bony stapes footplate	6	24 000	0.05	CW	0.18	6–12	0.5–0.7
or	20–22†	80 000–88 000	0.03–0.05	CW	ca. 0.5, 0.6, or 0.7	1	0.5–0.7
Fibrous neomembrane	1–2	4000–8000	0.05	CW	0.18	6–12	0.5–0.7
or	4–8†	16 000–32 000	0.03–0.05	CW	ca. 0.5, 0.6, or 0.7	1	0.5–0.7

*   The wattage data represent the actual power levels at the output of the delivery system. When the SurgiTouch scanner system (Lumenis) is used on the stapes footplate, additional single applications without the scanner (6 W, pulse duration 0.05 s) may be necessary to enlarge the opening (focal distance f = 250 mm, focal spot size = 0.18 mm [Acuspot 712]).
†   Laser energy delivered with rotating mirrors (SurgiTouch).

Safe and Effective Energy Parameters for CO_2 Laser Stapedotomy

The safe and effective parameters for CO_2 laser stapedotomy (type 40c with the Lumenis Acuspot 712 micromanipulator) have been determined based on data obtained in the petrous bone, in the cochlear model, and in experimental animals [57, 61, 63, 70] (Tables 2.**1**, 2.**2**).

The laser is operated in the CW mode. A power of 1–22 W and pulse duration of 0.03–0.05 s are recommended as the most effective settings for vaporizing soft tissue and bone with minimal thermal injury to surrounding tissues. The resulting power density ranges from 4000 W/cm² to 80,000 W/cm². A single laser application with the scanner system (SurgiTouch, Lumenis) will generally produce a precise footplate opening 0.5–0.7 mm in diameter (one-shot technique). If necessary, the diameter of the opening can be enlarged by firing additional pulses without a scanner. If a scanner system is not available, a series of short, low-power pulses are laid down in a slightly overlapping rosette pattern using a small beam diameter (multishot technique). A good beam profile allows for optimum tissue results with minimal thermal side effects.

Strict adherence to the recommended laser energy parameters will minimize the risk of thermal and/or acoustic damage to middle and inner ear structures.

Surgical Technique of CO_2 Laser Stapedotomy

The external auditory canal is infiltrated with 1 % lidocaine (Xylocaine) with 1:200,000 epinephrine, and the tympanomeatal flap is elevated to enter the middle ear. The canal bone covering the oval window niche is removed with a sharp House curette or diamond bur, preserving the chorda tympani. As in conventional surgery, sufficient access to the oval window is gained when the pyramidal process and tympanic segment of the facial nerve are clearly visible. Before the CO_2 laser is used, test firings are made on a wooden spatula or other suitable object to check for any malalignment between the HeNe aiming beam and the invisible CO_2 laser beam. Then the stapedial tendon, incu-

dostapedial joint, and crura are vaporized and the footplate is perforated with the CO_2 laser beam using noncontact technique. The stapedial tendon is vaporized with two or three separate pulses of 0.05 s duration at 2 W (power density 8000 W/cm²) (Fig. 2.**20**). In some cases it may be possible to preserve the tendon if anatomic conditions are favorable.

The incudostapedial joint is generally separated by conventional means in cases with complete stapes fixation. If the footplate is only partially fixed, laser-assisted separation of the joint is performed. The joint is opened with 8–14 pulses of 0.05 s duration at 6 W (power density 24,000 W/cm²), vaporizing the stapes capitulum (Fig. 2.**21**). Since the CO_2 laser beam often does not strike the joint precisely at a perpendicular angle, the joint should also be probed with a manual instrument, which is used to clear any remaining connections between the lenticular process and stapes capitulum.

The posterior crus, which is generally thicker, longer, and more curved, is transected close to the footplate with four to eight pulses of 0.05 s duration at 6 W (power density 24,000 W/cm²), the same settings used on the incudostapedial joint (Fig. 2.**22**). When this relatively high wattage is used to vaporize the joint and posterior crus, care

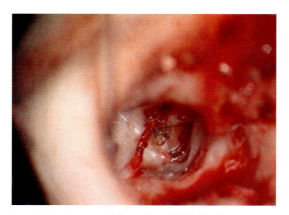

Fig. 2.**20**   The stapedial tendon is divided with two or three low wattage laser pulses (2 W).

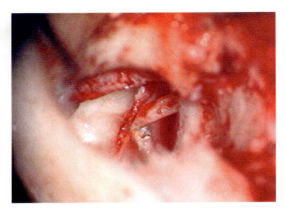

Fig. 2.**21** The incudostapedial joint is divided by vaporizing the stapes capitulum (6 W, pulse duration 0.05 s).

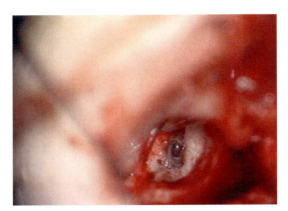

Fig. 2.**23** The stapes footplate is perforated with a single CO_2 laser application using the SurgiTouch scanner (20 W, pulse duration 0.04 s, scan diameter 0.6 mm).

should be taken that the beam does not accidentally strike middle ear structures that lie in the path of the beam (footplate, facial canal). This can be prevented by filling the middle ear with physiologic saline solution or covering these structures with moist gelatin sponge (Gelita or Spongostan). If the posterior crus remnant is still too long after the suprastructure has been removed, it can be vaporized to the level of the footplate using the same laser parameters to obtain better posterior exposure of the footplate.

The anterior crus of the stapes is fractured with a small hook using conventional technique. If all or part of the anterior crus is still visible, it is vaporized with the CO_2 laser beam using the same parameters as for the posterior crus. If this does not completely transect the crus, the vaporized site can be fractured using controlled pressure on the small hook. This virtually eliminates the danger of mobilizing the footplate or even partially or completely extracting it. The stapes superstructure is then extracted with a small forceps. Again, it is advisable to protect the surrounding structures (footplate, facial canal) by covering them with moist gelatin sponge or instilling physiologic saline solution.

After the suprastructure has been removed, the stapedotomy opening is created, usually placing it in the posterior half of the footplate. The goal is to create an approximately round, reproducible fenestra 0.5–0.7 mm in diameter, applying the beam either in a single application (one-shot technique) or in a slightly overlapping pattern (multishot technique), without causing significant thermal alteration of the peripheral zones.

The present author has been able to create a smooth, round fenestra 0.5–0.7 mm in diameter in approximately 70 % of cases with a single 20–22-W laser application of 0.03–0.05-s duration (Fig. 2.**23**). In cases where a single application did not make an opening of the desired diameter (≤0.3 mm), a second shot was applied to the same site with the scanner or multiple shots were applied without a scanner (approximately 15 % of cases each).

If a scanner is not available, the footplate can be perforated using the multishot technique. A beam 180 µm in diameter is used at a power of 6 W and pulse duration of 0.5 s. From six to 12 shots are needed to create a fenestra 0.5–0.7 mm in size, depending on the footplate thickness.

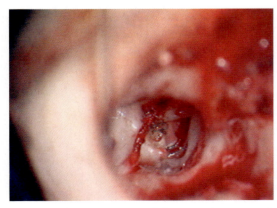

Fig. 2.**22** The posterior crus of the stapes is transected with four to eight laser pulses (6 W, pulse duration 0.05 s).

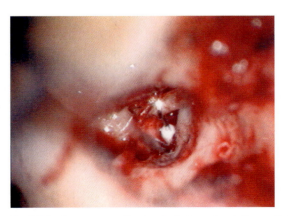

Fig. 2.**24** Appearance after implantation of a platinum–Teflon prosthesis.

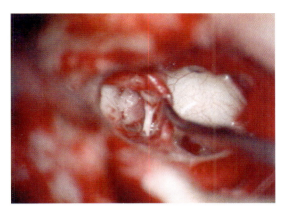

Fig. 2.**25** Intraoperative appearance of obliterative otosclerosis. Otosclerotic foci completely fill the oval window niche.

Care should be taken that the vestibule is filled with perilymph to ensure adequate protection for inner ear structures and prevent damage from direct irradiation. If the perilymph is inadvertently suctioned from the vestibule, no additional laser energy should be applied to the footplate. Lasing of the footplate is continued only after additional fluid has seeped into and adequately filled the vestibule. It may be necessary in some cases to fill the vestibule with physiologic saline solution. A platinum-Teflon piston 0.4–0.6 mm in diameter is then inserted into the fenestra and connected to the long process of the incus (Fig. 2.**24**). Finally the oval window niche is sealed with connective tissue or clotted blood.

Special Cases

Obliterative Otosclerosis

The incidence of obliterative otosclerosis (Fig. 2.**25**) is between 2 % and 10 % of all cases [162–165]. It was 5 % in the author's series. Drilling through a thick footplate obliterating the oval window niche can cause significant vibration-induced inner ear trauma. The CO_2 laser, on the other hand, can vaporize a fenestra in the stapes footplate, regardless of its thickness or degree of fixation, without mechanical trauma to the inner ear.

The settings on the SurgiTouch scanner are the same as for a laser stapedotomy. After the suprastructure is removed, the otosclerotic foci obliterating the oval window niche are uniformly removed over a broad front by laser application with the SurgiTouch scanner. This is continued until the lateral margins of the oval window can be clearly identified (Fig. 2.**26 a**). Lower power may have to be used at the periphery of the window niche to avoid accidentally entering the inner ear. Large amounts of char are produced as the bony material is vaporized. Since crystalline char reflects the CO_2 laser energy and reduces its ablative effect, it must be removed with a suitable instrument. The vestibule in the posterior part of the oval window niche is opened with the scanner (Fig. 2.**26 b**) using the same laser parameters as for a one-shot stapedotomy in a footplate without obliterative changes (see Table 2.**1**). If the diameter of the fenestra is too small to accommodate the prosthesis, the opening can be enlarged either by retreating the same site with the scanner or by applying a concentric pattern of laser flashes without a scanner. The prosthesis is placed in a routine fashion.

Overhanging Facial Nerve

An overhanging tympanic facial nerve segment, whether covered by bone or occasionally exposed, can be a serious obstacle to surgical access. If the facial nerve is covered by bone, the CO_2 laser beam can be carefully applied tangentially at low power (1–2 W), using short pulse lengths of 0.05 s, to remove the bone. Scanner settings of 4–5 W, 0.03–0.04 s pulse length, and 0.3–0.4 mm scan diameter are safe and effective. Occasionally this measure is sufficient to obtain a clearer view of the footplate. It is best to avoid completely freeing the facial nerve from its bony covering to protect it from a direct laser strike and prevent nerve prolapse through the resulting bone defect, which can hamper visibility.

In cases where the facial canal completely obstructs access to the oval window niche and removal of the frequently very thin bone will not significantly improve access, or if the tympanic facial nerve segment is not covered by bone, laser use should be suspended in favor of, e. g., a conventional stapedotomy with a curved perforator. Another option for difficult access is to redirect the CO_2 laser beam with a mirror. This may enable the surgeon to perforate a footplate that is not directly accessible to the laser beam.

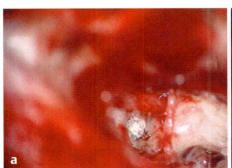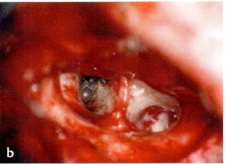

Fig. 2.**26** **a** Uniform vaporization of otosclerotic foci in the oval window niche with the SurgiTouch scanner after removal of the suprastructure. This process creates a large amount of whitish char with higher reflectivity, causing the CO_2 laser beam to become ineffective. **b** The vestibule is opened in the posterior part of the oval window niche.

Overhanging Promontory

Narrowing of the oval window niche by an overhanging promontory wall projecting into the niche generally poses only a minor surgical problem. Using the precautionary measures described earlier (covering the footplate with saline solution or moist gelatin sponge), the bony overhang can be ablated with a tangential beam using the parameters given above to provide a clearer view of the oval window niche.

During removal of the overhanging promontory bone, care is taken to avoid opening the scala tympani. The risk of opening the scala tympani and damaging the inner ear with the CO_2 laser beam, however, is far less than with a conventional instrument such as a diamond bur owing to complete absorption of the laser energy by the perilymph and the very low penetration depth of 0.01 mm. Thus, the inner ear structures are well protected from a direct CO_2 laser strike and are safe over a relatively large range of energies.

Inaccessible Footplate

If the footplate is not accessible, for example, due to an abnormal course of the facial nerve or a vascular anomaly, restoration of the sound conduction apparatus may require fenestration of the promontory using the technique described by Plester et al. [166]. Apart from using the CO_2 laser to make the fenestra, the surgery is done according to conventional technique. The experimentally determined laser parameters are the same as those recommended for a stapedotomy. The present author has no personal experience with CO_2 laser fenestration of the promontory, as he has been able to define the oval window niche in all cases.

Floating Footplate

In a conventional stapedotomy, it is not uncommon for manipulations of the stapes to accidentally mobilize the smallest of the ossicles and create a floating footplate, especially if the stapes is partially fixed. Often it is no longer

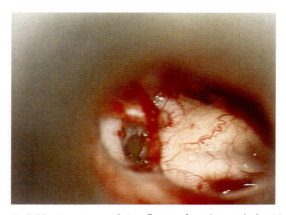

Fig 2.**27** Fenestra made in a floating footplate with the CO_2 laser and SurgiTouch scanner (one-shot application technique).

possible to perforate the footplate in these cases, necessitating a stapedectomy. The CO_2 laser, on the other hand, enables the otologic surgeon to create a fenestra of the desired diameter even in a floating footplate (Fig. 2.**27**). A platinum–Teflon piston can then be placed into the fenestra. The incidence of a floating footplate in laser-assisted surgery is very low, however, compared with a conventional stapedotomy. In the author's series the incidence was 0.5 %, and none of the cases required a stapedectomy.

Problems in Revision Procedures

Successful restoration of hearing in revision stapedotomies involves precise identification and correction of the causative abnormality without traumatizing the inner ear.

Conventional surgical procedures frequently result in unsatisfactory hearing and inner ear injuries. Numerous studies have shown that successful closure of the air–bone gap (≤10 dB) is achieved in less than half of patients who undergo a revision stapedotomy ([167–170], etc.), and 8–33 % of revision patients complain of poor hearing. The incidence of significant postoperative sensorineural hearing loss is 3–20 %, with up to a 14 % incidence of severe hearing loss.

Damage to the inner ear from excessive manipulation of the prosthesis and/or of the connective tissue occluding the oval window niche is recognized as a particular danger in conventional operations. Histopathologic studies of petrous bone specimens from stapedectomized patients have shown that adhesions often exist between the prosthesis and/or the neomembrane of the oval window and the inner ear (utricle and saccule) [171, 172]. Because of this, surgical manipulations in revision procedures can tear these fine inner ear structures, resulting in hearing loss and vertigo.

The otosurgeon faces a dilemma when exploring the middle ear of a patient after a failed stapedectomy. To determine the reasons for the conductive hearing loss, the surgeon must test the mobility and integrity of the entire ossicular chain and accurately evaluate the status of the oval window and the position of the prosthesis at the entrance to the vestibule. Often one is unable to determine the depth and lateral margins of the oval window or see the connective tissue covering the structures behind the oval window niche. When palpation of these structures is minimized to avoid inner ear trauma, the surgeon may be unable to identify the exact cause(s) of the conductive hearing loss and therefore cannot provide adequate treatment.

The old prosthesis should be removed with extreme care. If dizziness occurs, the prosthesis should be left in place to avoid permanent inner ear dysfunction. If the prosthesis can be extracted without causing significant inner ear trauma, the new prosthesis (frequently too short) is placed at the presumed center of the oval window niche.

Generally, the patient's hearing will initially improve if the oval window is free of residual disease and the surgeon's manipulation has not damaged the inner ear. In many cases, however, the revision does not correct the problem believed to be responsible for most failed stapedectomies: prosthetic migration. The new prosthesis may again migrate out of the oval window niche. The formidable problems that can arise in revision stapedectomies are reflected in the reported success rates of 30–50 %.

Technique of CO_2 Laser Revision Stapedotomy

The tympanomeatal flap is outlined and elevated, and the middle ear is inspected. The malleus and incus are probed with a needle to assess their integrity and mobility. Adhesions are frequently present and are vaporized with the CO_2 laser using the safe and effective laser parameters determined experimentally (see Table 2.**2**). With a beam diameter of 0.18 mm, it is sufficient to use a low power setting of 1–2 W with a pulse duration of 0.05 s. When the SurgiTouch scanner is used, settings of 4–8 W, pulse duration 0.03–0.05 s, and scan diameter 0.3–0.7 mm are adequate for soft-tissue ablation. These parameters are used to expose the prosthesis by vaporizing the soft tissue surrounding it (Fig. 2.**28 a, b**).

In patients with a wire prosthesis (e. g., platinum) attached to a connective tissue graft over the oval window, it is not dangerous to strike the wire directly with the laser beam. If the prosthesis is a piston with Teflon components (e. g., a platinum–Teflon piston), following stapedotomy it should not be struck directly with the beam because the Teflon cannot withstand high temperatures (> 300 °C) and its surface will swell into a "mushroom" shape without disintegrating or combusting.

The prosthesis is exposed by noncontact vaporization of the fibrous attachments. This technique avoids mechanical trauma to the inner ear. Next, the soft tissue covering the oval window niche is uniformly vaporized on a broad front until the lateral margins of the oval window are clearly visualized (Fig. 2.**28 c**). If the prosthesis is still embedded in connective tissue, the vaporization is continued until it has been completely freed. Once the distal end of the prosthesis has been cleared of all fibrous attachments, it is detached from the incus and extracted with a 90° hook 2 mm long. If dizziness occurs (under local anesthesia), the surgeon should stop all manipulations at once and reinspect

the distal end of the prosthesis for any remaining fibrous attachments that might be pulling on the inner ear.

The tissue at the center of the oval window is then uniformly vaporized to create a fenestra 0.5 mm or 0.7 mm in diameter. Vestibular perilymph should be visible through the opening. Depending on what is found in the oval window (a fibrous neomembrane and/or bony footplate), a 4–22-W beam with a pulse duration of 0.04 s is applied with a scanner system using one-shot technique, or a 1–6-W beam (pulse duration 0.05 s) is applied in a slightly overlapping pattern of six to12 shots without a scanner.

The length of the revision prosthesis is determined by measuring the distance from the lower surface of the incus to the vestibule and adding 0.2 mm. (The most common is 4.5–4.7 mm.) The prosthesis should extend 0.1–0.2 mm into the fenestra to help prevent recurrent migration. The platinum–Teflon piston is inserted into the fenestra and, if the incus is intact, attached to the neck of the incus. If the incus is badly eroded, a malleovestibulopexy will reestablish sound conduction. Finally, the oval window niche is sealed with connective tissue.

Author's Results with CO_2 Laser Stapedotomy

Results of Initial Operations

Between 1990 and 2002, 365 patients with otosclerosis were treated by CO_2 laser stapedotomy. Figure 2.**29** shows the mean bone conduction threshold at 0.5, 1, 2, 3, and 4 kHz before CO_2 laser stapedotomy and at 1.5–6 months postoperatively. Before surgery the bone conduction threshold was 0.5 kHz at 13 dB HL, 2 kHz at 28 dB HL (Carhart notch), and 4 kHz at 24 dB HL. By 1.5–6 months postoperatively, the mean bone conduction threshold showed improvement of 5 dB at 0.5 kHz, 9 dB at 2 kHz, and 2 dB at 4 kHz, indicating a statistically significant improvement in the bone conduction threshold at all frequencies (the Wilcoxon test, $P < 0.01$).

At a frequency of 4 kHz, five patients (2 %) showed a decline in postoperative bone conduction threshold to a maximum of 20 dB. None of the patients showed a decline greater than 20 dB. Two patients (1 %) showed a maximum 20-dB

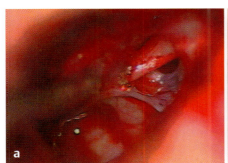
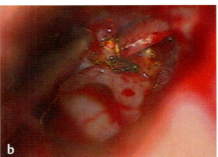
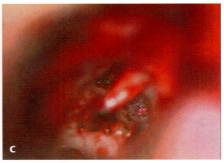

Fig. 2.**28   a** Adhesions between the prosthesis and middle ear mucosa. **b** Noncontact exposure of a wire-connective tissue prosthesis by vaporization of the surrounding soft tissue with the CO_2 laser beam.

c Uniform vaporization of the soft tissue covering the oval window niche. The margins of the oval window are clearly identified.

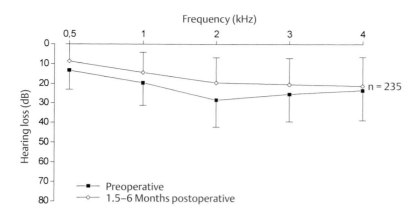

Fig. 2.**29** Hearing results after CO_2 laser stapedotomy. Mean bone conduction threshold: preoperatively and 1.5–6 months postoperatively (n = 235).

decrease in bone conduction threshold in the normal speech range (0.5, 1, 2, and 3 kHz). There were no instances of deafness.

Comparison of the mean pre- and postoperative air–bone gap in 213 patients who were followed for at least 1 year (1–9 years) is shown in Fig. 2.**30**. The air–bone gap improved steadily during the first year. After 1 year the air–bone gap was ≤20 dB in 98% of the patients (0–10 dB in 71%, 11–20 dB in 27%). Three patients (1%) developed an air–bone gap >30 dB and had to undergo revision. The air–bone gap following the revision was in the range of 11–20 dB.

The mean hearing loss for numbers by air conduction improved from 48 dB HL before surgery to 23 dB HL after surgery, with a follow-up period of 1 year or more.

Complications in Primary Operations

No intraoperative complications arose in any of the primary operations. Two patients (0.5%) experienced mild postoperative sensorineural hearing loss, and one patient had moderate sensorineural loss. Granulomas were found in two revision operations. One patient complained of tinnitus that had not been present before the surgery, and two patients reported exacerbation of preexisting tinnitus. Nine patients developed persistent dizziness caused by a

prosthesis that was too long, which resolved after a shorter revision prosthesis was inserted.

Another 13 patients underwent revision surgery due to recurrence of conductive hearing loss within a period of 6 months to 5 1/2 years. In six cases the prosthesis was displaced out of the stapedotomy opening. Prosthetic migration was combined with partial incus erosion in two cases and with total incus erosion in three cases. In two of six patients, the prosthesis was too short. In all cases the prosthesis was attached to the residual incus. Other reasons for conductive hearing loss without prosthetic migration were a too-short prosthesis in two cases and loosening of the eyelet in four cases. In one patient the eyelet was loose and the prosthesis was fixed to the incus by adhesions. Hearing improved after the adhesions were removed with the laser and the prosthesis was reattached to the incus.

Results of Revision Operations

Sixty-eight patients with otosclerosis underwent CO_2 laser revision stapedotomy. Twenty-one of the patients had undergone stapedectomy with insertion of a Schuknecht-type wire-connective tissue prosthesis, 45 had undergone stapedotomy with implantation of a platinum-Teflon piston, two had a gold prosthesis, one had a Causse Teflon prosthesis, and two had undergone stapes mobilization.

Analysis of the postoperative pure-tone audiograms of 46 patients at 1.5–6 months postoperatively showed a significant improvement in the average bone conduction threshold for 0.5, 1, 2, 3, and 4 kHz (the Wilcoxon test, $P < 0.05$) (Fig. 2.**31**). The average improvements were 4 dB at 0.5 kHz, 3 dB at 2 kHz, and 6 dB at 4 kHz.

Seventeen patients (25%) had a maximum decrease of 10 dB in their postoperative bone conduction threshold. Two patients (3%) had a postoperative hearing loss greater than 10 dB for at least one frequency (maximum of 35 dB in one case). One of these patients (1%) had hearing loss over the normal speech range (0.5, 1, 2, 3 kHz), and the other patient (1%) had hearing loss only at 4 kHz. No instances of early or late deafness were observed.

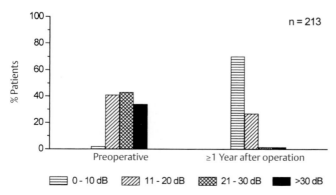

Fig. 2.**30** Hearing results after CO_2 laser stapedotomy. Distribution of patients with a postoperative air–bone gap of 0–10 dB, 11–20 dB, 21–30 dB, and >30 dB (n = 213).

Figure 2.**32** shows the average air–bone gap at 0.5, 1, 2, and 3 kHz in 30 patients ≥1 year (1–9 years) after surgery com-

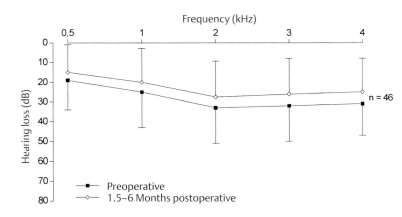

Fig. 2.**31** Hearing results after revision CO_2 laser stapedotomy. Average bone conduction threshold preoperatively and 1.5–6 months postoperatively (n = 46).

pared with preoperative findings. The air–bone gap improved steadily during the first year. At 1 year it was 0–10 dB in 60% of operated patients, 11–20 dB in 33%, and 21–30 dB in 7%. Thus, the air–bone gap was 20 dB or less in 93% of the patients. None of the patients had an air–bone gap >30 dB.

The analysis of speech audiograms in 30 patients showed that the mean air-conduction hearing loss for numbers improved from 49 dB HL to 32 dB HL by 1 year or more after the surgery.

Complications of Revision Operations

In one case the vestibule was opened prematurely at operation, with possible laser irradiation of the empty vestibule. Postoperatively the patient had a moderate pancochlear sensorineural hearing loss of approximately 40 dB with accompanying tinnitus. One woman developed a moderate pancochlear sensorineural hearing loss of approximately 40 dB 1 week after the operation, which subsequently improved to 15 dB. One patient underwent revision 6 months postoperatively due to an increase in sensorineural hearing loss. The hearing loss improved after adhesions between the prosthesis and tympanic membrane were cleared and the tympanic membrane was reinforced

posterosuperiorly with a perichondrial graft. None of the patients complained of persistent dizziness.

Laser Versus Conventional Surgery

Before a new technique can become established, its success rates must be compared with those of traditional techniques. This comparison is difficult to make, however, due to differences in recruitment and data analysis. For example, while the average air–bone gap in older studies was determined for frequencies of 0.5, 1, and 2 kHz, it is additionally determined for 3 kHz in more recent studies.

Nevertheless, a comparison of the results in major publications shows that the postoperative hearing gain after primary laser stapedotomy [15, 29, 38, 80, 84, 87, 148, 173, 174] does not differ from the good results of conventional surgery [73, 86, 149, 164, 175–183]. The results published in the literature clearly demonstrate, however, that complications after CO_2 laser stapedotomy are less frequent and less severe than after conventional operations [32, 84, 87, 149]. The present author's results are consistent with these findings.

Laser use in revision surgery offers significant advantages over conventional technique. The principal advantages are improved diagnostic and therapeutic precision, the ability to better stabilize the new prosthesis at the center of the oval window niche, and the reduction of inner ear trauma. Based on an improvement of the air–bone gap to 20 dB or less, the success rates with laser revision surgery were 70–92% compared with 49–85% with conventional surgery. The higher success rates and lower complication rates are statistically significant and do not depend on the type of laser system used [15, 32, 39, 79, 81, 125, 184–186].

The CO_2 laser appears to be suitable for use in stapes surgery. With advances in laser technology, one-shot stapedotomy can be done in most patients. With strict adherence to recommended settings, the laser helps to optimize this very exacting procedure and should reduce the incidence of inner ear damage. It is superior to conventional techniques, particularly in the surgery of obliterative otosclerosis and in revision procedures.

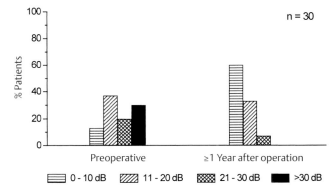

Fig. 2.**32** Hearing results after revision CO_2 laser stapedotomy. Distribution of patients with a postoperative air–bone gap of 0–10 dB, 11–20 dB, 21–30 dB, and >30 dB (n = 30).

■ Laser Use in the Inner Ear

Cochleostomy

A laser cochleostomy can be created for inserting the electrode of a cochlear implant. This technique is particularly effective for an ossified cochlea. In experimental studies the holmium:YAG laser was used to reopen the basal turn of artificially obliterated human cochlea in fresh cadavers [187, 188]. This allowed the intracochlear insertion of the stimulating electrode of a cochlear implant. CT and light microscopy confirmed recanalization of the basal turn of the cochlea without damage to surrounding structures.

The author has experimented with cochleostomies using the CO_2 laser and microprocessor-controlled scanners. The laser parameters are the same as for a stapedotomy (see Otosclerosis above), although some cases will require higher power densities and multiple laser applications because the bony wall of the cochlea is thicker than the stapes footplate. It is still too early to make a definitive assessment of this technique due to lack of clinical experience.

Peripheral Vestibular Disorders: Benign Paroxysmal Positional Vertigo and Endolymphatic Hydrops

Conventional labyrinthectomy has been proposed as a last recourse for the treatment of chronic, intractable peripheral vestibular disorders, although the indications are limited due to the resultant hearing impairment and vestibular compensation. It is already known that abnormalities of the inner ear fluids can cause macular dysfunction [189, 190]. Earlier studies also demonstrated involvement of the maculae in a setting of perilymphatic and endolymphatic hypertension [189]. Moreover, clinical observations show that macular dysfunction is often present in acute and recurring peripheral vestibular disorders. For this reason, the selective induction of macular damage without altering the function of the ampullary crest and cochlea would result in minimal surgical trauma and functional deficits. In experiments where the otolithic organs of guinea pigs were irradiated through the oval window with the argon laser after stapedectomy, morphologic studies revealed degeneration of the macula utriculi and macula sacculi [191]. The semicircular canals and cochlea remained intact, suggesting that it was possible to preserve hearing. This surgical procedure was first performed clinically in a 62-year-old woman who developed benign paroxysmal positional vertigo (BPPV) after the closure of a perilymph fistula [192]. The macula utriculi was lased with an argon beam through the stapedectomized oval window (1.5 W, pulse duration 0.5 s), and the oval window was subsequently sealed with perichondrium. A Teflon prosthesis was then inserted as in a conventional stapedotomy. Two years after the surgery, the patient was completely free of vertigo and her hearing was unchanged. Selective lasing of the macula sacculi is problematic, however, because the wall of the saccule contains pigment and may be perforated by an argon laser beam [193].

It has also been shown that irradiating the ampullary nerves with an argon laser beam through the oval window niche can selectively disrupt the nerves due to a local thermal effect [194].

Laser-assisted partitioning of the posterior semicircular canal was first carried out by Anthony in 1991 for the treatment of BPPV [195, 196]. In two patients the BPPV disappeared within 24 hours. In another 14 patients the BPPV resolved within 7 days in most cases. Six patients (43 %) had a transient sensorineural hearing loss and one diabetic patient (7 %) had a permanent hearing loss. Nomura et al. [193] found that argon laser treatment of the labyrinth in guinea pigs caused shrinkage of the membranous semicircular canal followed by occlusion due to fibrosis and ossification. Kartush and Sargent [197] fenestrated the posterior semicircular canal of four patients with a diamond drill through a transmastoid approach. A CO_2 laser pulse (power 0.5 W, duration 0.1 s, beam diameter 600 μm) was applied directly to the membranous semicircular canal causing the canal to shrink, before mechanically plugging it with fascia and small bone plates. All the patients were followed for at least one year, and all had complete resolution of their vertigo with no hearing loss referable to the procedure.

Antonelli et al. [198] investigated mechanical versus CO_2 laser-assisted occlusion of the posterior semicircular canal in a prospective study of six patients with intractable BPPV. While postoperative dysequilibrium resolved in all of the CO_2 laser-treated patients, who were hospitalized for an average of 2.8 days, dysequilibrium persisted in four of the six patients treated by mechanical canal occlusion and required an average hospital stay of 5.2 days. Hearing was not significantly different between the two groups, and neither group had clinically significant postoperative hearing loss. The authors concluded that the incidence of persistent dysequilibrium after posterior semicircular canal occlusion could be reduced by using the CO_2 laser to seal the membranous canal prior to occluding the bony canal.

Westhofen [199] described the selective ablation of the otolithic organs in guinea pigs with an argon laser beam applied through the intact footplate. The observation of vestibulospinal responses and the analysis of histomorphologic findings indicated functional obliteration of the maculae during the first few postoperative days and rapid vestibular compensation after four days. Given the limitations imposed by the animal model (guinea pig footplate thinner than in humans, difficult to detect vestibular disorders in the selected species), these results are not applicable to human patients. In a more recent animal study, Adamczyk and Antonelli [200] reported on the selective KTP laser-assisted ablation of all three semicircular canals in guinea pigs with experimentally induced endolymphatic hydrops following unilateral closure of the endolymphatic duct. The canals were ablated without the need for extensive fenestration of the bony labyrinth. Electrocochleographic and histologic studies showed no changes in the cochlea. This technique could prove useful in the treatment of severe, intractable Ménière's disease.

Tinnitus and Sensorineural Hearing Loss

Low-level laser therapy (LLLT, also known as LILT [low-intensity laser therapy]) is used exclusively for "biomodulation purposes." The lasers for this therapy emit at visible wavelengths (400–700 nm) in the milliwatt range, which is about 1/100 of the power output of surgical lasers. Because of their low wattage, these lasers have no damaging effects on the exposed tissue. Their sole function is to exert a stimulatory effect on cells and tissues. The mechanism of action is based on photochemical processes induced in the irradiated cells by the absorption of laser energy. Presumably this leads to the activation of endogenous porphyrins and cytochromes [201]. The stimulatory effects have also been related to an increase in mitochondrial ATP production [202–206]. The effects of LLLT have been confirmed in the treatment of wound healing problems [207]. Anti-inflammatory and analgesic effects have also been demonstrated [208, 209].

"Soft" lasers have been used in otology for approximately 20 years [210]. The indications range from chronic tinnitus to sensorineural hearing loss and vertigo. The laser energy is usually applied through the external auditory canal and/or from a retroauricular approach through the mastoid. The therapeutic response is believed to correlate chiefly with the total energy transfer. The higher the total applied energy, the greater the effect. Other relevant factors are the age of the patient and the duration of the disease [211]. The therapeutic results vary considerably from one study to the next, however, and are still a matter of controversy. At least from a physical standpoint, the efficacy of LLLT appears extremely dubious when the beam is directed through the intact mastoid, since the applied energies are not sufficient to penetrate the bone and reach the cells of the inner ear [212].

Most studies have shown no efficacy of LLLT for the above indications, regardless of the application modality, and attribute the sporadic positive results to a placebo effect [213, 214]. On the whole, although the final word on the use of soft lasers in otologic surgery has not yet been written, current data do not prove therapeutic efficacy.

■ Laser Use in the Internal Auditory Canal

Acoustic Neuroma

Glasscock et al. [215] were the first to note the advantages of argon laser use in the surgery of acoustic neuroma. Powers et al. [216] reported on the use of the argon laser in 68 neurosurgical procedures that included the removal of intracranial tumors. They listed the characteristics that make the argon laser a very useful instrument: availability of fiberoptic delivery; spot size focusable to 0.15 mm, free passage of argon laser light through media such as cerebrospinal fluid, and good hemostatic effect of the argon laser wavelength. The substantial clinical use of the CO_2 laser in the surgery of cerebellopontine angle tumors (n = 105)

was first described in 1983 [217, 218]. Technical modifications allowed the laser to be used with an operating microscope, providing the precision and control necessary for intracranial surgery.

Silverstein et al. [219] reported on the intraoperative monitoring of auditory evoked potentials during CO_2 laser-assisted acoustic neuroma surgery. Two patient groups had acoustic neuroma surgery with and without the CO_2 laser and were compared with regard to completeness of tumor removal, anatomic and functional preservation of the facial nerve, hearing preservation, morbidity and mortality, average hospital stay, and sequelae. Significantly better results, with a better quality of life, were documented in the CO_2 laser group [220]. More recent studies underscore these results [221, 222]. Clinical studies on the use of the KTP laser in acoustic neuroma surgery are less numerous. Nissen et al. [223] reported on a series of 115 patients. They noted the advantages of laser dissection over conventional technique, particularly in the removal of larger tumors. Postoperative functional evaluation of the facial nerve using the House–Brackmann grading system indicated satisfactory functional results (grade I or II) in 90.2% of patients with smaller tumors, in 72.2% with moderately large tumors, and in 75.0% with large tumors. These favorable results compared with conventional surgery demonstrate the advantages and safety of KTP laser use in the posterior cranial fossa.

Reports on the use of the Nd:YAG laser in acoustic neuroma surgery are rare. Kopera et al. [224] reported on 63 intracranial tumors, including 8 acoustic neurinomas, 32 meningiomas, 16 gliomas (11 glioblastomas), and 11 metastatic tumors, which underwent Nd:YAG laser-assisted removal. The ability of the Nd:YAG laser to debulk and devascularize tumors made it particularly useful for the treatment of vascular intracranial tumors such as meningiomas and metastases. The noncontact technique, minimal thermal collateral effects, better hemostasis, and higher precision allowed for the easier and less traumatizing removal of acoustic nerve tumors. The main advantages of Nd:YAG laser use included the reduction of mechanical trauma, less blood loss, and the more radical removal of intracranial tumors. Acoustic neuroma is difficult to shrink with this laser, however, due to the lack of contractile elements in the tumor. The principal advantage of laser use lies in the improved dissection technique.

A recent experimental and clinical study confirmed the suitability of the pulsed holmium:YAG laser for the removal of cranial and spinal meningiomas and neuromas. In 18 patients with hard fibrous or calcified spinal and cranial meningiomas and neuromas, the tumors were completely removed with the pulsed laser beam without causing additional neurologic deficits. The thermal effects measured with an infrared camera were negligible.

Nevertheless, the photoablative effect of the pulsed holmium:YAG laser, and the associated nonlinear processes in the tissue, make this laser unpredictable and hazardous for microsurgical use in this delicate region.

■ Conclusions

Continuing efforts to perfect the technique of middle ear surgery are based on the desire to minimize the critical aspects of these procedures, especially the dangers posed to the inner ear. Laser usage appears to be the ideal approach to achieving this concept. The goal is to optimize the technique of conventional surgery and reduce the incidence of inner ear damage through the precise, controlled, noncontact application of laser energy to middle ear structures.

Although the relatively new technological advance of laser use in middle ear surgery is gaining acceptance, it must be emphasized that the laser is only a tool, though a highly developed one, and is no substitute for the knowledge, experience, judgment, and manual skills of the surgeon. As H. P. House said, "It is not the instruments or technique that necessarily lead to success but rather the attentiveness and instrument-wielding hands of the surgeon."

Nevertheless, the use of the laser in middle ear surgery represents an optimum evolution of conventional operative technique in both primary and revision procedures, promising improvement in hearing results and reduction of complications. The purpose of this chapter was to review previous experience with laser use in otologic surgery and offer detailed descriptions of laser use for selected indications. The final word is not yet written, and as equipment continues to improve, other novel applications are sure to be discovered.

■ References

1 DiBartolomeo JR, Ellis M. The argon laser in otology. Laryngoscope 1980; 90: 1786–1796
2 Clarke TE. Electrolysis of exostoses of the ear. Br Med J 1973; 2: 656–657
3 Mülwert H, Voss O. Eine neue physicalische Behandlungsmethode chronischer Schwerhörigkeit und deren Ergebnisse. Acta Oto-Laryngol (Stockh.) 1928; 12: 63–71
4 Krejci F. Experimentelle Grundlagen einer extralabyrinthären chirurgischen Behandlungsmethode. Basel: 1952; 14: 18
5 Sjöberg A, Stahle J. Treatment of Meniere's disease with ultrasound; a follow-up on 117 cases using a new ultrasound apparatus with an electronystagmographical analysis of the caloric reaction. Arch Otolaryngol 1965; 82: 498–502
6 Yousuf M, Novotny GM. Cryosurgery: scientific basis and clinical application in otolaryngology. Ear Nose Throat J 1976; 55: 353–357
7 Stahle J, Högberg L. Laser and the Labyrinth: Some preliminary experiments on pegions. Acta Otolaryngol, (Stockh.) 1965; 60: 367–374
8 Stahle J, Högberg L, Engström B. The laser as a tool in inner-ear surgery. Acta Otolaryngol 1972; 73: 27–37
9 Sataloff J. Experimental use of laser in otosclerotic stapes. Arch Otolaryngol 1967; 85: 58–60
10 Kelemen G, Laor Y, Klein E. Laser induced ear damage. Arch Otolaryngol 1967; 86: 21–27
11 Wilpizeski C et al. Selective vestibular ablation in monkeys by laser irradiation. The Laryngoscope 1972; 82: 1045–1058
12 Escudero L et al. Argon laser in human tympanoplasty. Arch Otolaryngol 1979; 105: 252–253
13 Perkins RC. Laser stapedotomy for otosclerosis. Laryngoscope 1980; 90: 228–241
14 Silverstein H, Rosenberg S, Jones R. Small fenestra stapedotomies with and without KTP laser: a comparison. Laryngoscope 1989; 99: 485–488

15 Lesinski SG. Lasers for otosclerosis. Laryngoscope 1989; 99 (Suppl. 46): 1–24
16 Pfalz R, Bald N, Hibst R. Eignung des Erbium:YAG Lasers für die Mittelohrchirurgie. Eur Arch Otorhinolaryngol 1992; II (Suppl.): 250–251
17 Poe DS. Laser-assisted endoscopic stapedectomy: a prospective study. Laryngoscope 2000; 110: 1–37
18 Lyons GD, Webster DB, Mouney DF, Lousteau RJ. Anatomical consequences of CO_2 laser surgery of the guinea pig ear. Laryngoscope 1978; 88: 1749–1754
19 DiBartolomeo J. Argon and CO_2 lasers in otolaryngology: Which one, when, and why? Laryngoscope 1981; 91 (Suppl. 26): 1–16
20 Thoma J, Unger V, Kastenbauer E. Temperatur- und Druckmessungen im Innenohr bei der Anwendung des Argon-Lasers. Laryngo-Rhino-Otol 1981; 60: 587–590
21 Thoma J, Unger V, Kastenbauer E. Funktionelle Auswirkungen des Argon-Lasers am Hörorgan des Meerschweinchens. Laryngo-Rhino-Otol 1982; 61: 473–476
22 Thoma J. Experimentelle Untersuchungen zur Anwendbarkeit von Laserlicht zum Zweck der Stapedotomie. Habilitationsschrift an der Freien Universität Berlin, 1984
23 Thoma J, Mrowinski D, Kastenbauer E. Experimental investigations on the suitability of the carbondioxide laser for stapedotomy. Ann Otol Rhinol Laryngol 1986; 95: 126–131
24 Gantz BJ, Jenkins HA, Kishimoto S, Fisch U. Argon laser stapedotomy. Ann Otol Rhinol Laryngol 1982; 92: 25–26
25 Vollrath M, Schreiner C. Influence of argon laser stapedotomy on cochlear potentials. I. Alteration of cochlear microphonics (CM). Acta Otolaryngol (Stockh.) 1982; 385 (Suppl.): 1–31
26 Vollrath M, Schreiner C. The effects of the argon laser on temperature within the cochlea. Acta Otolaryngol (Stockh.) 1982; 93: 341–348
27 Vollrath M, Schreiner C. Influence of argon laser stapedotomy on cochlear potentials. III. Extracochlear record DC potential. Acta Otolaryngol (Stockh.) 1983; 96: 49–55
28 Vollrath M, Schreiber C. Influence of argon laser stapedotomy on inner ear function and temperature. Otolaryngol Head Neck Surg 1983; 91: 521–526
29 McGee TM. The argon laser in surgery for chronic ear disease and otosclerosis. Laryngoscope 1983; 93: 1177–1182
30 Lesinski SG. Laser stapes surgery (letter). Laryngoscope 1990; 100: 106–107
31 Lesinski SG. Lasers for otosclerosis – which one if any and why. Lasers Surg Med 1990; 10: 448–457
32 Lesinski SG, Newrock R. Carbon dioxide lasers for otosclerosis. Otolaryngol Clin North Am. 1993; 26: 417–441
33 Palva T. Argon laser in otosclerosis surgery. Acta Otolaryngol (Stockh.) 1987; 104: 153–157
34 Silverstein H, Bendet E, Rosenberg S, Nichols M. Revision stapes surgery with and without laser: a comparison. Laryngoscope 1994; 104: 1431–1438
35 McGee TM, Kartush JM. Laser stapes surgery (letter). Laryngoscope 1990; 100: 106–107
36 Bartels LJ. KTP laser stapedotomy: is it safe? Otolaryngol Head Neck Surg 1990; 103: 685–692
37 Vernick DM. Laser stapes surgery (letter). Laryngoscope 1990; 100: 106–107
38 Horn KL, Gherini S, Griffin GM. Argon laser stapedectomy using an Endo-Otoprobe system. Otolaryngol Head Neck Surg 1990; 102: 193–198
39 Gherini SG, Horn KL, Bowman CA, Griffin GM. Small fenestra stapedotomy using a fiberoptic hand-held argon laser in obliterative otosclerosis. Laryngoscope 1990; 100: 1276–1282
40 Gherini S, Horn KL, Causse JB, McArthur GR. Fiberoptic argon laser stapedotomy: is it safe? Am J Otol 1993; 14: 283–289
41 Fischer R, Schönfeld U, Jovanovic S, Scholz C. Experimenteller Vergleich zwischen kurzgepulsten und kontinuierlich strahlenden Lasern in der Stapeschirurgie – akustische und thermische Ergebnisse. Arch Otorhinolaryngol 1990; II (Suppl.): 224–227
42 Fischer R, Schönfeld U, Jovanovic S, Jaeckel P. Thermische Belastung des Innenohres durch verschiedene Lasertypen bei der Laser-Stapedotomie. Arch Otorhinolaryngol 1992; II (Suppl.): 251–253
43 Jovanovic S, Scholz C, Berghaus A, Schönfeld U. Experimenteller

Vergleich zwischen kurzgepulsten und kontinuierlich strahlenden Lasern in der Stapeschirurgie – histologisch-morphologische Ergebnisse. Arch Otorhinolaryngol 1990; II (Suppl.): 72–73

44 Jovanovic S, Berghaus A, Schönfeld U, Scherer H. Bedeutung experimentell gewonnener Daten für den Klinischen Einsatz verschiedener Laser in der Stapeschirurgie. Eur Arch Otorhinolaryngol 1991; II (Suppl.): 278–280

45 Jovanovic S, Schönfeld U, Berghaus A, Fischer R, Beuthan J, Prapavat V, Jaeckel P, Anft D, Döring M, Bierhals W. Eignung verschiedener Laser in der Stapeschirurgie. In: Wissenschaftswoche. Forschungsprojekte am Klinikum Steglitz, 1991: 123–125

46 Jovanovic S, Schönfeld U, Berghaus A, Fischer R, Beuthan J, Jäckel P, Anft D, Prapavat V, Döring M, Bierhals W. CO_2-Laser-Stapedotomie – klinische Erfahrungen. In: Wissenschaftswoche. Forschungsprojekte am Klinikum Steglitz, 1992: 202–203

47 Jovanovic S, Prapavat V, Schönfeld U, Berghaus A, Beuthan J, Scherer H, Müller G. Experimentelle Untersuchung zur Optimierung der Parameter verschiedener Lasersysteme zur Stapedotomie. Lasermedizin 1992; 8: 174–181

48 Jovanovic S, Berghaus A, Scherer H, Schönfeld U. Klinische Erfahrungen mit dem CO_2-Laser in der Stapeschirurgie. Eur Arch Otorhinolaryngol 1992; II (Suppl.): 249–250

49 Jovanovic S, Anft D, Schönfeld U, Tausch-Treml R, Berghaus A, Prapavat V, Scherer H, Müller G. Tierexperimentelle Untersuchungen zur Laserstapedotomie. In: Wissenschaftswoche. Forschungsprojekte am Klinikum Steglitz, 1993: 100–101

50 Jovanovic S, Anft D, Schönfeld U, Tausch-Treml R. Tierexperimentelle Untersuchungen zur Eignung verschiedener Lasersysteme für die Stapedotomie. Eur Arch Otorhinolaryngol 1993; II (Suppl.): 38–39

51 Jovanovic S, Schönfeld U, Fischer R, Scherer H. CO_2 laser in stapes surgery. Proc SPIE 1993; 1876: 17–27

52 Jovanovic S, Schönfeld U, Application of the CO_2 laser in stapedotomy. Adv Oto-Rhino-Laryngol 1995; 49: 95–100

53 Jovanovic S, Anft D, Schönfeld U, Berghaus A, Scherer H. Tierexperimentelle Untersuchungen zur CO_2-Laser-Stapedotomie. Laryngo-Rhino-Otol 1995; 74: 26–32

54 Jovanovic S, Anft D, Schönfeld U, Berghaus A, Scherer H. Experimental studies on the suitability of the erbium laser for stapedotomy in an animal model. Eur Arch Otorhinolaryngol 1995; 252: 422–442

55 Jovanovic S, Schönfeld U, Fischer R, Döring M, Prapavat V, Müller G, Scherer H. Temperaturmessungen im Innenohr-Modell bei Laserbestrahlung. Lasermedizin 1995; 11: 11–18

56 Jovanovic S, Schönfeld U, Prapavat V, Berghaus A, Fischer R, Scherer H, Müller G. Die Bearbeitung der Steigbügelfußplatte mit verschiedenen Lasersystemen, Teil I: Kontinuierlich strahlende Laser. HNO 1995; 43: 49–158

57 Jovanovic S, Schönfeld U, Prapavat V, Berghaus A, Fischer R, Scherer H, Müller G. Die Bearbeitung der Steigbügelfußplatte mit verschiedenen Lasersystemen, Teil II: Gepulste Laser. HNO 1995; 43: 223–233

58 Jovanovic S, Schönfeld U. Application of the CO_2-laser in stapedotomy. Adv Otorhinolaryngol 1995; 49: 95–100

59 Jovanovic S, Sedlmaier B, Schönfeld U, Scherer H, Müller G. Die CO_2-Laser-Parazentese – tierexperimentelle und klinische Erfahrungen. Lasermedizin 1995; 11: 5–10

60 Jovanovic S, Schönfeld U, Fischer R, Döring M, Prapavat V, Müller G, Scherer H. Thermische Belastung des Innenohres bei der Laser-Stapedotomie. Teil I: Kontinuierlich strahlende Laser. HNO 1995; 43: 702–709

61 Jovanovic S, Schönfeld U, Fischer R, Döring M, Prapavat V, Müller G, Scherer H. Thermische Belastung des Innenohres bei der Laser-Stapedotomie. Teil II: Gepulste Laser. HNO 1996; 44: 6–13

62 Jovanovic S, Schönfeld U, Prapavat V, Berghaus A, Fischer R, Scherer H, Müller GJ. Effects of continuous wave laser systems on stapes footplate. Lasers Surg Med 1996; 19: 424–432

63 Jovanovic S. Der Einsatz neuer Lasersysteme in der Stapeschirurgie. In: Müller GJ, Berlien HP (eds). Fortschritte der Lasermedizin 14. Landsberg: Ecomed, 1996

64 Jovanovic S, Hensel H, Schönfeld U, Scherer H. Ergebnisse nach Revisions-Stapedotomien mit dem CO_2-Laser. HNO 1997; 45: 251

65 Jovanovic S, Schönfeld U, Prapavat V, Berghaus A, Fischer R, Scherer H, Müller G. Effects of pulsed laser systems on stapes footplate. Lasers Surg Med 1997; 21: 341–350

66 Jovanovic S, Schönfeld U, Scherer H. CO_2 Laser in Revision. Stapes Surgery SPIE Proceed 1997; 2970: 102–108

67 Jovanovic S, Schönfeld U, Hensel H, Scherer H. Clinical experiences with the CO_2-laser in revision stapes surgery. Lasermedizin 1997; 13: 37–40

68 Jovanovic S, Schönfeld U, Fischer R, Döring M, Prapavat V, Müller G, Scherer H. Thermic effects in the "vestibule" during laser stapedotomy with pulsed laser systems. Lasers Surg Med 1998; 23: 7–17

69 Jovanovic S, Schönfeld U, Scherer H. Laseranwendungen in der Mittelohrchirurgie – Gegenwart und Zukunft. HNO 1998; 46: 385

70 Jovanovic S, Anft D, Schönfeld U, Berghaus A, Scherer H. Influence of CO_2 laser application of the guinea-pig cochlea on compound action potentials. Am J Otol 1999; 20: 166–173

71 Jovanovic S, Jamali J, Anft D, Schönfeld U, Scherer H, Müller G. Influence of pulsed lasers on the morphology and function of the guinea-pig cochlea. Hearing Res 2000; 144: 97–108

72 Jovanovic S. CO_2-Laser in stapes surgery. In: Oswal V. Remacle M, Jovanovic S, Krespi J (Hrsg.). Principles and Practice of Lasers in Otolaryngology, Head and Neck Surgery. Den Haag: Kugler Verlag, 2002: 335–357

73 Hodgson RS, Wilson DF. Argon laser stapedotomy. Laryngoscope 1991; 101: 230–233

74 Pfalz R, Lindenberger M, Hibst R. Mechanische und thermische Nebenwirkungen des Argon-Lasers in der Mittelohrchirurgie (in vitro). Eur Arch Otorhinolaryngol 1991; II (Suppl.): 281–282

75 Pfalz R, Hibst R, Bald N. Suitability of different lasers for operations ranging from the tympanic membrane to the base of the stapes. Adv Otorhinolaryngol 1995; 49: 87–94

76 Lim RJ. Safety of carbon dioxide laser for stapes surgery. Lasers Surg Med 1992; 4: 61

77 Strunk CL, Quinn FB, Bailey BJ. Stapedectomy techniques in residency training. Laryngoscope 1992; 102: 121–124

78 Schönfeld U, Fischer R, Jovanovic S, Scherer H. „Lärmbelastung" während der Laser-Stapedotomie. Eur Arch Otolaryngol 1994; II (Suppl.): 244–246

79 Haberkamp TJ, Harvey SA, Khafagy Y. Revision stapedectomy with and without the CO_2-laser: An analysis of results. Am J Otol 1996; 17: 225–229

80 Vernick DM. A comparison of the results of KTP and CO_2 laser stapedotomy. Am J Otol 1996; 17: 221–224

81 Wiet RJ, Kubek DC, Lemberg P, Byskosh AT. A meta-analysis review of revision stapes surgery with argon laser: effectiveness and safety. Am J Otol 1997; 18: 66–171

82 Nissen RL. Argon laser in difficult stapedotomy cases. Laryngoscope 1989; 108: 1669–1673

83 Nissen A. Laser applications in otologic surgery. ENT Journal 1995; 74: 477–480

84 Shabana YK, Allam H, Pedersen CB. Laser stapedotomy. J Laryngol Otol 1999; 113: 413–416

85 Häusler R, Schar PJ, Pratisto H, Weber HP, Frenz M. Advantages and dangers of erbium laser application in stapedotomy. Acta Otolaryngol 1999; 119: 207–213

86 Häusler R. Fortschritte in der Stapeschirurgie. Laryngo-Rhino-Otol 2000; 79 (Suppl. 2): 95–139

87 Buchman CA, Fucci MJ, Roberson JB, de la Cruz, Jr A. Comparison of argon and CO_2 laser stapedotomy in primary otosclerosis surgery. Am J Otolaryngol 2000; 21: 227–230

88 Huber A, Linder T, Fisch U. Is the Er:YAG laser damaging to inner ear function? Otol Neurotol 2001; 22: 311–315

89 Lippert BM, Gottschlich S, Kulkens C, Folz BJ, Rudert H. Experimental and clinical results of Er:YAG laser stapedotomy. Lasers Surg Med 2001; 28: 11–17

90 Keck T, Wiebe M, Rettinger G, Riechelmann H. Safety of the erbium:yttrium-aluminium-garnet laser in stapes surgery in otosclerosis. Otol Neurotol 2002; 23: 21–24

91 Garin P, van PK, Jamart J. Hearing outcome following laser-assisted stapes surgery. J Otolaryngol 2002; 31: 31–34

92 Yung MW. A study of the intraoperative effect of the Argon and KTP-laser in stapes surgery. Clin Otolaryngol 2002; 27: 279–282

93 Lesinski SG. Causes of conductive hearing loss after stapedectomy or stapedotomy: a prospective study of 279 consecutive surgical revisions. Otol Neurotol 2002; 23: 281–288

94 Silverstein H, Jackson LE, Conlon WS, Rosenberg SI, Thompson Jr JH. Laser stapedotomy minus prosthesis (laser STAMP): absence of refixation. Otol Neurotol 2002; 23: 52–157

95 Thedinger BS. Applications of the KTP laser in chronic ear surgery. Am J Otol 1990; 11: 79–84

96 Hamilton J. The KTP laser in cholesteatoma. In: Oswal V, Remacle M, Jovanovic S, Krespi J. (eds.). Principles and Practice of Lasers in Otorhinolaryngology and Head and Neck Surgery. Den Haag: Kugler Plublications, 2002: 317–324

97 Schindler RA, Lanser MJ. The surgical management of cholesteatoma. In: Tos M, Thomsen J, Peitersen E (Hrsg). Cholesteatoma and Mastoid Surgery Proceedings of the Third International Congress on Cholesteatoma and Mastoid Surgery held in Copenhagen, Denmark June 5–9, 1988. Amsterdam, Berkeley, Milano: 1989 Kugler & Gedini Publications, 2002: 769–778

98 Scholz C, Grothues-Spork M. Die Bearbeitung von Knochen mit dem Laser. In: Berlien HP, Müller G (Hrsg). Angewandte Lasermedizin, Lehr- und Handbuch für Praxis und Klinik. Landsberg, München, Zürich: ecomed, 1989; 1. Auflage, 5. Ergänzungslieferung 1992, II-3.11.1: S1–S23

99 Nuss RC, Fabian RL, Sarkar R, Puliafito C. Infrared laser bone ablation. Lasers Surg Med 1988; 8: 381–391

100 Charlton A, Dickinson MR, King TA, Freemont AJ. Erbium:YAG and holmium:YAG laser ablation of bone. Lasers Med Sci 1990; 5: 365–373

101 Pfalz R. Eignung verschiedener Laser für Eingriffe vom Trommelfell bis zur Fußplatte (Er:YAG-, Argon-, CO_2-s.p.-, Ho:YAG-Laser), Laryngo-Rhino-Otol 1995; 74: 21–25

102 Pratisto H, Frenz M, Ith M, Romano V, Felix D, Grossenbacher R, Altermatt H, Weber H. Temperature and pressure effects during erbium laser stapedotomy. Lasers Surg Med 1996; 18: 100–108

103 Nagel D. The Er:YAG laser in ear surgery: first clinical results. Lasers Surg Med 1997; 21: 79–87

104 Bretlau P. Argon laser stapedotomy vs Erbium laser stapedotomy. Zürich: Otology 2000, XXII Annual Meeting of the Politzer Society, 1999

105 Pfander F. Das Knalltrauma. Berlin, Heidelberg, New York: Springer Verlag, 1975

106 Parkin J. Lasers in tympanomastoid surgery. Otolaryngol Clin N Am 1990; 23: 1–5

107 Kumar BN, Walsh RM, Courtney-Harris RG, Wilson PS. Treatment of chronic otitis externa by KTP/532 laser. J Laryngol Otol 1997; 111: 1126–1129

108 Cohen D, Siegel G, Krespi J, Schechter Y, Slatkine M. Middle ear laser office ventilation (LOV) with a CO_2-laser flashscanner. J Clin Laser Med Surg 1998; 16: 07–109

109 Coma I, Aragon J, Rodriguez Adrados F. CO_2-laser tympanostomy without ventilation tubes. Acta Otorrinolaryngol Esp 1999; 50: 101–105

110 Garin P, Remacle M. Laser-assisted myringotomy combined with adenoidectomy in children: preliminary results. Acta Otorhinolaryngol Belg 1999; 53: 105–108

111 Marchant H, Bisschop P. Value of laser CO_2 myringotomy in the treatment of seromucous otitis. Ann Otolaryngol Chir Cervicofac 1998; 115: 347–351

112 Sedlmaier B, Jivanjee A, Gutzler R, Huscher D, Jovanovic S. Ventilation time of the middle ear in otitis media with effusion (OME) after CO_2 laser myringotomy. Laryngoscope 2002; 112: 661–668

113 Sedlmaier B, Jovanovic S. Die Behandlung der akuten Otitis media mit dem CO_2-Laser. HNO 2000; 557–560

114 Sedlmaier B, Jivanjee A, Gutzler R, Huscher D, Jovanovic S. Die Dauer der Mittelohrbelüftung nach Lasermyringotomie mit dem CO_2-Laser Otoskop Otoscan. HNO 2001; 49: 447–453

115 Saito H, Miyamoto K, Kishimoto S, Higashitsuji H, Kitamura H. Burn perforation as a method of middle ear ventilation. Arch Otolaryngol 1978; 104: 79–81

116 Tolsdorff P. Bipolare Thermoparazentese – Grundlagen und Klinik. HNO 1998; 4: 368

117 Sedlmaier B, Blödow A, Jovanovic S, Nagli L, Eberle H. Effects of different IR laser systems on the tympanic membrane. Proc Spie, 1997; 2970B-24, session 5

118 Sedlmaier B, Blödow A, Schönfeld U, Jovanovic S. Das CO_2-Laserotoskop – ein neues Applikationssystem für die Parazentese. HNO 1998; 46: 870–875

119 Garin P, Ledeghen S, Prooyen-Keyser S, Remacle M. Office-based CO_2-laser-assisted tympanic membrane fenestration addressing otitis media with effusion. J Clin Laser Med Surg 2001; 19: 185–187

120 Sedlmaier B, Tagl P, Gutzler R, Schönfeld U, Jovanovic S. Experimental and clinical experiences with the Er:YAG laser otoscope. HNO 2000; 48: 816–821

121 Armstrong B. New treatment for chronic secretory media. Arch Otolaryngol 1954; 59: 653–654

122 Pulitzer A. Diseases of the Ear. Lea and Febiger, 1869; fifth edition: 282–302

123 Midgley EJ, Dewey C, Pryce K, Maw AR. The frequency of otitis media with effusion in British pre-school children: a guide for treatment. ALSPAC Study Team. Clin Otolaryngol 2000; 25: 485–491

124 Goode RL. CO_2-laser myringotomy. Laryngoscope 1982; 92: 420–423

125 Silverstein H, Kuhn J, Choo D, Krespi YP, Rosenberg SI, Rowan PT. Laser-assisted tympanostomy. Laryngoscope 1996; 106: 1067–1074

126 Buckingham RA. Cholesteatoma and chronic otitis media following middle ear intubation. Laryngoscope 1981; 91: 1450–1456

127 Gates GA, Avery C, Prihoda TJ, Holt GR. Delayed onset post-tympanotomy otorrhea. Otolaryngol Head Neck Surg 1988; 98: 111–114

128 Münker G. Ergebnisse der Behandlung des sekretorischen Mittelohrkatarrhs durch Adenotomie und Paukenröhrchen – eine Zehn-Jahres-Übersicht. Arch Ohr-Nase-Kehlkopfheilkunde 1976; 213: 403–406

129 Gates GA, Avery CA, Cooper JC, Prihoda TJ. Chronic secretory otitis media: effects of surgical management. Ann Otol Rhinol Laryngol 1989; 138 (Suppl.): 2–32

130 McKennan KX. "Tissue welding" with the argon laser in middle ear surgery. Laryngoscope 1990; 100: 1143–1145

131 Pyykkö I, Poe D, Ishizaki H. Laser-assisted myringoplasty, technical aspects. Acta Otolaryngol (Stockh.) 2000; 543: 135–138

132 Saeed SR, Jackler R. Lasers in surgery for chronic ear disease. Otolaryngol Clin N Am 1996; 29: 245–255

133 Sands J, Napolitano N. Use of the argon laser in the treatment of malleus fixation. Arch Otolaryngol Head Neck Surg 1990; 116: 975–976

134 McGee TM. Laser appications in ossicular surgery. Otolaryngol Clin N Am 1990; 23: 7–20

135 Park MS, Min HK. Laser soldering and welding for ossicular reconstruction: an *in vitro* test. Otolaryngol Head Neck Surg 2000; 122: 803–807

136 Sheehy JL, Brackmann DE, Graham MD. Cholesteatoma surgery: residual and recurrent disease. A review of 1024 cases. Ann Otol Rhinol Laryngol 1977; 86: 451–462

137 Gyo K, Sasaki Y, Hinohira Y, Yanagihara N. Residue of middle ear cholesteatoma after intact canal wall tympanoplasty: surgical findings at one year. Ann Otol Rhinol Laryngol 1996; 105: 615–619

138 Jahnke K, Khatib M, Rau U. Long-term results following cholesteatoma surgery. Laryngol Rhinol Otol (Stuttg) 1985; 64: 238–242

139 Mitrovic M, Haralampiev K, Dzinic M. Problems in diagnosis and treatment of cholesteatoma in children. Int J Pediatr Otorhinolaryngol 1991; 21: 149–153

140 Ogawa H, Ohtani I, Akaike T. Examination for prediction of residual cholesteatoma. Nippon Jibiinkoka Gakkai Kaiho 1998; 101: 1–8

141 Reimer A, Andreasson L, Harris S. Surgical treatment of cholesteatoma: a comparison of closed and open techniques in an follow-up of 164 ears. Clin Otolaryngol 1987; 12: 447–454

142 Roger G, Denoyelle F, Chauvin P, Schlegel-Stuhl N, Garabedian EN. Prediçtive risk factors of residual cholesteatoma in children: a study of 256 cases. Am J Otol 1997; 18: 550–558

143 Rosenfeld RM, Moura RL, Bluestone CD. Predictors of residual-

recurrent cholesteatoma in children. Arch Otolaryngol Head Neck Surg 1992; 118: 384–391

144 Stangerup SE, Drozdziewicz D, Tos M. Cholesteatoma in children, predictors and calculation of recurrence rates. Int J Pediatr Otorhinolaryngol 1999; 49: S69–S73

145 Vartiainen E. Factors associated with recurrence of cholesteatoma. J Laryngol Otol 1995; 109: 590–592

146 Raslan WWRJRLP. Lessening cholesteatoma residual with laser: an experimental study. In: Proceedings of the Third International Conference on Cholesteatoma and Mastoid Surgery. Amsterdam: Kugler and Ghedini Publications, 1989: 761–767

147 Robinson PJ, Grant HR, Brown SG. Nd:YAG laser treatment of a glomus tympanicum tumour. J Laryngol Otol 1993; 107: 236–237

148 Beatty TW, Haberkamp TJ, Khafagy YW, Bresemann JA. Stapedectomy training with the carbon dioxide laser. Laryngoscope 1997; 107: 1441–1444

149 Rauch SD, Bartley ML. Argon laser stapedectomy: comparison to traditional fenestration techniques. Am J Otol 1992; 13: 556–560

150 Causse JB, Gherini S, Horn KL. Surgical treatment of stapes fixation by fiberoptic argon laser stapedotomy with reconstruction of the annular ligament. Otolaryngol Clin North Am 1993; 26: 395–416

151 Schlenk E, Profeta G, Nelson JS, Andrew JJ, Berns MW. Laser assisted fixation of ear prosthesis after stapedectomy. Lasers Surg Med 1990; 10: 444–447

152 Segas J, Georgiadis A, Christodoulou P, Bizakis J, Helidonis E. Use of the excimer laser in stapes surgery and ossiculoplasty of middle ear ossicles: Preliminary report of an experimental approach. Laryngoscope 1991; 101: 186–191

153 Kautzky M, Trödhan A, Susani M, Schenk P. Infrared laser stapedotomy. Eur Arch Otorhinolaryngol 1991; 248: 449–451

154 Hommerich CP, Hessel S. Untersuchungen mit dem Holmium:YAG-Laser an Amboß und Steigbügel. Eur Arch Otorhinolaryngol 1991; II (Suppl.): 280

155 Hommerich CP, Schmidt-Elmendorff A. Experimentelle CO_2-, Holmium:YAG- und Erbium:YAG-Laseranwendung an der Steigbügelfußplatte. Eur Arch Otorhinolaryngol 1993; II (Suppl.): 39–40

156 Stubig IM, Reder PA, Facer GW, Rylander HG, Welch AJ. Holmium:YAG laser stapedotomy: preliminary evaluation. Proc SPIE 1993; 1876: 10–19

157 Zrunek M, Kautzky M, Hübsch P. Experimentelle Laserchirurgie bei ossifizierter Cochlea. Eur Arch Otorhinolaryngol 1993; II (Suppl.): 37–38

158 Shah KU, Poe DS, Rebeiz EE, Perrault DF, Pankratow MM, Shapshay SM. Erbium laser in middle ear surgery: *in vitro* and *in vivo* animal study. Laryngoscope 1996; 106: 418–422

159 Nagel D. Laser in der Ohrchirurgie. HNO 1996; 44: 553–554

160 Arnold W, Niedermeyer HP, Altermatt HJ, Neubert WJ. Pathogenesis of otosclerosis. "State of the art". HNO 1996; 44: 121–129

161 Riechelmann H, Tholen M, Keck T, Rettinger G. Perioperative glucocorticoid treatment does not influence early post-laser stapedotomy hearing thresholds. Am J Otol 2000; 21: 809–812

162 Schuknecht H. Stapedectomy. Boston: Little, Brown, 1971

163 Raman R, Mathew J, Idikula J. Obliterative otosclerosis. J Laryngol Otol 1991; 105: 899–900

154 Hough JV, Dyer RK. Stapedectomy. Causes of failure and revision surgery in otosclerosis. Otolaryngol Clin North Am 1993; 26: 453–470

155 Fisch U. Tympanoplasty, mastoidectomy, and stapes surgery. Stuttgart, New York: Thieme, 1994

156 Plester D, Hildmann H, Steinbach E. Atlas der Ohrchirurgie. Stuttgart: Kohlhammer, 1989

167 Crabtree JA, Britton B, Powers WH. An evaluation of revision stapes surgery. Laryngoscope 1980; 90: 224–227

168 Lippy WH. Stapedectomy revision. Am J Otol 1980; 2: 15–21

169 Sheehy JL, Nelson RA, House HP. Revision stapedectomy: A review of 258 cases. Laryngoscope 1981; 91: 43–51

170 Glasscock ME. Revision stapedectomy surgery. Otolaryngol Head Neck Surg 1987; 96: 141–148

171 Hohmann A. Inner Ear Reactions to stapes surgery (Animal Experiments). In: Schuknecht HF (ed). Otosclerosis. Boston: Little Brown & Co., 1962: 305–317

172 Linthicum F. Histologic evidence of the cause of failure in stapes surgery. Ann Otol Rhinol Laryngol 1971; 80: 67–77

173 Molony TB. CO_2-laser stapedotomy. J La State Med Soc 1993; 145: 405–408

174 Antonelli PJ, Gianoli GJ, Lundy LB, LaRouere MJ, Kartush JM. Early post-laser stapedotomy hearing thresholds. Am J Otol 1998; 19: 443–446

175 Moon CN, Hahn MJ. Partial vs total footplate removal in stapedectomy: a comparative study. Laryngoscope 1984; 94: 912–915

176 Levy R, Shvero J, Hadar T. Stapedotomy technique and results: ten years' experience and comparative study with stapedectomy. Laryngoscope 1990; 100: 1097–1099

177 Backous DD, Coker NJ, Jenkins HA. Prospective study of resident-performed stapedectomy. Am J Otol 1993; 14: 451–454

178 Strunk CL, Quinn FB. Stapedectomy surgery in residency: KTP-532 laser versus argon laser. Am J Otol 1993; 14: 13–117

179 Somers T, Govaerts P, Marquet T, Offeciers E. Statistical analysis of otosclerosis surgery performed by Jean Marquet. Ann Otol Laryngol 1994; 103: 945–951

180 Glasscock ME, Storper IS, Haynes DS, Bohrer PS. Twenty-five years of experience with. Laryngoscope 1995; 105: 899–904

181 Persson P, Harder H, Magnuson B. Hearing results in otosclerosis surgery after partial stapedectomy, total stapedectomy and stapedotomy. Acta Otolaryngol (Stockh.) 1997; 117: 94–99

182 Ramsay H, Karkkainen J, Palva T. Success in surgery for otosclerosis: hearing improvement and other indicators. Am J Otolaryngol 1997; 18: 23

183 Shea PF, Ge X, Shea JJ. Stapedectomy for far-advanced otosclerosis. Am J Otol 1999; 20; 425–429

184 Lesinski SG, Stein JA. Lasers in revision stapes surgery. Otolaryngol Head Neck Surg 1992; 3: 21–31

185 McGee TM, Diaz-Ordaz EA, Kartush JM. The role of KTP laser in revision stapedectomy. Otolaryngol Head Neck Surg 1993; 109: 839–843

186 Horn KL, Gherini S, Franz DC. Argon laser revision stapedectomy. Am J Otol 1994; 15: 383–388

187 Kautzky M, Susani M, Hubsch P, Kursten R, Zrunek M. Holmium:YAG laser surgery in obliterated cochleas: an experimental study in human cadaver temporal bones. Eur Arch Otorhinolaryngol 1994; 251: 165–169

188 Kautzky M, Susani M, Franz P, Zrunek M. Flexible fiberoptic endoscopy and laser surgery in obliterated cochleas: human temporal bone studies. Lasers Surg Med 1996; 18: 271–277

189 Gulya AJ, Schuknecht HF. Anatomy of the Temporal Bone with Surgical Implications. New York, London: The Parthenon Publishing Group, 1995

190 Westhofen M. Otolith disease – experimental findings and clinical implications. In: Ernst A, Marchbanks R, Samil M (Hrsg.). Intracranial and intralabyrinthine fluids: Basic aspects and clinical applications. Berlin, Heidelberg: Springer Verlag, 1996: 263–278

191 Okuno T, Nomura Y, Young YH, Hara M. Argon laser irradiation of the otolithic organ. Otolaryngol Head Neck Surg 1990; 103: 926–930

192 Nomura Y, Okuna T, Mizuno M. Treatment of vertigo using laser labyrinthectomy. Acta Otolaryngol 1993; 113: 261–262

193 Nomura Y, Ooki S, Kukita N, Young YH. Laser labyrinthectomy. Acta Otolaryngol (Stockh) 1995; 115: 158–161

194 Nomura Y, Okuno T, Young YH, Hara M. Laser labyrinthectomy in humans. Acta Otolaryngol. 1991; 111: 319–326

195 Anthony PF. Partitioning of the labyrinth: application in benign paroxysmal positional vertigo. Am J Otol 1991; 12: 388–393

196 Anthony PF. Partitioning the labyrinth for benign paroxysmal positional vertigo: clinical and histologic findings. Am J Otol 1993; 14: 334–342

197 Kartush JK, Sargent EW. Posterior semicircular canal occlusion for benign paroxysmal positional vertigo CO_2-laser-assisted technique: preliminary results. Laryngoscope 1995; 105: 268–274

198 Antonelli PJ, Lundy LB, Kartush JM, Burgio DL, Graham MD. Mechanical versus CO_2-laser occlusion of the posterior semicircular canal in humans. Am J Otol 1996; 17: 416–420

199 Westhofen M. Treatment of otolith disease concepts and new development of laser microsurgery. In: Reid A, Marchbanks RJ, Ernst A (Hrsg.). Physiology and Pathophysiology. London: Whurr Publishers, 1998: 221–230

200 Adamczyk M, Antonelli PJ. Selective vestibular ablation by KTP laser in endolymphatic hydrops. Laryngoscope 2001; 111: 1057–1062

201 Sroka R, Schaffer M, Fuchs C, Pongratz T, Schrader-Reichard U, Busch M, Schaffer P, Dühmke E, Baumgartner R. Licht induzierte Biomodulation von Normal- und Tumorzellen (Abstract). Lasermedizin 1999; 3: 68

202 Passarella S, Ostuni A, Atlante A, Quagliarello E. Increase in the ADP/ATP exchange in rat liver mitochondria irradiated in-vitro by Helium-Neon laser irradiation. Biomech Biophys Res Comm 1988; 156: 978–986

203 Rigau J, Trelles MA, Calderhead RG, Mayayo E. Changes in fibroblast proliferation and metabolism following *in vitro* Helium-Neon laser irradiation. LLLT 1991; 3: 25–33

204 Wilden L, Karthein R. Import of radiation phenomena of electrons and therapeutic low-level laser in regard to the mitochondrial energy transfer. J Clin Laser Med Surg 1998; 16: 159–165

205 Wilden L, Karthein R. Zur Wirkung von Low Level Laser Strahlung auf den zellulären Energietransfer. Lasermedizin 2000; 15: 33

206 Stadler I, Evans R, Kolb B, Naim JO, Narayan V, Buehner N, Lanzafame RJ. *In vitro* effects of low-level laser irradiation at 660 nm on peripheral blood lymphocytes. Lasers in Surg and Med 2000; 3: 255–261

207 Mester E, Szende B, Spiry B. Effect of laser rays on wound healing. Am J Surg 1971; 122: 532–535

208 Walker J. Relief from chronic pain by low-energy laser irradiation. Neurosci Lett 1983; 43: 339–344

209 Rochkind S, Nissan M, Lubart M. A single transcutaneous light irradiation to injured peripheral nerve. Comparative study with five different wavelengths. Lasers Med Sci 1989; 4: 259–263

210 Ribari O. The stimulating effect of low-power laser rays: experimental examinations in otorhinolaryngology. Rev Laryngol 1981; 102: 531–533

211 Wilden L, Ellerbrock D. Verbesserung der Hörkapazität durch Low-Level-Laser-Licht (LLLL). Lasermedizin 1999; 14: 129–138

212 David R, Nissan M, Cohen I, Soudry M. Effect of low-power He-Ne Laser on fracture healing in rats. Lasers in Surg and Med 1996; 4: 458–464

213 Mirz F, Zachariae R, Andersen SE et al. The low-power laser in the treatment of tinnitus. Clin Otolaryngol 1999; 24: 346–354

214 Nakashima T, Ueda H, Misawa H et al. Transmeatal low-power laser irradiation for tinnitus. Otol Neurotol 2002; 23: 296–300

215 Glasscock, 3rd ME, Jackson CG, Whitaker SR. The argon laser in acoustic tumor surgery. Laryngoscope 1981; 91: 1405–1416

216 Powers SK, Edwards MS, Boggan JE, Pitts LH, Gutin PH, Hosobuchi Y, Adams JE, Wilson CB. Use of the argon surgical laser in neurosurgery. J Neurosurg 1984; 60: 523–530

217 Robertson JH, Clark WC, Robertson JT, Gardner LG, Shea MC. Use of the carbon dioxide laser for acoustic tumor surgery. Neurosurgery 1983; 12: 286–290

218 Gardner G, Robertson JH, Clark WC, Bellott Jr AL, Hamm CW. Acoustic tumor management-combined approach surgery with CO_2-laser. Am J Otol 1983; 5: 87–108

219 Silverstein H, Norrel H, Hyman SM. Simultaneous use of CO_2-laser with continuous monitoring of eighth cranial nerve action potential during acoustic neuroma surgery. Otolaryngol Head Neck Surg 1984; 92: 80–84

220 Cerullo LJ, Mkrdichian EH. Acoustic nerve tumor surgery before and since the laser: comparison of results. Lasers Surg Med 1987; 7: 224–228

221 Deruty R, Pelissou-Guyotat I, Mottolese C, Amat D. Routine use of the CO_2-laser technique for resection of cerebral tumours. Acta Neurochir (Wien) 1993; 123: 43–45

222 Eiras J, Alberdi J, Gomez J. Laser CO_2 in the surgery of acoustic neuroma. Neurochirurgie. 1993; 39: 16–23

223 Nissen AJ, Sikand A, Welsh JE, Curto FS. Use of the KTP-532 laser in acoustic neuroma surgery. Laryngoscope 1997; 107: 118–121

224 Kopera M, Majchrzak H, Idzik M. Use of the Nd:YAG laser in surgical treatment of intracranial tumors. Neurol Neurochir Pol 1992; 1: 237–242

3 Lasers in Rhinology

B. M. Lippert

■ Contents

■ Abstract

To date, several laser systems (argon, KTP, diode, Nd:YAG, Ho:YAG, Er:YAG, CO_2) have been used to treat a variety of rhinologic disorders. The advantages of laser use in the nose and paranasal sinuses include good intraoperative visibility owing to markedly improved hemostasis, high precision tissue removal, less tissue trauma resulting in reduction of postoperative edema, and less postoperative pain. Intranasal packing can be dispensed with in many cases. Knowledge of the biophysical effects of the laser system used, along with careful patient selection, can lead to excellent therapeutic results. We feel that laser therapy has gained an established place in the treatment of turbinate hyperplasia, recurrent epistaxis including Rendu–Osler–Weber disease, hemangiomas and vascular malformations, choanal atresia, circumscribed benign lesions, and rhinophyma. Laser surgery of the nasal septum, paranasal sinuses, and lacrimal ducts, on the other hand, is still questionable as an alternative to conventional techniques.

■ Introduction: Laser Systems in Rhinology

The first laser was described by Theodor Maiman in 1960. By the 1970s, the CO_2 laser was already being used clinically for microsurgery of the larynx. In subsequent years other laser systems such as the argon laser, neodymium:yttrium aluminum garnet (Nd:YAG) laser, ruby laser, holmium (Ho):YAG laser, erbium (Er):YAG laser, diode laser, and assorted dye lasers have been applied in the treatment of various diseases of the head and neck [1].

Intranasal use of laser was first reported in 1977 by Lenz et al. [2], who reduced the hypertrophic mucosa of the inferior turbinate with an argon laser. While the precise cutting properties of the laser are of foremost importance in the larynx and oropharynx, coagulative effects and the ability to ablate bone are additional important properties in the nose and paranasal sinuses [3].

A laser ideally suited for rhinologic applications should meet the following requirements (which will vary according to the specific indication):
• equal ability to ablate bone and mucosa;
• shallow penetration depth (<1 mm), allowing precise tissue ablation;
• almost bloodless tissue ablation;
• ability to coagulate vessels >0.5 mm in diameter;
• minimal thermal damage to adjacent tissues;
• laser beam can be transmitted through a flexible carrier.

None of the laser systems commonly used in medicine meet all these criteria. Consequently, laser selection often represents a trade-off between the physician's requirements for a certain disease and the capabilities of the available laser devices [4]. The laser systems most commonly employed in rhinology are briefly described below.

Argon Laser

The argon laser emits blue-green light at wavelengths of 488 nm and 514 nm. These wavelengths are preferentially absorbed by melanin and hemoglobin [1]. Selective absorption by blood accounts for the excellent coagulation properties of the argon laser, which can seal vessels up to 1 mm in diameter. The beam can be delivered through a microscope, handpiece, and optical fibers. Tissue ablation requires high energy densities, which can be delivered even through thin flexible fibers (50 µm). The argon laser can also ablate thin bone.

KTP Laser

The potassium-titanyl-phosphate (KTP) laser is a frequency-doubled Nd:YAG laser. Doubling the frequency reduces the wavelength (of Nd:YAG) by half to 532 nm. The green light is absorbed chiefly by tissue pigments, similar to the argon laser beam. The KTP laser is a trade-off between the CO_2 and Nd:YAG lasers with regard to tissue effects. It is considerably more powerful than the argon laser, and its beam can be delivered through flexible fibers [5].

PDT Laser

Lasers used for photodynamic therapy (PDT) have a wavelength appropriate for the type of photosensitizer used. Hematoporphyrin derivatives or 5-δ-aminolevulinic acid (5-ALA) are generally used for photosensitization and are stimulated by wavelengths of 630 nm and 635 nm, respectively. This is accomplished with diode lasers tuned to the appropriate wavelength [6].

Diode Lasers

Diode lasers emit light in the near-infrared range of the spectrum (805–980 nm). Depending on its wavelength, the light may be strongly absorbed by water (980 nm) or may bind selectively to hemoglobin (805 nm). The diode laser is intermediate between the argon and Nd:YAG lasers. The laser light can be transmitted through a flexible carrier and is particularly useful for endoscopic surgery. The treatment parameters can be modulated to produce coagulative and vaporizing effects on the mucosa and to ablate cartilage and bone [7].

Nd:YAG Laser

The Nd:YAG laser is a solid-state laser with an yttrium-aluminum garnet crystal. It emits a beam in the near-infrared spectrum with a wavelength of 1064 nm and is absorbed more strongly by blood than by the surrounding tissue. Unlike the argon or KTP laser, the energy is not selectively absorbed by hemoglobin. The coagulation properties of the Nd:YAG laser result from strong scattering by cellular blood constituents. The beam is weakly absorbed by water, enabling it to penetrate the tissue surface and travel for about 4 mm before it is absorbed due to scattering. A penetration depth up to 10 mm can be achieved through heat conduction. If the target area is very dry, the laser can vaporize and coagulate the tissue surface. The fiber tip can be precharred to modulate the optical penetration depth in tissue and achieve controlled vaporization in the contact mode. The Nd:YAG laser can coagulate vessels up to 1.5 mm in diameter. The laser light is transmitted through a flexible carrier, allowing for numerous endoscopic applications [8].

Ho:YAG Laser

The Ho:YAG laser is a pulsed laser system with a wavelength of 2050–2130 nm. The laser energy is emitted in single pulses through a flexible carrier. The high energy, which is applied in the millisecond range, leads to focal superheating of water in tissues, causing explosive tissue vaporization with the expulsion of lased tissue fragments. This process causes very little thermal injury to the surrounding structures. Based on its strong absorption by water, the Ho:YAG laser is useful for the precise ablation of bone and soft tissue. Thus, unlike the CO_2 laser, the Ho:YAG laser can also coagulate tissue and provide effective intraoperative hemostasis [4].

Er:YAG Laser

The Er:YAG laser emits at a wavelength of 2940 nm. It is more strongly absorbed by bone than the Ho:YAG laser, allowing precise, largely athermal bone ablation. However, the hemostatic effect is relatively poor [3].

CO$_2$ Laser

The CO_2 laser emits infrared light at a wavelength of 10,600 nm. Its strong absorption by tissue water allows precise incision of the mucosa with little thermal damage beyond the vaporization zone. The penetration depth is less than 0.1 mm. At the same time, the CO_2 laser has limited coagulation properties and can seal blood vessels only up to 0.5 mm in diameter [1]. Since bone contains relatively little water, the CO_2 laser is not well suited for bone ablation, and rapid overheating occurs. The CO_2 laser beam is usually delivered through a microscope with a micromanipulator or through a special focusing handpiece. Microprocessor-controlled scanner systems are also available for ablating tissue over a larger area [3]. Since the beam can only be directed straight ahead, its intranasal applications are limited. Flexible carriers in the form of hollow waveguides or infrared fibers are too thick for intranasal use with power loss of 60–70% due to autoabsorption [4].

Successful laser surgery is impossible without knowledge of the biophysical effects of various laser systems on tissue. The treatment outcome and the risk of intraoperative and postoperative complications depend upon selection of the laser system best suited for a particular disease. Moreover, special instruments have been developed for intranasal laser use that facilitate the application of laser energy while

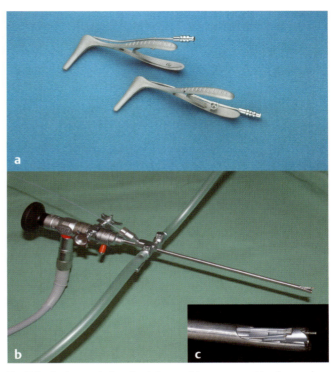

Fig. 3.**1** Instrumentation for intranasal laser use. **a** Nasal speculum with built-in suction. **b** Laser rhinoscope with built-in channels for viewing scope, laser fiber, and suction. **c** Tip of the laser rhinoscope with an Albarran lever for positioning the fiber tip.

improving the safety of the procedure. A basic prerequisite for good intranasal vision is effective smoke evacuation during laser use. Special specula with built-in suction have been developed for this purpose, along with special laser applicators and a "laser rhinoscope" (Fig. 3.**1**) with a built-in suction channel and laser fiber [5, 7–9].

The important applications of laser in rhinologic surgery are described in the sections below and also critically evaluated based on a review of the literature and personal experience.

■ Intranasal Laser Applications

Turbinate Reduction

Chronic nasal airway obstruction is one of the most common problems seen by the ENT physician. A large percentage of these patients have enlarged inferior nasal turbinates secondary to allergic or vasomotor rhinitis [10]. In patients with turbinate hyperplasia, the site of greatest narrowing in the nose is typically located at the head of the inferior turbinate. The more posterior portions of the nose have considerably less impact on nasal airflow [10]. Conservative treatment measures are often beneficial for only a limited time, and many cases require surgical treatment.

Many different operative techniques have been used for inferior turbinate reduction [11] and the sheer number of techniques suggests that an ideal method has not yet been found. Drawbacks of all conventional techniques include varying degrees of intraoperative and postoperative bleeding, potentially severe mucosal injury, and uncertain long-term results. There have also been numerous reports of the development of atrophic rhinitis [12].

Since the introduction of lasers in otorhinolaryngology, various laser systems have been used for the reduction of hyperplastic nasal turbinates [10, 13]. Thermal damage to the nasal mucosa from the laser energy causes scarring of the mucosal epithelium and in the submucosa, reducing the swelling capacity and secretory functions of the turbinate [14, 15]. Laser surgery of hypertrophic inferior turbinates is appropriate only if the obstruction is largely due to severe mucosal swelling [16]. Hence, the preoperative intranasal examination should always be supplemented by focal decongestion of the turbinate mucosa. If the patient notes significant improvement of nasal breathing after the decongestion, it may be concluded that the airway obstruction has a predominantly mucosal cause. If the obstruction is due to an enlarged or deviated bony turbinate, a conventional surgical technique such as a submucous turbinectomy or inferior turbinoplasty is preferred.

Confusing terms such as "submucous laser conchotomy" [17] or "laser turbinectomy" [18] are often used to describe the laser techniques. Since the laser affects only the turbinate mucosa, it is more accurate to use terms such as "laser turbinate reduction," "laser mucotomy" [19], or "laser cautery" [20]. It should be noted, however, that the widely used term "laser turbinectomy" refers strictly to treatment of the mucosa [10].

The first laser turbinate reduction was carried out in 1976 by Lenz et al. [2] using the argon laser. Under local anesthesia, the argon laser is used for linear cautery (Fig. 3.**2 a**) along the free border of the inferior turbinate. A 90° side-firing laser probe, sheathed in a protective quartz tube, is drawn along the inferior turbinate in the posterior-to-anterior direction. Patchy areas of fibrin exudation appear during the initial days after the surgery, followed by transient crust formation. Wound healing takes 3–6 weeks depending on the extent of collateral tissue destruction. Laser-induced subepithelial fibrosis is not complete until about 1 year postoperatively [21, 22]. More than 80 % of patients showed improved nasal breathing after argon laser cautery, and no serious complications were observed [23]. Although the technique has since been used successfully in more than 10,000 patients, the argon laser has not gained wide popularity because of its high acquisition costs and limited applications in otolaryngology.

The KTP laser has biophysical properties similar to those of the argon laser. Levine [14] reported on 21 patients with turbinate hypertrophy treated with the KTP laser. The laser energy was applied in contact to the anterior two-thirds of the inferior turbinate. The cautery lines were laid down in a cross-hatched pattern (Fig. 3.**2 b**) to eliminate any untreated islands of epithelium that could lead to reepithelialization. An approximately 85 % success rate has been reported with this technique for improvement of nasal breathing [14, 24].

The Nd:YAG laser induces marked fibrosis in the mucosa with atrophy of the mucous glands and shrinkage of the venous plexus [15, 21, 22]. Due to the deep penetration of the Nd:YAG laser energy, these tissue changes are more pronounced than with an argon or KTP laser. This results in a stiffer inferior turbinate with a limited potential for swelling [25]. Because the laser energy is delivered through a fiberoptic cable, the full length of the turbinate can be treated under endoscopic control [26].

Various contact techniques have been described for the Nd:YAG laser, including linear vaporization of the entire turbinate mucosa [27], cross-hatching of the mucosa [26], vaporization of the inferior free edge of the turbinate (Fig. 3.**2 c**) [28], deep longitudinal incision of the mucosa [25], and complete excision of the turbinate mucosa with partial exposure of the turbinate bone (Fig. 3.**2 d**) at a very high power setting [29]. Interstitial or submucous Nd:YAG laser treatment of the turbinate produces an approximately 3–4-mm-deep coagulation zone surrounding the laser fiber inserted into the turbinate. This technique causes very little damage to the respiratory ciliated epithelium [17]. The surface of the mucosa can also be spared by noncontact application of the Nd:YAG laser beam at low power. This has a negligible effect on mucociliary clearance [26]. The noncontact Nd:YAG laser energy is applied at such a low power setting (Fig. 3.**2 e**) that it causes only visible blanching of the mucosal surface [26, 30]. Based on personal experience, it is unwise to denature or carbonize the turbinate mucosa

Fig. 3.**2** Schematic lateral view of laser techniques for reducing the inferior turbinate. **a** Linear cautery: parallel strips are coagulated along the full length of the inferior turbinate with a contact fiber. **b** Cross-hatched pattern of laser application. **c** Contact cautery along the free edge of the turbinate. **d** Laser vaporization of the mucosa, exposing the anterior bony portion of the turbinate. **e** Diffuse application using non-contact technique. **f** CO_2 laser spot applications on the head of the turbinate.

with laser energy applied at a high dosage, as the severe mucosal damage results in considerable postoperative fibrin exudation and crusting requiring several weeks of an intensive postoperative regimen [26, 31]. It also increases the risk of synechia formation. The efficacy of combining interstitial photocoagulation with Nd:YAG laser cautery of the mucosal surface, as described by Vagnetti et al. [32], is uncertain.

The results of Nd:YAG laser treatment are generally good. The long-term success rates are 60–80%, despite a variety of surgical techniques and are comparable with those with conventional procedures [17, 25, 26, 33, 34]. The complication rate after Nd:YAG laser surgery is low. In particular, there have been no reports of serious intraoperative or postoperative bleeding [17, 25]. Fibrin exudation occurs postoperatively, regardless of the technique used. This can lead to synechia formation, which must be prevented by regular postoperative care [17, 26].

The tissue effects of the diode laser are very similar to the Nd:YAG laser. To date, few reports have been published on turbinate surgery with diode lasers. Min et al. [35] used a diode laser (810 nm) in the treatment of 53 patients with vasomotor rhinitis. The results were very satisfactory in terms of relieving nasal airway obstruction. In another 30 patients treated endoscopically with a diode laser (940 nm), nasal breathing improved in 85% [33]. Hopf et al. [7] and Janda et al. [36] reported comparably good results in a series of 50 patients each, with very low complication rates. DeRowe et al. [37] reported considerably poorer results with only 41% of their patients showing postoperative improvement in nasal breathing. It is still too early to evaluate the long-term efficacy of diode lasers in inferior turbinate reduction surgery. Some advantages are already apparent, such as low procurement costs and convenience of use, suggesting that the diode laser will gain an established place in otorhinolaryngology [8].

The pulsed Ho:YAG laser represents a compromise between superficial mucosal ablation and coagulation, with a superficial effect sparing deeper structures [36]. Fiberoptic delivery of the laser energy makes all intranasal regions accessible to treatment [38]. Recent published reports on inferior turbinate reduction with the Ho:YAG laser are contradictory, with success rates ranging from 52% [39] to 86% [40]. Even with largely athermal tissue ablation, fibrin deposits and crusts form after the surgery, but these can be separated without difficulty between 3 and 6 weeks [41]. Postoperative complications such as pain or bleeding were observed in 3–4% of cases [36]. Some patients complained of transient perinasal dysesthesia for 2–3 weeks [39].

The CO_2 laser can reduce turbinate mucosa by excision or vaporization [2]. A variety of CO_2 laser techniques have been described in the literature. While Selkin [16] made linear incisions in the thickened anterior turbinate mucosa, Elwany and Harrison [42] almost completely vaporized the mucosa on the anterior third of the turbinate. Fukutake et al. [43] vaporized all the inferior turbinate mucosa, and Englender [19] carried out laser mucotomy on the anterior two-thirds of the inferior turbinate. A scanner system can apparently be used for the char-free ablation of superficial tissue layers [44]. Based on comparative studies, we have adopted the single-spot technique (Fig. 3.**2 f**) for almost all CO_2 laser turbinate reductions in recent years [45]. This technique involves the application of separate laser spots to the head of the turbinate, causing shrinkage of the mucosa and subsequent scarring. Good results have also been achieved with endoscopically controlled CO_2 laser application via a handpiece or waveguide [37, 46, 47].

Histologic and electron microscopic studies after CO_2 laser vaporization have shown a markedly decreased number of seromucinous glands in the respiratory epithelium, increased connective tissue fibrosis, and a reduced number of blood vessels [15, 43, 48]. The higher the power setting and the more mucosa removed, the greater is the scarring. Extensive epithelial scars lead to marked functional impairment of the turbinate mucosa, creating a tendency for recurrent crusting [49]. On the other hand, a moderate degree of scarring is desirable, especially in allergic rhinitis, to suppress allergic reactions in the submucosa [43, 50].

In the great majority of cases, CO_2 laser turbinate reduction surgery can be done under local anesthesia on an outpatient basis [45, 51]. Intranasal packing is not strictly necessary due to the low risk of bleeding [19, 34]. Postoperative fibrin formation and crusting occur as a result of mucosal thermal injury, emphasizing the necessity of postoperative care [8, 19, 49]. Wound healing takes 3–6 weeks, depending on the extent of mucosal injury (Fig. 3.**3**). The long-term results are good, regardless of the technique used, with reported success rates ranging from 65% to 93% [18, 20, 34, 44, 45, 52, 53]. There is no significant difference between patients with and without allergy with regard to treatment outcomes [34].

On the basis of published data and comprehensive personal experience, we now consider laser reduction surgery to be the treatment of choice for inferior turbinate hypertrophy with a mucosal cause. The laser surgery is less traumatizing, has fewer adverse side effects, and it can be done on an ambulatory basis using local anesthesia. Generally there is no need for intranasal packing. The type of laser system used is of minor importance when due attention is given to recommended treatment parameters. The results of laser surgery are comparable or even superior to those of conventional procedures. The treatment is easily applied to children owing to the low degree of tissue trauma. Meticulous postoperative care, especially to prevent synechiae, is recommended in all procedures, especially when concomitant surgery has been done on the nasal septum.

Septal Surgery

The use of lasers in septal surgery is a very controversial issue [54]. Advocates of laser septoplasty point out that laser surgery makes it unnecessary to mobilize the mucosa, cartilage, and bone as in traditional septoplasties. It can also reduce the possible complications of conventional septoplasty such as bleeding, septal perforation, and instability leading to external nasal deformity. Another advantage is the preservation of the vomeronasal organ. The laser

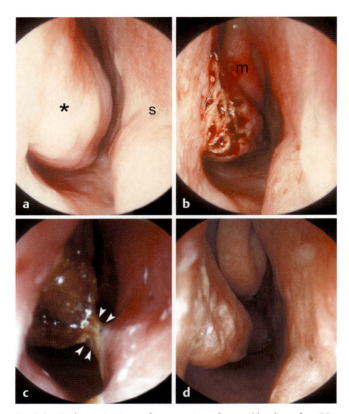

Fig. 3.**3** Endoscopic views of progression of wound healing after CO_2 laser turbinate reduction using the single-spot technique. **a** Bulky inferior turbinate (*) causing significant nasal airway obstruction. **b** Appearance immediately after laser application. **c** Crusting 3 weeks postoperatively, with risk of synechia formation (arrows). **d** By 4 weeks postoperatively, epithelialization is almost complete. The nasal airway has been expanded, and the middle turbinate is clearly visible (s, nasal septum; m, middle turbinate).

systems used in septal surgery include the CO_2 laser [55–57], Nd:YAG laser [58], and diode laser [8].

The great majority of surgical experience with laser septoplasty has been reported for the CO_2 laser. Kamami et al. [56, 57] applied the CO_2 laser beam (scanner system, 10 W, superpulse, continuous-wave [CW] mode) through a specially developed handpiece. The scanner minimizes thermal damage to the cartilage. Mucoperichondrial resection is done in a strictly horizontal plane from anterior to posterior. The vertical extent of the resection should not exceed 2–3 mm to avoid creating an excessive wound surface. Very satisfactory results were achieved with this technique in more than 700 patients [56, 57]. Krespi and Kacker [55, 59] used the same technique to treat 150 patients. Improvement in nasal airway obstruction was described in 96 % of cases. Scherer et al. [58] used the Nd:YAG laser or diode laser for the treatment of limited septal pathologies. The laser energy was applied with a contact fiber introduced through a special endoscope, using high power settings (30–60 W) and short application times (0.02–0.5 s). Linear cautery of the mucosa was first done above and below the spur to minimize bleeding during resection. Deviated cartilage segments can usually be removed without difficulty. Bone, on the other hand, is trans-

formed by the laser beam into a "porcelain-like substance" that shatters when touched by the fiber and can be pushed aside. Only the tip of the spur is removed. It is important to avoid thermal injury to the base of the spur on the septum to prevent necrosis of the vomer or perpendicular plate. In 150 patients treated under topical anesthesia, there was only one case of septal perforation. Point coagulation at low power can also be used to decongest bulky cavernous tissue on the nasal septum [8].

When discussing the value and benefits of laser septoplasty, it is important to distinguish among the different types of septal deformity. Laser-assisted septal surgery is confined to removing a ridge or spur chiefly on the anterior portions of the septum. An S-shaped septal deformity with an ascending ridge should still be corrected using conventional techniques [54, 60]. Exceptions are patients with coagulation disorders or a serious underlying medical disease. It should be added that it is important to consider the wound surfaces that are created when a laser septoplasty is done concurrently with turbinate reduction. Combining the procedures increases the risk of synechia formation, requiring a meticulous regimen of postoperative wound care.

Paranasal Sinuses

The laser was first used in paranasal sinus surgery by Lenz et al. [61], who used an argon laser to create a window between the inferior meatus and maxillary sinus. More than a decade later, Ohyama [62] reported on the initial use of the Nd:YAG laser in the maxillary sinus. Abnormal tissue was removed from the maxillary sinus, and the natural ostium enlarged from the inside, using an Nd:YAG laser passed through a flexible endoscope inserted into the sinus via the canine fossa. Other clinical applications of the Nd:YAG laser as well as KTP, Ho:YAG, and diode lasers followed [4, 5, 8, 9, 38, 58, 63–65]. The CO_2 laser does not have a role in paranasal sinus surgery, although successful applications have been reported in the literature [66, 67]. Its disadvantage is that the beam cannot be delivered into the nose through a flexible cable. Currently available flexible waveguide systems for the CO_2 laser are either too bulky or absorb too much of the laser energy [68]. This led Sato and Nakashima [67] to use a specially curved laser handpiece for resecting choanal polyps in seven children.

The role of laser surgery in the treatment of chronic sinusitis and chronic polypous sinusitis is a controversial topic in the literature [7, 58, 69, 70]. Conventional intranasal sinus surgery under endoscopic–microscopic control is still considered the treatment method of choice [71]. Laser use is expected to achieve almost bloodless tissue ablation resulting in a clearer intraoperative view—of particular important in intranasal sinus surgery. Other possible advantages are less tissue trauma eliminating the need for nasal packing and reducing the costs of postoperative care. Most experience in this area has been reported for the Nd:YAG and Ho:YAG lasers.

In patients whose middle meatus is obstructed by a small number of polyps or an excretory duct is obstructed due to an isolated swelling, Scherer et al. [58] perform endoscopically controlled Nd:YAG laser surgery to relieve the obstruction. "Spot welding" with the laser can shrink the obstructing tissue with moderate subsequent scarring, relieving the obstruction. Isolated polyps can be removed by laser on an outpatient basis under topical anesthesia and is largely painless and bloodless. The polyps are shrunk with a high-power beam (20–30 W, short exposure time) using noncontact technique. A low-power contact technique is used for severing the polyp stalk and removing mucosa. Rarefying osteitis is prevented by using low power settings in close proximity to bone [58]. One modification is to apply physiologic saline solution during use of the Nd:YAG laser ("water-laser technique"). The fluid is heated by the sapphire tip, helping further to reduce bleeding [69].

As early as 1993, Zhang [72] did a prospective study comparing conventional surgical techniques with Nd:YAG laser therapy in 102 patients with chronic polypous sinusitis. Recurrence rates were lower after the laser therapy, and postoperative bleeding was reduced. Scherer and his group [7, 58] also used the Nd:YAG and diode laser in selected patients for removing the uncinate process, opening the ethmoid bulla, or marsupializing a frontal or ethmoid mucocele.

In contrast to the primary surgical treatment of chronic sinusitis, where bony structures must be removed to gain access, revision sinus surgery generally does not require additional bone removal to obtain an adequate view of the operative site. Prompt intervention is important to allow good endoscopic access to the site of recurrent disease [8, 73]. Ilgner et al. [73] carried out a total of 128 Nd:YAG laser-assisted endoscopic procedures in 86 patients with recurrent polyps following conventional sinus surgery. In 63 patients, no further disease was seen after the revision procedure. Only six cases had intraoperative bleeding that reduced visibility. Two patients reported paresthesia in the area of the nasolabial fold. There were no injuries to the periorbita, anterior skull base, or major vessels. Similar results were reported by Hopf et al. [7], who have increasingly used diode lasers in recent years.

In contrast to thermal laser systems, which can lead to thermal necrosis and delayed wound healing, the Ho:YAG laser permits the almost athermal removal of bone and mucosa while providing effective hemostasis [4, 63]. Its biophysical properties appear to make it particularly suitable for paranasal sinus surgery [65]. Gleich et al. [64] used the Ho:YAG laser in 29 patients with chronic sinusitis, combining the laser with conventional technique. The laser was especially useful in opening the anterior wall of an ethmoid mucocele for marsupialization. No complications occurred. Kautzky et al. [63], however, felt that laser-assisted surgery was not better than a purely conventional procedure due to the prolonged operating time.

Metson [4] undertook a randomized, controlled study comparing the Ho:YAG laser with conventional surgery in the treatment of chronic and chronic polypous sinusitis. Thirty-two patients underwent endoscopic sinus surgery using the Ho:YAG laser on one side of the nose and conventional endoscopic instrumentation on the other side. The laser was used to reduce the middle turbinate, resect

the uncinate process, open the ethmoid bulla, exenterate the anterior and posterior ethmoid cells, and enlarge the maxillary sinus ostium. No differences were noted in the postoperative results. Mucosal edema was increased on the laser-treated side, while crust formation was greater on the conventionally treated side; both conditions resolved in about 2 months. The main benefit of laser surgery was improved intraoperative hemostasis, resulting in better visibility. Metson [4] considers the Ho:YAG laser to be particularly helpful in revision surgery, as it can remove diseased tissue close to the orbit and skull base without exerting the tensile forces that occur with conventional instrumentation. On the other hand, Qadir and Kennedy [74] found that use of the Ho:YAG laser in experimental animals could easily cause optic nerve injury. Another drawback is that aerosolized tissue particles are expelled from the ablation zone of the Ho:YAG laser, which can fog the endoscope and obstruct vision [64].

To summarize previous experience with laser applications in sinus surgery, it may be said that conventional intranasal techniques are still the treatment methods of choice at the present time. Laser techniques can be considered an adjunct to conventional instrumentation. Laser use in the paranasal sinuses has basically two valid indications: (i) the removal of polyps in patients who refuse conventional surgery or are poor candidates for general anesthesia, and (ii) the treatment of circumscribed recurrent polyposis following prior intranasal surgery [7, 8].

Lacrimal Duct Surgery

The cardinal symptom of all diseases of the lacrimal drainage system is epiphora (excessive lacrimation). Due to their anatomic proximity, diseases of the lacrimal passages may also relate to pathology of the nose and paranasal sinuses, emphasizing the need for cooperation between the ophthalmologist and ENT physician [75]. Diagnosis of the mechanical obstruction is based on lacrimal irrigation and imaging procedures (dacryocystography with contrast medium, digital subtraction dacryocystography, radionuclide dacryocystography, ultrasonography, computed tomography (CT), magnetic resonance imaging), which are applied according to individual requirements. Endoscopic examination should not be limited to examining the nasal cavity and the opening of the nasolacrimal duct but should include the lacrimal passages themselves [76].

Surgery is the only appropriate treatment for frank lacrimal obstruction. External dacryocystorhinostomy (DCR) was first described by Toti in 1904 [77], while intranasal surgical techniques date back to West [78]. Over the years, the introduction of the operating microscope and of endoscopes with high-intensity illumination has led to modifications and advances in intranasal procedures. Techniques in which antegrade illumination of the lacrimal sac is combined with microscopically or endoscopically assisted intranasal dissection of the nasal mucosa, bone, and lacrimal sac have yielded particularly good results [79]. Various laser systems have been used in recent years for the treatment of lacrimal obstruction [80–84]. Three main techniques have evolved: laser-assisted transcanalicular DCR,

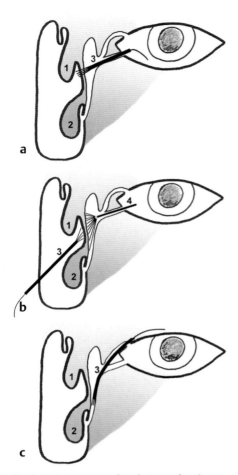

Fig. 3.**4** Laser-assisted techniques for the treatment of lacrimal obstruction. **a** Laser-assisted transcanalicular dacryocystorhinostomy (DCR). **b** Laser-assisted endonasal DCR with translacrimal illumination. **c** Laser-assisted dacryoplasty (1, middle turbinate; 2, inferior turbinate; 3, flexible laser fiber; 4, fiberoptic light source).

intranasal laser-assisted DCR, and laser dacryoplasty (Fig. 3.**4**).

Laser-Assisted Transcanalicular Dacryocystorhinostomy

This technique is used mainly in the treatment of infrasaccal or postsaccal lacrimal stenosis. After the endoscope has been placed in the lacrimal sac, it is rotated toward the bone (laser beam position checked intranasally), and the laser is fired to create a rhinostomy window measuring at least 5 × 5 mm. The lacrimal sac mucosa, bone, and nasal mucosa are divided in one step (Fig. 3.**4 a**). This is followed by the insertion of a silicone stent, which is left in place for 3–6 months [85]. Early approaches to laser-assisted transcanalicular DCR were described by Massaro et al. [80], Gonnering et al. [86], and Christenbury [87]. The main problem was creating a rhinostomy of adequate size. In 1993, Reifler [88] reported a clinical success rate of 68.4% using the KTP laser. Patel et al. [84] reported on the transcanalicular revision of a conventional external DCR using the Nd:YAG laser. The success rate was only 46%. Both laser applications were carried out without endoscopic control. Based on their biophysical properties, the KTP and Ho:YAG are the most suitable lasers for transcanalicular DCR. The success rates achieved with these laser systems range from 70% to 90%, making them comparable to conventional techniques [85, 89–91].

Laser-Assisted Intranasal Dacryocystorhinostomy

In laser-assisted intranasal DCR (Fig. 3.**4 b**), the lacrimal sac is illuminated with a light probe inserted through the inferior canaliculus, while an intranasal laser is used to perforate the bone and lacrimal sac [92].

Laser-Assisted Dacryoplasty

In laser-assisted dacryoplasty (Fig. 3.**4 c**), the lacrimal passages are recanalized with an intracanalicular inserted laser. This technique can be used to correct bland stenoses at the level of the canaliculi or lacrimal sac [93]. Dacryoendoscopy is a necessary prelude to laser dacryoplasty, as the endoscopic findings will dictate the therapeutic procedure that should be done in the same sitting [76, 92]. A modified three-channel Jünemann catheter is passed down the lacrimal duct, providing access for inserting a 0.3- or 0.5-mm scope and a 325- or 375-μm laser fiber. The irrigation channel is used to clear away blood and cellular debris. After the duct has been recanalized, a bicanalicular silicone tube is inserted for 3–6 months to prevent postoperative adhesions [76].

The Er:YAG laser appears to be particularly well suited for this technique. Since its wavelength is strongly absorbed by water, the laser treatment induces a mild fibroblastic reaction and slight scarring that should lower the incidence of recurrence [82, 92]. The Er:YAG laser can be used on circumscribed membranous intrasaccal and postsaccal stenoses, punctate canalicular stenoses, and membranous recurrent stenoses after a prior DCR. External surgery is preferred for mucoceles and posttraumatic stenoses. The power output of the laser is too low to perform a rhinotomy for laser-assisted DCR [76, 93]. Laser-assisted dacryoplasty has a reported success rate of 75–80% [76, 93, 94]. This is below the 85–90% success rate of external DCR, which continues to be the gold standard for surgery of the lacrimal drainage system [95].

The main problem in laser-assisted lacrimal surgery is the thermally induced fibroblastic reaction with the formation of granulation tissue, predisposing to restenosis. This is particularly common in children [92]. Intraoperative mitomycin C may be of value for inhibiting fibroblastic activity and the formation of granulation tissue [96]. Another controversial issue is the necessity and duration of stent insertion. While silicone intubation promotes granulation formation on the one hand [97], Boush et al. [98] found that considerably better results were achieved after intubation.

To summarize the experience to date with laser-assisted lacrimal surgery, the advantages of endoscopically controlled transcanalicular DCR are the absence of a skin incision, the ability to treat the site directly, the relatively short operating time, the ability to perform out the surgery on an outpatient basis, and the low rate of postoperative complications. But because conventional DCR (external or intranasal) has a higher than 90 % success rate [83, 92] and the laser technique is much more cost-intensive, laser use cannot presently be justified solely by its lower degree of invasiveness.

Choanal Atresia

Congenital unilateral or bilateral choanal atresia is the most common malformation involving the nasal cavity and nasopharynx. It was first described by Johann Röderer in 1755 [99]. Congenital choanal atresia has a reported incidence of 1–2 in 10,000 births. Unilateral atresia is considerably more common than bilateral cases. The closure of the choanae may be partial or complete. Females predominate by a 2:1 ratio [100]. The atresia is bony in approximately 90 % of cases and membranous in approximately 10 % [101], although more recent publications cite a 29 % incidence of pure bony atresias and a 71 % incidence of mixed bony–membranous forms [102, 103].

Bilateral choanal atresia constitutes a life-threatening emergency, as the infant cannot breathe effectively through the mouth during the first 3 weeks of life. The only recourse is emergency intubation or tracheotomy. Unilateral choanal atresia, on the other hand, is often manifested during the first year of life by chronic unilateral catarrh [104]. The diagnosis is based on the clinical manifestations and endoscopic examination. Adjunctive studies are intranasal intubation and testing of nasal patency with a Politzer bag. Thin-slice axial CT scanning is also indicated [103, 104]. It provides information on the nature and thickness of the atresia and is helpful in planning treatment. Radiographic contrast examination of the nasal cavities has become a less important study [105].

The timing of treatment for unilateral choanal atresia is controversial. On the one hand, early surgical intervention can prevent possible sequelae such as impaired eustachian tube ventilation and rhinosinusitis. On the other hand, the surgical procedure becomes technically easier as the child grows. The ideal time for surgical correction is between the sixth and twelfth year of life [101]. The first successful operation for choanal atresia was reported in 1853 by Emmert [106], who pierced a unilateral atresia plate with a transnasal trocar in a 7-year-old child. Since then, a variety of surgical methods have been devised. The transpalatine and transnasal endoscopic approaches are currently the most widely practiced surgical techniques [100]. The transpalatine approach provides excellent topographic orientation and yields good long-term results [101]. Refinements in the endoscope and operating microscope and continual improvements in endoscopic instrumentation have led to an increasing preference for transnasal techniques in recent years [102, 107].

In 1978, Healy et al. [108] first described the use of the CO_2 laser for repair of unilateral choanal atresia. The laser was used transnasally to vaporize an opening in the atresia plate. In subsequent years the KTP, Ho:YAG, Nd:YAG and diode lasers have also been used with good results. Regardless of the type of laser used, the operation is done under general anesthesia. The nasal mucosa is decongested by inserting a cotton pledget soaked in 0.1 % naphazoline nitrate. Tzifa and Skinner [100] used a 5 % cocaine solution for decongestion. Transnasal exposure is maintained with a modified ear speculum or a self-retaining nasal speculum [27]. If direct access to the atretic choana through the inferior turbinate is difficult, reduction of the turbinate has proved useful [100]. The nasopharynx is packed with moist cotton to protect the mucosa from accidental laser exposure. The atresia plate is lased from the medial side. A small hole is vaporized in the plate until the moist cotton in the nasopharynx can be seen. This opening is then progressively enlarged, working mainly toward the vomer. The need for stent placement is discussed below.

Postoperative nasal hygiene is essential for a successful outcome [109]. The regimen consists of intensive nasal care with decongestant nose drops, inhalation, and saline irrigation, generally performed by the parents themselves. If a stent has been placed, it should be suctioned several times daily to maintain patency. Regular endoscopic examinations are scheduled for the early detection of granulation tissue formation, which promotes restenosis. Granulations can also be removed by laser surgery and are additionally treated by local steroid therapy [14].

CO_2 laser treatment is carried out under microscopic control (Fig. 3.**5**). One drawback is that the CO_2 laser beam can only be directed straight ahead. At present it cannot be transmitted through thin optical fibers, and certain conditions impede CO_2 laser surgery such as septal deviation, enlarged inferior turbinates, or a high arched hard palate [110]. Nevertheless, the CO_2 laser has proved its practical value and has yielded good therapeutic results [27, 108, 110, 111]. Due to the limited ability of the CO_2 laser to divide bone, Johnson [27] additionally uses a diamond bur to enlarge the choana. Dedo [111] modifies the pure CO_2 laser procedure by dissecting anterior and posterior mucosal flaps, which are rotated into the newly created opening.

Tzifa and Skinner [100] and Pototschnig et al. [103] felt that the KTP laser was better for the treatment of choanal atresia since it could be transmitted through optical fibers. The deflectable fiber minimizes the risk of injury to the skull base and carotid artery. Another advantage of this laser system is its wavelength, which enables the surgeon to cut tissue and bone while also producing good hemostasis. Pototschnig et al. treated 13 patients with the KTP laser (3–5 W, CW mode, contact technique) without complications. Satisfactory results have also been reported with the intranasal use of the Ho:YAG laser [64, 112], Nd:YAG laser [113], and diode laser [7], although only small numbers of patients have been treated with these devices.

Regardless of the method used, removal of the atresia plate always creates a circular wound area with a strong contractile tendency, similar to surgery of the trachea and frontal sinuses [104, 114]. Restenosis most commonly occurs during the first 12 months [104]. Stents are inserted

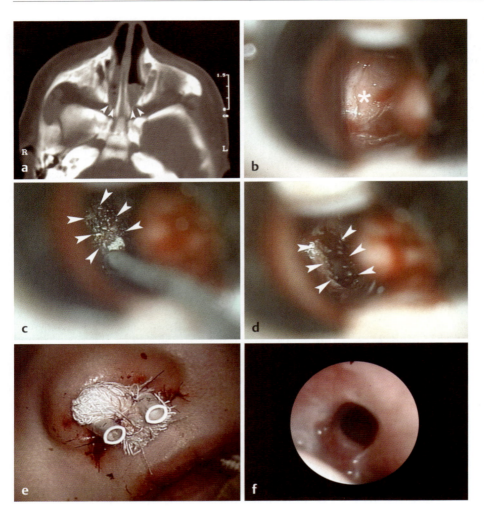

Fig. 3.5 Bilateral choanal atresia in a 2-week-old infant. **a** Axial computed tomography (CT) scan demonstrates bilateral closure of the choanae (arrows). **b** Microscopic view of the membranous stenosis (*) through the left nasal cavity. **c** CO_2 laser vaporization of the membranous atresia plate (arrows) using a backstop. **d** Opened and enlarged choana (arrows). **e** Silicone stent with protection of the columella. **f** Flexible endoscopic view of the patent choana at 3 months, with healthy-looking mucosa.

postoperatively to inhibit restenosis and facilitate nasal breathing. The necessity, size, material, and duration of stent placement are controversial issues in the literature. Most authors recommend placing a stent for 2 weeks to 6 months after the laser repair [103, 110, 112, 115]. This is particularly advised in newborns and patients with bilateral atresia. On the other hand, small children in particular have great difficulty tolerating the necessary postoperative nasal care [116]. For this reason, Illum [105], Panwar and Martin [117], and Tzifa and Skinner [100] do not insert a stent after the laser repair, and these authors have not observed an increased incidence of restenosis. Possible complications resulting from stent placement include ulcerations of the nasal septum, columella or alar cartilage, formation of intranasal synechiae, and sinusitis [100, 110]. Also, the stent itself can promote the formation of granulation tissue [108].

Intranasal laser surgery has become an established modality for the treatment of unilateral and bilateral choanal atresia. The operation is easy and quick to do and is well tolerated with a shorter hospital stay. Stent placement is unnecessary in older children and adults but is still recommended in newborns with bilateral stenosis due to the miniscule size of the passages. The rate of restenosis is comparable to that seen in conventional transnasal techniques, regardless of the type of laser used.

Nasopharynx

Aside from choanal atresia, very few reports have been published on laser applications in the nasopharynx. Available reports deal with the use of argon, KTP, Nd:YAG, diode and CO_2 lasers introduced by the transnasal or transoral route [118]. Possible indications for the laser treatment of benign diseases are adenoids, hyperplastic nasopharyngeal mucosa, cysts, papillomas, and scar adhesions. Hopf et al. [7] used Nd:YAG and diode lasers in adolescents to remove adenoids and hyperplastic mucosa from around the eustachian tube eminence under local anesthesia. This should be done only after histologic examination has ruled out a malignant tumor. Since adequate topical anesthesia cannot be obtained in this region, the authors feel that the procedure should not be used in children. Giannoni et al. [119] described the development of nasopharyngeal stenosis following adenoidectomy with the KTP laser, attributable to the use of excessive power settings leading to massive fibrin exudation. In another report, the CO_2 laser was used successfully to divide scar adhesions in the nasopharynx, which occasionally develop following conventional ade-notomy, tonsillectomy or uvulopalatopharyngoplasty [120]. Lasers have also been used in the treatment of recurrent papillomatosis. Dedo and Yu [121] described the successful removal of recurrent papillomas in the nose and nasopharynx by periodic vaporization with the CO_2 laser.

Laser treatment of nasopharyngeal tumors has been attempted rarely. Gunkel et al. [122] described the microendoscopically controlled resection of a nasopharyngeal teratoma in a newborn girl with the CO_2 laser. Scholtz et al. [123] and Nakamura et al. [124] combined the KTP laser with endoscopic surgery to resect a juvenile nasopharyngeal fibroma. These authors note the advantages of laser surgery in coagulating blood vessels and shrinking the tumor mass, allowing for a more confident and complete resection.

Laser surgery of malignant nasopharyngeal tumors is limited to palliative indications [8, 118, 125]. In cases where a malignant recurrence is affecting quality of life due to nasal airway obstruction, impaired eustachian tube ventilation, or recurrent bleeding, the laser can be used in a minimally invasive procedure to debulk the tumor and alleviate these complaints (Fig. 3.**6**). The Nd:YAG laser is good for this purpose, as it can be delivered through a fiberoptic cable under endoscopic control. The power should not be set too high, as this may cause necrotic changes in the skull base region and carotid artery [8]. Another possible application of lasers is debulking tumors in preparation for radiotherapy or chemotherapy.

Epistaxis, Hereditary Hemorrhagic Telangiectasia

Approximately 60% of the population have one or more nosebleeds during their lifetime. Most cases are self-limiting and require no specific treatment, but approximately 6% will require medical attention. The tortuous vascular channels in the Kieselbach area on the anterior nasal septum are the most frequent source of bleeding (Fig. 3.**7**). Other, less common sources of epistaxis are telangiectatic granulomas, benign and malignant tumors, vascular malformations, and hereditary hemorrhagic telangiectasia (HHT) [126].

As early as in the mid-1970s, Lenz and Eichler [127] found that the argon laser beam could occlude small blood vessels in experimental animals. However, laser therapy is not appropriate in the acute stages of a severe nosebleed. Profuse bleeding obscures the treatment site and prevents selective vascular coagulation. The best options for these cases are still electrocoagulation, anterior and posterior intranasal packing, and vascular ligation or embolization [128].

The laser systems with the most favorable biophysical properties for treating epistaxis are the argon, KTP, and Nd:YAG lasers. Another recent option for vascular coagulation are the diode lasers. While lasers have little role in the acute treatment of nosebleed, they are useful in special situations for preventing recurrent bouts of epistaxis. The goal of laser therapy is to occlude blood vessels through light absorption. During laser use, the treatment parameters should be carefully adjusted to induce blanching of the

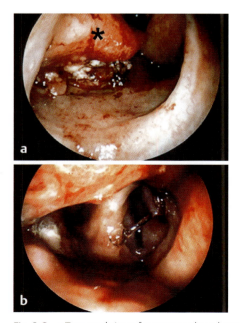

Fig. 3.**6** **a** Transoral view of a recurrent lymphoepithelial carcinoma (*) with a 90° endoscope, following radiotherapy and brachytherapy. The right choana is completely obstructed by tumor tissue. **b** The tumor has been debulked with the Nd:YAG laser, restoring the patency of the right choanal passage.

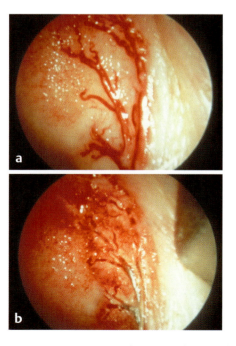

Fig. 3.**7** Prominent vascular tree on the Kieselbach area, a source of recurrent nosebleeds (**a**) before and (**b**) after treatment with the Nd:YAG laser.

target area. The power density should be increased in small increments to avoid inducing a "popcorn effect," i. e., sudden rupture of the vessels by expanding gas bubbles without prior, slow coagulation of the vessel walls [129]. Multiple treatments may be necessary, depending on the size and location of the vessels. To avoid accidental septal perforation, the bilateral treatment of ectatic vessels at corresponding sites should be avoided if at all possible.

In contrast to local causes of epistaxis, HHT is a systemic disease of the vascular connective tissue. The term "hereditary hemorrhagic telangiectasia" was coined in 1909 by Hanes [130]. It is also called Rendu–Osler–Weber disease, after the authors who first described it. HHT has an autosomal dominant mode of inheritance. Gene mutations have been described on chromosomes 9q, 3p, and 12p. There is no sex predilection, and all races are affected [131, 132]. The disease is characterized by the presence of dark red, pinhead to rice grain sized angiodysplastic lesions, which appear in the second or third decade of life in approximately 50 % of patients [133] and become more numerous with age [131]. The lesions may be ubiquitously distributed. The skin and mucosa of the head are the sites of predilection. The nasal and oral mucosa, lower lip, cheek, and auricle are particularly affected. The vessel walls of angiodysplasias are exceptionally fragile due to an imperfectly formed layer of smooth muscle cells and elastic fibers, and they can bleed easily and profusely in response to mechanical stresses [134]. Accordingly, recurrent epistaxis from the anterior part of the nose is the cardinal symptom of Rendu–Osler–Weber disease and is the first presenting symptom in 90 % of cases [131]. Besides small telangiectasias, the lesions of HHT can consist of vascular aneurysms and arteriovenous fistulas [134]. The sites of occurrence include pulmonary and intracranial lesions, which can lead to life-threatening complications [131]. As a result, all patients affected by HHT should undergo appropriate screening examinations [135].

A number of different procedures have been used in the treatment of HHT including vascular embolization, brachytherapy, dermoplasty, cryosurgery, topical and systemic estrogens, and electrocoagulation [128]. Despite the many options, no treatment modality to date has completely resolved recurrent epistaxis despite repeated use [136]. Consequently, the goal of treatment in HHT is to reduce the frequency and severity of epistaxis to improve the patient's quality of life and eliminate the need for blood transfusions. These goals can be accomplished with laser therapy.

Most reports on the laser treatment of HHT are based on the use of the Nd:YAG laser [137–139]. There have also been reports on the CO_2 laser [140, 141], argon laser [127, 142, 143], KTP laser [5], flashlamp-pulsed dye laser [144, 145], and diode laser [146]. Patients should be hospitalized and treated under general anesthesia [143]. The endotracheal tube ensures airway patency in the event of heavy intraoperative bleeding [136]. Also, intranasal manipulations such as cotton insertion or the injection of local anesthetic can easily injure the angiodysplasias and cause bleeding that will hamper or prevent subsequent laser treatment. Various parameters for the treatment of HHT with laser are given in the literature [137–139, 146]. Since

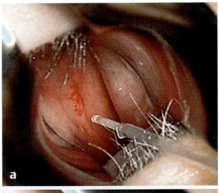
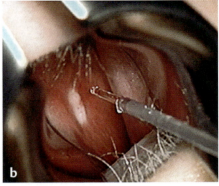

Fig. 3.**8** Typical telangiectasia of the endonasal mucosa in Rendu–Osler–Weber disease before (**a**) and immediately after (**b**) diode laser coagulation (940 nm), with typical blanching of the treated area.

setting the power too high can rupture the vessels and cause them to bleed, it is best to start with a low power setting and gradually increase it according to individual tissue response. Angiodysplasias are usually lased at a distance of 2–5 mm using a centripetal technique, i. e., starting at the periphery and moving towards the center [143]. The angiodysplastic vessels blanch as they are photocoagulated (Fig. 3.**8**).

Avoid intranasal packing at the end of the operation as it can cause significant trauma to the inherently fragile nasal mucosa, with an increased risk of bleeding during pack removal. Good results have been obtained by instilling a corticosteroid ointment into the nasal cavity at the end of the operation. This ointment pack will compress smaller bleeding sites and also prevent drying and crusting of the nasal mucosa [139, 146].

The therapeutic results achieved with argon and KTP lasers have been satisfactory in most patients [142, 146, 147]. Levine [5] observed a marked decline in the frequency and severity of epistaxis following intranasal KTP laser therapy. We have also noted a marked decrease in the frequency and intensity of bleeding in most of our patients, which is consistent with the results of other authors [136, 137, 147]. Control of epistaxis persists for varying lengths of time after the surgery, with many patients requiring additional treatment at 4–8 months [128, 143]. The Nd:YAG laser offers several advantages over the argon and KTP lasers. For example, the Nd:YAG laser energy penetrates more deeply in tissues, providing a deeper level of vascular coagulation and subsequent fibrosis [129]. Often the superficial telangiectasias are accompanied by a very pronounced network of subepithelial arteriovenous malformations which are not accessible to argon and KTP lasers, especially in the region of the inferior turbinates [148]. If slight bleeding occurs during laser treatment, the Nd:YAG laser can often obliterate the bleeding sites owing to its greater penetration depth [144].

Diode lasers might be a promising alternative. Hopf et al. [146] treated eight patients with the diode laser (940 nm) on an outpatient basis using local anesthesia. With the patient in a semi-sitting position, the laser light was applied under endoscopic control using a noncontact technique (10–25 W, pulsed mode). The authors reported very satisfactory results, although the number of patients was too small for a definitive evaluation. The CO_2 laser is unsuitable for the treatment of telangiectasias because of its biophysical properties [1, 136, 149]. "Yellow light lasers," which are very selectively absorbed by hemoglobin, have been disappointing in the treatment of recurrent epistaxis [144, 145]. It may be that the low penetration depth of these lasers provides only a superficial occlusion of vascular lesions.

The complication rate after laser treatment is low. There were no instances of severe intraoperative or postoperative bleeding in our patients. It should be noted that heavy bleeding very often cannot be controlled by laser treatment alone and will require conventional bipolar coagulation [143]. One risk of laser therapy is that a septal perforation may develop during the postoperative course [8, 142]. This risk can be substantially reduced by treating the nasal septum in two stages [137]. A regimen of postoperative nasal care is effective in preventing the formation of intranasal synechiae.

Lasers with a good coagulating action, such as the argon, KTP, Nd:YAG, and diode lasers, are very effective for controlling local epistaxis from convoluted vessels and also in the treatment of HHT. The treatments are less traumatizing and painful than other operative techniques and can be repeated as often as needed. The hospital stay is short, and the laser surgery has little if any adverse effect on the quality of life. Laser techniques cannot permanently cure Rendu–Osler–Weber disease, but in many cases they can significantly improve epistaxis by reducing the intensity and frequency of bleeding. Multiple treatments are often required. It should be emphasized that a meticulous postoperative care regimen that includes a soft nasal ointment is an essential part of the treatment of HHT with laser surgery.

Benign Tumors

A number of reports have been published on intranasal laser applications for benign tumors of the nose. Advantages of laser therapy are hemostasis with good intraoperative visibility, minimal tissue trauma, the ability to carry out the surgery under local anesthesia, and generally the absence of a surgical defect requiring repair. Lasers (CO_2, KTP,

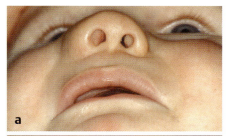
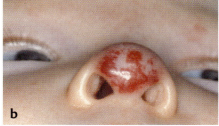

Fig. 3.**9**　**a** Vascular malformation of the right nasal sidewall with intranasal and extranasal components. **b** Capillary hemangioma of the nasal tip.

argon, Nd:YAG, and diode) have been used on a variety of intranasal lesions such as pyogenic granulomas, hemangiomas and vascular malformations, columellar cysts, granulations, polyps, verrucae, and papillomas [5, 8, 16, 150]. Levine [5] treated circumscribed inverted papillomas of the maxillary sinus using an endoscope and the KTP laser. There is no question, however, that the treatment of choice for inverted papillomas of the nose and paranasal sinuses is complete surgical resection through an intranasal or open rhinosurgical approach using conventional instruments. The intranasal resection of these tumors should be left to experienced surgeons using nonlaser techniques [151]. Lasers are most frequently used in the treatment of hemangiomas and vascular malformations, and these applications are described below in some detail.

Vascular anomalies are among the most frequent abnormalities encountered in infants and small children [152, 153]. Our understanding of vascular anomalies was greatly advanced by the studies of Mulliken and Glowacki [154], who developed a classification system based on the biological and clinical behavior of these lesions. This classification defines two major categories of vascular anomalies: hemangiomas and vascular malformations. Hemangiomas are not congenital and only appear days or weeks after birth. In contrast, vascular malformations are already present at birth, although some are so small that they may go undetected for years. Hemangiomas are also distinguished by rapid, proliferative growth during the first 2 years of life [153]. This is followed by a phase of regression occasionally completed by the second or third year of life but often continuing until the tenth year [155]. Vascular malformations, on the other hand, grow proportionately with the child and never undergo spontaneous regression.

Approximately 80 % of all hemangiomas are located in the head and neck region, but isolated intranasal involvement is relatively rare. Lesions may also occur in the paranasal sinuses [156, 157], nasal septum [158], and turbinates [8]. Common symptoms are nasal airway obstruction and recurrent epistaxis. Diagnosis is established by the history and typical endoscopic findings. Imaging studies such as CT, magnetic resonance imaging, or angiography are also necessary in many cases to define the extent of the nasal vascular anomalies [159, 160]. Purely intranasal vascular anomalies are much less common than lesions having both intranasal and extranasal components and have infiltrated the bony nasal skeleton (Fig. 3.9). These lesions are particularly challenging from a therapeutic standpoint.

In contrast to the wait-and-see approach widely advocated in the past, current preference is for early treatment of lesions showing definite progression. Early treatment seems particularly warranted in problem locations and in patients with functional complications. In many respects the laser is ideal for treating hemangiomas and vascular malformations owing to good absorption of the laser energy by hemoglobin, making it possible to photocoagulate vessels. Laser treatment is almost bloodless, causes few side effects, and yields very satisfactory functional and cosmetic results [159, 161]. The effect of the laser is not based on the thermal destruction of hemangioma cells. The laser acts, rather, by halting the progression of the lesions and accelerating their regression. Lasers can induce the involution of hemangiomas in the majority of cases [153].

Some laser systems work on the principle of selective photothermolysis (e.g., pulsed dye lasers, pulsed frequency-doubled Nd:YAG lasers, argon and KTP lasers), while others produce nonspecific coagulation (CW Nd:YAG and diode lasers). The latter have deep penetration and can coagulate tissues of almost any structure [155]. The laser is usually applied under endoscopic or microscopic control using a noncontact technique. The laser parameters are set to induce blanching of the angiomatous tissue. Interstitial Nd:YAG laser therapy is also effective for treating components that cannot be adequately treated by superficial lasing. This therapy requires advancing the laser fiber into the deeper tissues through a puncture needle [161, 162].

Lasers are excellent for treating easily accessible circumscribed hemangiomas or vascular malformations, such as turbinate lesions (Fig. 3.10). The diode, Nd:YAG, argon, and KTP lasers have yielded good results for this application. When the more deeply penetrating Nd:YAG and diode lasers are used, special care must be taken to protect adjacent structures such as the orbit and skull base from accidental injury. In the literature, conventional surgical treatment is advocated for hemangiomas in the paranasal sinuses [156, 157]. Possible extranasal angiomatous components are accessible to laser treatment, similar to cutaneous hemangiomas and vascular malformations at other sites (see also Chapter 7, Lasers in Dermatology) [161, 163].

In the great majority of cases, laser surgery is followed by intranasal swelling combined with fibrin exudation and crusting. A meticulous postoperative regimen with saline irrigation and nasal ointment is recommended to prevent synechia formation. Wound healing is complete in about 6–8 weeks. Laser therapy can produce areas of persistent hypo- and hyperpigmentation on the external nose as well as thermally induced scars [153]. These complications depend directly on the laser parameters used. To avoid cosmetically objectionable scars, intranasal adhesions, and cartilage damage, which can be particularly disfiguring in children, we follow the principle of "better too little than too much," undertaking if necessary a second stage of treatment after the nose has healed.

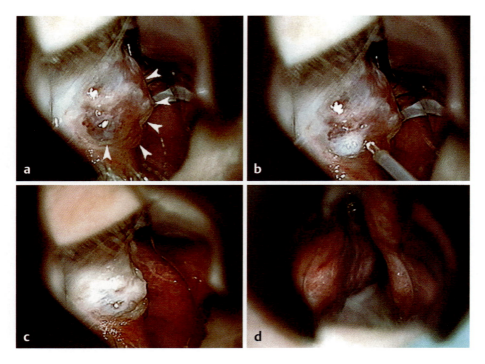

Fig. 3.10 Vascular malformation of the inferior turbinate (arrows) in a 56-year-old woman, causing marked nasal airway obstruction and recurrent epistaxis. **a** Initial appearance. **b** Blanched area immediately after Nd:YAG laser treatment. **c** Appearance at the end of the operation. **d** Healed site 3 months postoperatively. The patient has been free of complaints for 1 year.

The juvenile growth pattern of critical anatomic structures such as the cartilaginous nasal framework requires a skeptical attitude toward laser use on intranasal and extranasal vascular malformations. In the case of very fast-growing lesions, particularly capillary hemangiomas during the first months of life, a conventional surgical procedure, preceded if necessary by superselective embolization, should be preferred over laser therapy to avoid the risk of unpredictable tissue defects [159]. This particularly applies to vascular lesions of the nasal tip, where prolonged mass effect from a hemangioma can lead to disfigurement and conventional resection by an experienced surgeon can yield excellent cosmetic results [164, 165].

It should be added that some fast-growing capillary hemangiomas can be successfully treated with steroids (e. g., prednisone, 2–4 mg/kg per day) [166]. This does not mean, however, that cortisone is the treatment of choice for all hemangiomas. This type of therapy should be discontinued after 8–10 days at the latest if the lesion continues to enlarge [159]. Also, it is known that steroids are effective only during the proliferative phase [167]. Cortisone therapy or, in rare cases, interferon therapy may be tried in cases where hemangioma growth is unresponsive to laser application [152, 153].

Based on personal experience, we consider laser therapy to be the method of first choice for the treatment of intranasal and extranasal hemangiomas and vascular malformations. Laser systems that selectively absorb hemoglobin and can photocoagulate vessels are particularly effective. These devices can provide very satisfactory cosmetic and functional results in the majority of cases. It is difficult to define standard laser parameters for this application, and the outcome depends greatly on the experience of the operator. It should also be noted that vascular anomalies in this region occasionally require a very complex treatment protocol including embolization and conventional surgical resection.

Malignant Tumors

Primary curative treatment of malignant tumors of the nose and paranasal sinuses relies on conventional surgical excision, radiotherapy, or a combination of both. Laser use is not indicated. Lasers may be used with purely palliative intent, however, in patients with inoperable recurrent disease. In many cases lasers can improve the patient's quality of life by debulking tumors causing nasal obstruction and recurrent bleeding.

Publications on the use of laser techniques are limited to a few case reports. Jones [66] used the Ho:YAG and argon lasers to debulk inoperable residual or recurrent tumors of the skull base. Other authors have reported on the palliative intranasal use of CO_2, KTP, and Nd:YAG lasers for plasmacytoma, olfactory neuroma, sinus histiocytosis, adenocarcinoma, and squamous cell carcinoma [7, 16, 66, 118, 150, 168–171]. Interstitial Nd:YAG laser application has also been used successfully for the palliative treatment of inoperable recurrent carcinomas and adenoid cystic carcinomas of the paranasal sinuses [172, 173].

Synechiae

Intranasal synechiae are most commonly located between the middle or inferior turbinate and the nasal septum or between the middle turbinate and lateral nasal wall. Most of these synechiae develop as a sequel to intranasal surgery of the septum, turbinates, or paranasal sinuses, or as post-traumatic lesions. Synechiae can also form in the choanal region following a conventional adenotomy, tonsillectomy, or uvulopalatopharyngoplasty and other mucosal injuries [119]. Synechiae always develop from wound surfaces with associated fibrin coatings and crusting. As noted earlier, intranasal laser use is usually followed by significant fibrin exudation predisposing to synechia formation unless suitable postoperative care is provided [60, 110, 119].

Lasers are excellent instruments for dividing granulation tissue, scar adhesions, and membranous stenoses [120]. The CO_2, argon, Ho:YAG, KTP, diode, and Nd:YAG lasers have all been successfully used for this purpose [5, 7, 60, 65]. In many cases it is enough simply to divide the tissue. In some cases it is also advisable to vaporize the peripheral tissue to gain additional space. Stent insertion is generally unnecessary, but regular postoperative care with removal of fibrin deposits should be maintained to prevent recurrence. The topical application of cortisone ointment has proved beneficial [7].

■ Extranasal Laser Applications

Lasers have been increasingly used in recent years to treat diseases of the external nose. Most of these procedures fall under the heading of cosmetic surgery (laser skin resurfacing), but lasers have also become a mainstay in the treatment of hemangiomas and vascular malformations [161]. The various extranasal laser applications are discussed more fully in Chapter 7 (Lasers in Dermatology). Here, laser use in the treatment of rhinophyma is described. Laser-assisted PDT of basal cell carcinoma and other carcinomas is discussed in the section on PDT below.

Laser Treatment of Rhinophyma

The term "rhinophyma" was coined by von Hebra in 1845 [174]. Rhinophyma (alternative names: bulbous nose, drinker's nose) is the end stage of acne rosacea, appearing as a benign, slowly progressive disfigurement of the external nose. The development of rhinophyma is based on an inflammatory hyperplasia of the sebaceous glands combined with connective-tissue hyperplasia and scarring. In rare cases basal or squamous cell carcinoma may develop in the setting of rhinophyma [175]. The condition has been attributed to excessive alcohol consumption. Other possible etiologic factors are regular coffee consumption, eating very spicy foods, intestinal disorders, vitamin deficiency, androgenic regulatory dysfunction, angioneuropathy, poor hygiene, nonspecific exogenous irritants, and saprophytic parasitic growth of *Demodex folliculorum* [176].

Rhinophyma is always treated surgically [176]. Intervention is usually prompted by cosmetic concerns, but bulky rhinophyma can also cause nasal airway obstruction that is very troublesome for the patient. A variety of operative techniques have been described for removing the hyperplastic sebaceous glands, such as decortication with a scalpel or disposable razor blade, cryosurgery, electrosurgery, and dermabrasion [177]. The procedures differ in terms of providing partial or complete tissue ablation. Complete ablation techniques require the use of free autologous skin grafts to cover the surgical defect and are not recommended because of their unfavorable cosmetic results.

Various laser systems (Nd:YAG, argon, Er:YAG, CO_2 lasers) have increasingly been used in recent years for the treatment of rhinophyma. The main advantages of laser tissue ablation are bloodless surgery with good intraoperative visibility and the ability to carry out the surgery on an ambulatory basis under local anesthesia [176, 178, 179]. In laser ablations as in other procedures, the excised tissue should always be sent for histologic examination to ensure that the occasional subclinical basal or squamous cell carcinoma is not missed [175].

Most reports on laser treatment of rhinophyma deal with the use of the CO_2 laser [180–182]. Various techniques have been described in the literature. Ordinarily the hyperplastic skin is vaporized with a defocused target beam set at 10–15 W. The power setting should be reduced in proximity to cartilage structures to avoid thermal damage to the cartilaginous nasal framework. Smaller bleeding sites are controlled with bipolar electrocautery. Sedlmaier et al. [183] use the CO_2 laser with a scanner system (SilkTouch or FeatherTouch) for precise, controlled tissue ablation with virtually no collateral thermal effects. Additionally, a better hemostatic effect is obtained than with the traditional CO_2 laser beam, since the scanned beam produces intravascular thrombosis in small vessels before the vessels are opened [183]. Carbonaceous debris is carefully wiped away with saline solution at the end of the operation, and a dressing is applied over a petrolatum or antibiotic ointment. The ointment is continued until reepitheli-

alization is complete [182, 183]. This takes from 4 weeks to 8 weeks, depending on the size of the treated area [177, 180, 182, 183]. Acyclovir and an antibiotic should be given systemically during the first postoperative week to prevent viral and bacterial infections. Direct exposure to sunlight should be avoided for 3–5 months. Some authors recommend applying a cortisone-containing cream [184] to reduce possible postoperative scarring and prevent erythema.

The complication rate after rhinophyma ablation with the CO_2 laser is low. Rates of 10–16 % are stated in the literature comparable with those reported with conventional techniques [177, 180, 182, 185]. Typical complications after rhinophyma ablation are scarring leading to functional and cosmetic compromise (Fig. 3.**11**). The development of a nasocutaneous fistula has also been described due to injury to the cartilaginous skeleton [182].

The course of wound healing after Er:YAG laser use is comparable with that after nonlaser cutting surgery owing to the biophysical tissue effects of the laser [186]. On the other hand, the Er:YAG laser has only minimal coagulative properties, and so bleeding can occur during tissue ablation. Orenstein et al. [176] treated six patients with the Er:YAG laser under local anesthesia. The tissue is vaporized in layers. After each pass the ablation products are wiped away with a moist cloth containing saline and epinephrine. Generally this will provide adequate hemostasis, and most cases will not require electrocautery. In contrast to CO_2 laser treatment, reepithelialization is complete in only 1–2 weeks. Postoperative erythema persists for approximately 4 weeks.

Little experience has been reported on rhinophyma ablation with argon and Nd:YAG lasers. The main problem with these laser systems is the considerable thermal damage to adjacent tissues and to the cartilage. This results in prolonged wound healing, pain, and scarring with a poor cosmetic outcome [175, 187].

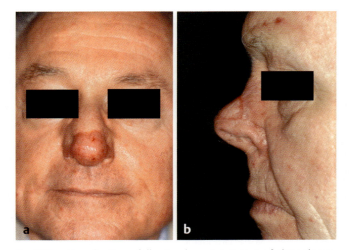

Fig. 3.**11**   Complications following laser treatment of rhinophyma. **a** Persistent erythema of the nasal tip 5 months after CO_2 laser treatment. **b** Poor cosmetic result caused by scarring due to excessive depth of CO_2 laser ablation.

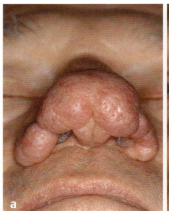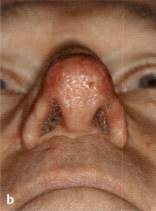

Fig. 3.**12**   Typical rhinophyma with predominantly right-sided nasal airway obstruction before (**a**) and after (**b**) CO_2 laser ablation.

We can summarize the experience to date by noting that both the CO_2 laser and the Er:YAG laser are effective in the treatment of rhinophyma (Fig. 3.**12**). The advantages of laser treatment are good intraoperative visibility due to reduced bleeding and the ability to ablate the rhinophyma tissue precisely and in layers, particularly when a scanner system is used. The postoperative results and complication rates are comparable to those of conventional techniques. Disadvantages of laser ablation are the need for more costly and complex equipment and delayed wound healing, which requires a longer period of postoperative care.

■ Photodynamic Therapy

The photodynamic effect is based on the selective uptake of light-sensitive substances called photosensitizers by tumors. The photosensitizer is exposed to light at a specific wavelength. The absorption of light excites the sensitizer to a higher energy state, and the associated energy transfer to molecular oxygen induces the formation of singlet oxygen. These radical products are capable of destroying cell membranes and other vital structures by photo-oxidation. Besides cellular damage, a breakdown of tumor vascularity occurs within minutes after light exposure. When both effects are combined, they are capable of destroying the tumor [188]. The key advantage of PDT over conventional therapeutic modalities is that it selectively destroys the tumor while sparing normal adjacent tissue. Additionally, the photosensitizer can be administered repeatedly without limitation, making it possible to repeat the therapy as often as desired.

Intranasal Photodynamic Therapy

The primary treatment for nasopharyngeal carcinomas is radiotherapy. But effective treatment options are no longer available to many patients presenting with residual or recurrent disease. PDT provides an additional option in these cases [189–191]. Kulapaditharom and Boonkitticharoen [189] treated 13 patients with recurrent cancer using PDT with hematoporphyrin derivatives. Six patients with a T1 or T2 tumor had 2-year disease-free survival. Tong et al. [190] also documented a good response rate of recurrent tumors to PDT (5 mg/kg bodyweight HpD, 200 J/cm^2). Lofgren et al. [192] carried out PDT in five patients with circumscribed recurrent nasopharyngeal tumor, administering a hematoporphyrin derivative and then activating the drug with laser light under topical anesthesia. Three patients had no evidence of disease at 4-year follow-up.

Another possible application of PDT is in the treatment of recurrent papillomatosis of the intranasal mucosa. Though benign, virus-induced papillomatosis can be a very troublesome condition and can even be life-threatening in rare cases. In the past, no primary curative therapy has been available and treatment has been limited to symptomatic removal by conventional surgery or, preferably, laser techniques. To date, PDT has been used mainly for the successful treatment of laryngeal and tracheal papillomas [6].

The following protocol has been developed at our center for PDT of recurrent papillomatosis using 5-ALA: the patient is given 20–40 mg/kg body weight of ALA orally about 2 hours before the operation. ALA itself is not photodynamically active, but it undergoes intracellular conversion to the photoactive dye protoporphyrin IX. In an initial diag-

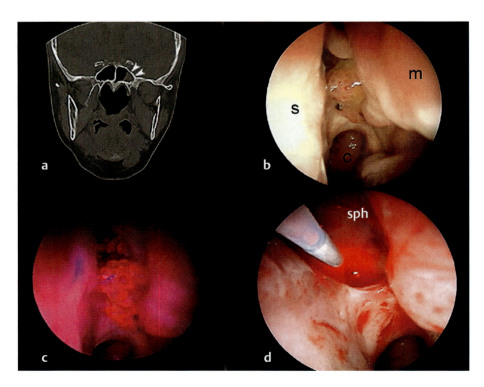

Fig. 3.**13** Photodynamic diagnosis and therapy of recurrent mucosal papillomatosis in the left sphenoid sinus. **a** Recurrent papilloma on the lateral wall of the sphenoid sinus (arrows) in a coronal computed tomography scan. **b** Initial appearance at white-light endoscopy. **c** Typical red fluorescence after 5-δ-aminolevulinic acid administration. **d** After the papillomas are removed, photodynamic therapy is undertaken by irradiating the area with 635-nm laser light (s, nasal septum; m, middle turbinate; c, choana; sph, sphenoid sinus).

nostic step, the increased uptake of protoporphyrin IX in the papilloma cells is used for fluorescent endoscopy of the nose and paranasal sinuses (Fig. 3.**13**). The mucosal areas affected by papillomatosis are clearly visualized by fluorescent endoscopy [193]. Since the 635-nm excitation beam has but a shallow penetration depth, the papillomas are initially removed by excision or ablation with a surgical laser. A biopsy sample is taken at this time for histologic confirmation. PDT is carried out after all papillomas have been grossly removed and the carbonaceous debris has been wiped away. The wound bed and adjacent mucosa are irradiated with laser light delivered through fibers with a low-divergent output, applying a total energy dose of 100 J/cm². To date, three patients have been successfully treated according to this protocol.

Extranasal Photodynamic Therapy

Resection of premalignant and malignant lesions of the external nose and adjacent facial skin is problematic from a functional and esthetic standpoint. Plastic reconstructive options are limited, especially in patients with recurrent disease after surgery or radiotherapy and patients with multifocal disease. Given this situation, PDT represents a valuable alternative treatment.

PDT with systemically administered hematoporphyrin derivatives has yielded good oncologic and cosmetic results in the treatment of localized, superficial basal cell carcinomas and spindle cell carcinomas. One disadvantage of this photosensitizer is that it photosensitizes the skin for a period of weeks, which can significantly affect the patient's quality of life [194].

Generalized photosensitization in PDT can be avoided by the topical administration of ALA [195]. A 10–20% ALA cream or gel is applied to the skin lesion and then covered with an occlusive dressing for 4–6 hours. Excitation of the tumor with blue light (370–440 nm) induces a typical red fluorescence that delineates the tumor boundaries. The tumor area is then lased at a wavelength of 600–800 nm, applying a total dose of 100–150 J/cm² [196]. Patients consistently report a sunburn-like pain during laser application [197]. No side effects besides erythema of the treated area have been described [198].

The successful PDT of premalignant and malignant lesions with topically administered ALA was first described in 1990 by Kennedy et al. [195]. Studies in recent years have reported cure rates of 79–100% for superficial basal cell carcinomas [195, 197, 199–203]. Much less favorable results have been reported for thicker lesions and nodular forms [199, 202, 203]. Actinic keratosis, which progresses to squamous cell carcinoma in up to 60% of cases, and Bowen's disease can also be successfully treated with local ALA PDT. The cure rates after one treatment range from 70% to 90% [202–206]. Actinic keratosis of the facial skin responds considerably better to PDT than similar lesions on the trunk or extremities [204].

Since the treatments practiced at different centers are by no means standardized, it is little wonder that response rates ranging from 50% to 100% have been reported in the literature [196]. Based on available data, however, it is reasonable to conclude that PDT with ALA is now an effective alternative in the treatment of actinic keratosis, superficial basal cell carcinoma, and Bowen's disease [206]. Essential advantages of PDT are its excellent cosmetic and functional results and lack of invasiveness. Due to the lack of histologic control, PDT is not currently recommended for the treatment of invasive squamous cell carcinoma [205].

■ Summary and Outlook

In the past few decades, laser surgery has evolved into an important therapeutic modality in otorhinolaryngology. At many institutions, CO_2 laser surgery has become the method of choice for resecting localized carcinomas of the upper aerodigestive tract. A number of laser systems have been successfully used in treating various diseases of the nose and paranasal sinuses, but laser therapy cannot yet be considered an established modality for many disorders. Especially in rhinologic applications, lasers offer several advantages over conventional techniques such as improved visualization due to better hemostasis, high-precision tissue ablation, minimal collateral tissue trauma resulting in less postoperative edema, and a reduction in postoperative pain. Intranasal packing, which is often difficult for patients to tolerate, can be omitted in many cases.

Given the rich vascularity of the nasal mucosa and the proximity of vulnerable structures such as the orbit and skull base, lasers used for intranasal surgery must meet certain requirements. Ideally, the laser should be equally effective in ablating bone and mucosa. It should provide good hemostasis, cause no collateral damage, and should be deliverable through a flexible carrier. The laser systems used in rhinology (argon, KTP, diode, Nd:YAG, Ho:YAG, Er:YAG, CO_2) meet the above criteria only to a degree, but very good therapeutic results can still be achieved when the biophysical effects of the various lasers are taken into account. We feel that laser therapy has an established place in the treatment of turbinate hyperplasia, recurrent epistaxis including Osler disease, hemangiomas and vascular malformations, choanal atresia, circumscribed benign lesions, and rhinophyma. Lasers are still questionable as a tool for nasal septal and sinus surgery and intranasal lacrimal duct surgery, but good results can be achieved by an experienced surgeon in carefully selected patients.

Further technical advances in laser systems may help to expand the range of indications for laser use in rhinology. This potential is illustrated by computer-assisted laser systems, which precisely define the area of tissue ablation while sparing adjacent structures. In addition, manufacturers are developing laser devices for clinical use that combine multiple wavelengths in one unit, resulting in cost savings and enabling the physician to select the optimum wavelength for a particular disease. Interest is also focusing on ways to develop better flexible carriers for the CO_2 laser. Although the CO_2 laser is the workhorse of otolaryngology, bulky carriers still limit its capacity for endonasal use.

■ Acknowledgements

The author expresses thanks to Mr. M. Schmidt for his help in processing the digital image data, Prof. Dr. J. A. Werner for critically reviewing the manuscript, and the Karl Storz company for its support in the printing of the color illustrations.

■ References

1 Lippert BM, Werner JA, Rudert H. Laser tissue effects with regard to otorhinolaryngology. Otolaryngol Pol 1994; 48: 505–513

2 Lenz H, Eichler J, Knof J, Salk J, Schäfer G. Endonasales Ar+-Laser-Strahlführungssystem und erste klinische Anwendungen bei der Rhinopathia vasomotorica. Laryngorhinootologie 1977; 56: 749–755

3 Oswal V, Hopf JUG, Hopf M, Scherer H. Endonasal laser applications. In: Oswal V, Remacle M (Hrsg). Principles and practice of lasers in otorhinolaryngology and head and neck surgery. The Hague, The Netherlands: Kugler Publications, 2002; 163–186

4 Metson R. Holmium:YAG laser endoscopic sinus surgery: a randomized controlled study. Laryngoscope 1996; 106: 1–18

5 Levine HL. Endoscopy and the KTP/532 laser for nasal sinus disease. Ann Otol Rhinol Laryngol 1989; 98: 46–51

6 Lippert BM, Werner JA. Photodynamische Therapie in der HNO-Heilkunde. In: Szeimies RM, Jocham D, Landthaler M (Hrsg). Klinische Fluoreszenzdiagnostik und Photodynamische Therapie. Berlin: Blackwell, 2002: 236–251

7 Hopf JUG, Hopf M, Koffroth-Becker C. Minimal invasive Chirurgie obstruktiver Erkrankungen der Nase mit dem Diodenlaser. Lasermedizin 1998/99; 14: 106–115

8 Werner JA, Rudert H. Der Einsatz des Nd-YAG-Lasers in der Hals-, Nasen-, Ohrenheilkunde. HNO 1992; 40: 248–258

9 Sroka R, Rosler P, Janda P, Grevers G, Leunig A. Endonasal laser surgery with a new laser fiber guidance instrument. Laryngoscope 2000; 110: 332–334

10 Lippert BM, Werner JA. Die Behandlung der hypertrophen unteren Nasenmuschel, Teil I. HNO 2000; 48: 170–181

11 Hol MK, Huizing EH. Treatment of inferior turbinate pathology: a review and critical evaluation of the different techniques. Rhinology 2000; 38: 157–166

12 Lippert BM, Werner JA. Die Behandlung der hypertrophen unteren Nasenmuschel, Teil II. HNO 2000; 48: 267–274

13 Janda P, Sroka R, Baumgartner R, Grevers G, Leunig A. Laser treatment of hyperplastic inferior nasal turbinates: a review. Lasers Surg Med 2001; 28: 404–413

14 Levine HL. The potassium-titanyl-phosphate laser for treatment of turbinate dysfunction. Otolaryngol Head Neck Surg 1991; 104: 247–251

15 Wexler DB, Berger G, Derowe A, Ophir D. Long-term histologic effects of inferior turbinate laser surgery. Otolaryngol Head Neck Surg 2001; 124: 459–463

16 Selkin SG. Pitfalls in intranasal laser surgery and how to avoid them. Arch Otolaryngol Head Neck Surg 1986; 112: 285–289

17 Emmerling O, di Martino E, Westhofen M. Ergebnisse der submukösen Lasercochotomie mit dem Nd:YAG-Laser. HNO 1999; 47: 338

18 Langerholm S, Harsten G, Emgard P, Olsson B. Laser-turbinectomy: long-term results. J Laryngol Otol 1999; 113: 529–531

19 Englender M. Nasal laser mucotomy (L-mucotomy) of the interior turbinates. J Laryngol Otol 1995; 109: 296–299

20 McCombe AW, Cook J, Jones AS. A comparison of laser cautery and submucosal diathermy for rhinitis. Clin Otolaryngol 1992; 17: 297–299

21 Lenz H, Preußler H. Histologische Veränderungen des respiratorischen Schleimhautepithels der unteren Nasenmuscheln nach Argon-Laserstrichkarbonisation (Laser-Muschel-Kaustik) bei Rhinopathia vasomotorica. Larynorhinootologie 1986; 65: 438–444

22 von Glass W, Hauerstein T. Wound healing in the nose and paranasal sinuses after irradiation with the argon laser. Arch Otorhinolaryngol 1988; 245: 36–41

23 Lenz H. Acht Jahre Laserchirurgie an den unteren Nasenmuscheln bei Rhinopathia vasomotorica in Form der Laserstrichkarbonisation. HNO 1985; 33: 422–425

24 Kunachak S, Kulapaditharom B, Prakunhungsit S. Minimally invasive KTP laser treatment of perennial allergic rhinitis: a preliminary report. J Otolaryngol 2000; 29: 139–143

25 Olthoff A, Martin A, Liebmann F. Nd:YAG-Laserbehandlung der unteren Nasenmuscheln im Kontaktverfahren bei der hyperreflektorischen und allergischen Rhinopathie. Laryngorhinootologie 1999; 78: 240–243

26 Lippert BM, Werner JA. Nd:YAG-laserlichtinduzierte Nasenmuschelreduktion. Laryngorhinootologie 1996; 75: 523–528

27 Johnson LP. Nasal and paranasal sinus applications of lasers. In: Davis RK (Hrsg). Lasers in Otolaryngology – Head and Neck Surgery, Philadelphia: Saunders, 1990: 145–155

28 Jovanovic S, Dokic D. Die Nd:YAG-Laserchirurgie in der Behandlung der allergischen Rhinitis. Laryngorhinootologie 1995; 74: 419–422

29 Ohyama M, Yamashita K, Furuta S, Nobori T, Daikuzono N. Applications of the Nd:YAG Laser in Otorhinolaryngology. In: Joffe SN, Oguro Y (Hrsg.). Advances in Nd:YAG Laser Surgery. Berlin, Heidelberg, New York: Springer, 1988: 156–165

30 Lippert BM. Experimentelle und klinische Untersuchungen zur biophysikalischen Wirkung und klinischen Anwendbarkeit verschiedener Lasersysteme im Kopf-Hals-Bereich. Aachen: Shaker, 1998

31 Lippert BM, Werner JA, Hoffmann P, Rudert H. CO_2- und Nd:YAG-Laser-Vergleich zweier Verfahren zur Nasenmuschelreduktion. Arch Otorhinolaryngol 1992; Suppl. II: 116–117

32 Vagnetti A, Gobbi E, Algieri GM, D'Ambrosio L. Wedge turbinectomy: a new combined photocoagulative Nd:YAG laser technique. Laryngoscope 2000; 110: 1034–1036

33 Tauber St, Janda P, Sroka R, Grevers G, Leunig A. Der Dioden- und Ho:YAG-Laser zur Mukotomie bei Nasenmuschelhyperplasie: eine klinische Bewertung, HNO 1999; 47: 338

34 Lippert BM, Werner JA. Long-term results after laser turbinectomy. Lasers Surg Med 1998; 22: 126–134

35 Min YG, Kim HS, Yun YS, Kim CS, Jang YJ, Jung TG. Contact laser turbinate surgery for the treatment of idiopathic rhinitis. Clin Otolaryngol 1996; 21: 533–536

36 Janda P, Sroka R, Betz CS, Grevers G, Leunig A. Die Laserkonchotomie mit Ho:YAG und Dioden-Laser zur Behandlung von hyperplastischen Nasenmuscheln. Laryngorhinootologie 2002; 81: 484–490

37 DeRowe A, Landsberg R, Leonov Y, Katzir A, Ophir D. Subjective comparison of Nd:YAG, diode, and CO_2 lasers for endoscopically guided inferior turbinate reduction surgery. Am J Rhino 1998; 12: 209–212

38 Shapshay SM, Rebeiz EE, Bohigian RK. Holmium:Yttrium Aluminium Garnet Laser-assisted endoscopic sinus surgery:clinical experience. Laryngoscope 1992; 102: 1177–1180

39 Serrano E, Percodani J, Yardeni E, Lombard L, Laffitte F, Pessey JJ. The holmium:YAG laser for treatment of inferior turbinate hypertrophy. Rhinology 1998; 38: 77–80

40 Leunig A, Janda P, Sroka R, Baumgartner R, Grevers G. Ho:YAG laser treatment of hyperplastic inferior nasal turbinates. Laryngoscope 1999; 109: 1690–1695

41 Oswal VH, Bingham BJG. A pilot study of the Holmium YAG laser in nasal turbinale and tonsil surgery. J Clin Laser Med Surg 1992; 3: 211–216

42 Elwany S, Harrison R. Inferior turbinectomy: comparison of four techniques. J Laryngol Otol 1990; 104: 206–209

43 Fukutake T, Yamashita T, Tomoda K, Kumazawa T. Laser surgery for allergic rhinitis. Arch Otolaryngol Head Neck Surg 1986; 112: 1280–1282

44 Papadakis CE, Skoulakis CE, Nikolidakis AA, Velegrakis GA, Bizakis JG, Helidonis ES. Swiftlase inferior turbinoplasty. Am J Rhinol 1999; 13: 479–482

45 Lippert BM, Werner JA. CO_2 laser surgery of hypertrophied inferior turbinates, Rhinology 1997; 35: 33–36

46 Jähne M, Wöllmer W, Ussmüller J. Erste Anwendungen des

Wave-Guide bei der CO_2-laserchirurgischen Verkleinerung der hyperplastischen Nasenmuscheln. Laryngorhinootologie 2002; 81: 289–292

47 Elwany S, Thabet H. Endoscopic carbon dioxide laser turbinoplasty. J Laryngol Otol 2001; 115: 190–193

48 Elwany S, Abel Salaam S. Laser surgery for allergic rhinitis: the effect on seromucinous glands. Otolaryngol Head Neck Surg 1999; 120: 742–744

49 Lippert BM, Werner JA. Comparison of carbon dioxide and neodymium:yttrium-aluminium-garnet lasers in surgery of the inferior turbinate. Ann Otol Rhinol Laryngol 1997; 106: 1036–1042

50 Takeno S, Osada R, Furukido K, Yajin K. Analysis of local cytokine gene expression in patients with allergic rhinitis treated with CO_2-laser surgery. Laryngoscope 2000; 110: 1968–1974

51 Testa B, Mesolella M, Squeglia C, Testa D, Motta G. Carbon dioxide laser turbinate surgery for chronic obstructive rhinitis. Lasers Surg Med 2000; 27: 49–54

52 Katz S, Schmelzer B, Vidts G. Treatment of the obstructive nose by CO_2-laser reduction of the inferior turbinates: technique and results. Am J Rhinol 2000; 14: 51–55

53 Tanigawa T, Yashiki T, Hayashi K, Sato T. Carbon dioxide laser vaporization for turbinate: optimal conditions and indications. Auris Nasus Larynx 2000; 27: 137–140

54 Rettinger G. Septal and turbinate surgery: What are the best methods. Laryngorhinootologie 2000; 79: S258

55 Krespi YP. Laser-assisted surgery of the nasal septum. Lasers Surg Med 1999; 11: 68

56 Kamami W. Laser-assisted outpatient septoplasty results on 120 patients. J Clin Laser Med Surg 1997; 15: 123–129

57 Kamami YV, Pandraud L, Bougara A. Laser-assisted outpatient septoplasty: results in 703 patients. Otolaryngol Head Neck Surg 2000; 122: 445–449

58 Scherer H, Reichert K, Schildhauer S. Die Laserchirurgie des mittleren Nasenganges bei der rezidivierenden Sinusitis. Laryngorhinootologie 1999; 78: 50–53

59 Krespi J, Kacker A. Laser-assisted septoplasty. In: Oswal V, Remacle M (Hrsg). Principles and pracice of lasers in otorhinolaryngology and head and neck surgery. The Hague, The Netherlands: Kugler Publications, 2002: 389–392

60 Lippert BM, Werner JA. CO_2-laser in rhinology. Med Laser Appl 2002; 17: im Druck

61 Lenz H, Eichler J, Schäfer G, Salk J, Bettges G. Production of an nasoantral window with an Ar laser. J Maxillofac Surg 1977; 5: 314–317

62 Ohyama M. Laser polypectomy. Rhinol Suppl 1989; 8: 35–43

63 Kautzky M, Bigenzahn W, Steurer M, Susani M, Schenk P. Holmium:YAG-Laserchirurgie. Anwendungsmöglichkeiten bei entzündlichen Nasennebenhöhlenerkrankungen. HNO 1992; 40: 468–471

64 Gleich LL, Rebeiz EE, Pankratov MM, Shapshay SM. The holmium:YAG laser-assisted otolaryngologic procedures. Arch Otolaryngol Head Neck Surg 1995; 121: 1162–1166

65 Feyh J. Endoscopic surgery of the nose and paranasal sinuses with the aid of the holmium:YAG laser. Adv Otorhinolaryngol 1995; 49: 122–124

66 Jones N. Lasers in rhinology. J Laryngol Otol 2000; 114: 824–826

67 Sato K, Nakashima T. Endoscopic sinus surgery for chronic sinusitis with antrochoanal polyp. Laryngoscope 2000; 110: 1581–1583

68 Stasche N, Hörmann K, Christ M, Schmidt H. Carbon dioxide laser delivery systems in functional paranasal surgery. Adv Otorhinolaryngol 1995; 49: 114–117

69 Zenner HP. Neue Technologien für die endonasale Nasennebenhöhlenchirurgie. HNO 1997; 45: 347–352

70 Vollrath M. Ambulante Entfernung von Nasenpolypen durch Laserverfahren? Dtsch Med Wochenschr 1997; 122: 347

71 Stammberger H. Unsere endoskopische Operationstechnik der lateralen Nasenwand – Ein endoskopisch-chirurgisches Konzept zur Behandlung entzündlicher Nasennebenhöhlenerkrankungen. Laryngorhinootologie 1985; 64: 559–566

72 Zhang B. Comparison of results of laser and routine surgery therapy in treatment of nasal polyps. Chin Med J 1993; 106: 707–708

73 Ilgner J, Emmerling O, Biesterfeld S, Westhofen M. Clinical experience with power-regulated contact laser surgery for the paranasal sinuses and the anterior skull base. Laryngorhinootologie 2002; 81: 346–350

74 Qadir R, Kennedy D. Use of the holmium:yttrium aluminium garnet (ho:YAG) laser for cranial nerve decompression: an in vivo study using the rabbit model. Laryngoscope 1993; 103: 631–636

75 Iro H, Waldfahrer F. Endonasale Tränenwegschirurgie aus HNO-ärztlicher Sicht. Ophthalmologe 2001; 98: 613–616

76 Meyer-Rüsenberg HW, Emmerich KH, Lüchtenberg M, Steinhauer J. Endoskopische Laserdakryoplastik. Ophthalmologe 1999; 96: 332–334

77 Toti A. Nuovo metodo conservatore de cura radicale delle suppurazioni croniche del sacco lacrimale (dacriocistorinostomia). Clin Moderna 1904; 10: 385–387

78 West J. Eine neue Methode zur Operation des Tränensackes von der Nase aus. Arch Laryngol Rhinol 1911; 24: 62–64

79 Michel O, Rüßmann W. Indikationen und Praxis der simultanen Ophthalmo-Rhino-Chirurgie. Eur Arch Otorhinolaryngol 1993; 1: 255–271

80 Massaro BM, Gonnering RS, Harris GJ. Endonasal laser dacryocystorhinstomy. A new approach to nasolacrimal duct obstruction. Arch Ophthalmol 1990; 108: 1172–1176

81 Eloy P, Trussart C, Jouzdani E, Collet S, Rombaux P, Bertrand B. Transcanalicular diode laser assisted dacryocystrhinostomy. Acta Otorhino Laryngol Belg 2000; 54: 157–163

82 Carversaccio M, Frenz M, Schar P, Hausler R. Endonasal and transcanalicular Er:YAG laser dacryocystorhinostomy. Rhinology 2001; 39: 28–32

83 Hartikainen MD, Grenman R, Puukka P, Seppä H. Prospective radomized comparison of external dacryocystorhinostomy and endonasal laser dacryocystorhinostomy. Ophthalmology 1998; 105: 1106–1113

84 Patel BCK, Phillips B, McLeish WM, Flaharty P, Anderson RL. Transcanalicular neodym:YAG laser for revision of dacryocystorhinostomy. Ophthalmology 1997; 104: 1101–1197

85 Müllner K, Wolf G. Endoskopische Behandlung von Tränenwegsstenosen mit Hilfe eines KTP-Lasers – Erster Erfahrungsbericht. Klin Monatsbl Augenheilkd 1999; 215: 28–32

86 Gonnering RS, Lyon DB, Fischer JC. Endoscopic laser-assisted lacrimal surgery. Am J Ophthalmol 1991; 111: 152–157

87 Christenbury JD. Translacrimal laser dacryocystorhinostomy. Arch Ophthalmol 1992; 110: 170–171

88 Reifler DM. Results of endoscopic KTP laser assisted dacryocystorhinostomy. Ophthal Plast Reconstr Surg 1993; 9: 231–236

89 Woog JJ, Metson R, Puliafito CA. Holmium:YAG endonasal laser dacryocystorhinostomy. Am J Ophthalmol 1993; 116: 1–10

90 Müllner K, Wolf G, Luxenberger W, Hofmann T. Laserassistierte transkanalikuläre Dakryozystorhinostomie. Ophthalmologe 2001; 98: 174–177

91 Moore EM, Bentley CR, Oliver JM. Functional and anatomic results after two types of endoscopic endonasal dacryocystorhinostomy: surgical and holmium laser. Ophthalmology 2002; 109: 1575–1582

92 Emmerich KH, Meyer-Rusenberg HW. Endoskopische Tränenwegschirurgie. Ophthalmologe 2001; 98: 607–612

93 Emmerich KH, Lüchtenberg M, Meyer-Rüsenberg HW, Steinhauer J. Dacryoendoskopie und Laserdacryoplastik: Technik und Ergebnisse. Klin Monatsbl Augenheilkd 1997; 211: 375–379

94 Steinhauer J, Norda A, Emmerich KH, Meyer-Rüsenberg HW. Lasercanaliculoplastik. Ophthalmologe 2000; 97: 692–695

95 Emmerich KH, Busse H, Meyer-Rüsenberg HW, Hörstenmeyer CG. External dacryocystorhinostomy: indications, method, complications and results. Orbit 1997; 16: 25–29

96 You YA, Fang CT. Intraoperative mitomycin C in dacryocystorhinostomy. Ophthal Plast Reconstr Surg 2001; 17: 115–119

97 Unlu HH, Toprak B, Aslan A, Guler C. Comparison of surgical outcomes in primary endoscopic dacryocystorhinostomy with and without silicone intubation. Ann Otol Rhinol Laryngol 2002; 111: 704–709

98 Boush GA, Lemke BN, Dortzbach RK. Results of endonasal laser

assisted dacryocystorhinostomy. Ophthalmology 1994; 105: 955–959

99 Otto AW. Lehrbuch der Pathologie, Anatomie des Menschen und der Tiere. Berlin: Rucker, 1830

100 Tzifa KT, Skinner DW. Endoscopic repair of unilateral choanal atresia with the KTP laser: a one stage procedure. J Laryngol Otol 2001; 115: 286–288

101 Jung H. Congenital choanal atresia and surgical correction. Laryngorhinootol 1994; 73: 586–590

102 Brown OE, Pownell P, Manning SC. Choanal atresia: a new anatomic classification and clinical management applications. Laryngoscope 1996; 106: 97–101

103 Pototschnig C, Volklein C, Appenroth E, Thumfart WF. Transnasal treatment of congenital choanal atresia with the KTP laser. Ann Otol Rhinol Laryngol 2001; 100: 335–339

104 Rudert H. Kombiniert transseptale-transnasale Chirurgie einseitiger Choanalatresien ohne Verwendung von Platzhaltern. Laryngorhinootologie 1999; 78: 697–702

105 Illum P. Congenital choanal atresia treated by laser surgery. Rhinology 1986; 24: 205–209

106 Emmert C. Lehrbuch der Chirurgie. Stuttgart: FVR Dann, 1853

107 Park AH, Brockenbrough J, Stankiewicz J. Endoscopic versus traditional approaches to choanal atresia. Otolaryngol Clin North Am 2000; 33: 77–90

108 Healy GM, McGill T, Strong MS, Jako GJ, Vaughan CR. Management of choanal atresia with carbon dioxide lasern. Ann Otol Rhinol Laryngol 1978; 87: 658

109 Masing H, Steiner W. Treatment of choanal atresia. Laryngorhinootologie 1984; 63: 181–183

110 Muntz HR. Pitfalls to laser correction of choanal atresia. Ann Otol Rhinol Laryngol 1987; 96: 43–46

111 Dedo HH. Transnasal mucosal flap rotation technique for repair of posterior choanal atresia. Otolaryngol Head Neck Surg 2001; 124: 674–682

112 Meer A, Tschopp K. Choanal atresia in premature dizygotic twins – a transnasal approach with Holmium:YAG-laser. Rhinology 2000; 38: 191–194

113 Furuta S, Itoh K, Shima T, Ohyama M. Laser beam in treating congenital atresia in three patients. Acta Otolaryngol (Stockh) 1994; 517: 33–35

114 Wiatrak BJ. Unilateral choanal atresia: initial presentation and endoscopic repair. Int J Ped ORL 1998; 48: 27–35

115 Fong M, Clarke K, Cron C. Clinical applications of the holmium:YAG laser in disorders of the paediatric airway. J Otolaryngol 1999; 28: 337–343

116 Holzmann D, Ruckstuhl M. Unilateral choanal atresia: surgical technique and long-term results. J Laryngol Otol 2002; 116: 601–604

117 Panwar SS, Martin FW. Transnasal endoscopic holmium:YAG laser correction of choanal atresia. J Laryngol Otol 1996; 110: 429–431

118 Hidaka H, Ikeda K, Oshima T, Ohtani H, Suzuki H, Takasaka T. A case of extramedullary plasmacytoma arising from the nasal septum. J Laryngol Otol 2000; 114: 53–55

119 Giannoni C, Sulek M, Friedman EM, Duncan, 3rd NO. Acquired nasopharyngeal stenosis: a warning and review. Arch Otolaryngol Head Neck Surg 1998; 124: 163–167

120 van Duyne J, Coleman, Jr JA. Treatment of nasopharyngeal inlet stenosis following uvulopalatopharyngoplasty with the CO_2-laser. Laryngoscope 1995; 105: 914–918

121 Dedo HH, Yu KC. CO_2-laser treatment in 244 patients with respiratory papillomas. Laryngoscope 2001; 111: 1639–1644

122 Gunkel AR, Sturm C, Simma B, Thumfart WF. Transoral CO_2-laser resection of extensive nasal and oropharyngeal teratoma. Lryngerhinootologie 1996; 75: 239–241

123 Scholtz AW, Appenroth E, Kammen-Jolly K, Scholtz JU, Thumfart WF. Juvenile nasopharyngeal angiofibroma: management and therapy. Laryngoscope 2001; 111: 681–687

124 Nakamura H, Kawasaki M, Higuchi Y, Seki S, Takahashi S. Transnasal endoscopic resection of juvenile nasopharyngeal angiofibroma with the KTP laser. Eur Arch Otorhinolaryngol 1999; 256: 212–214

125 Yamashita K, Ogawa A. The use of Nd:YAG laser in the management of nasopharyngeal pathology. J Jpn Laser Med 1984; 4: 229–230

126 Godbersen GS. Indications, risks and results of laser therapy for recurrent epistaxis. Adv Otorhinolaryngol 1995; 49: 109–113

127 Lenz H, Eichler J. Wirkung des Argon-Lasers auf die Gefäße, Mikro- und Makrozirkulation der Schleimhaut der Hamsterbackentasche. Eine intravitalmikroskopische Studie. Laryngorhinootologie 1975; 54: 612–619

128 Werner JA, Geisthoff UW, Lippert BW, Rudert H. Behandlung der rezidivierenden Epistaxis bei Morbus Rendu-Osler-Weber. HNO 1997; 45: 673–681

129 Jaques SL. Laser-tissue interactions. Photochemical, photothermal and photomechnical. Surg Clin North Am 1992; 72: 531–558

130 Hanes FM. Multiple hereditary telangiectases cause hemorrhage (hereditary hemorrhagic telangiectasia). Johns Hopkins Hosp Bull 1909; 20: 63–73

131 Porteous MEM, Burn J, Proctor SJ. Hereditary haemorrhagic telangiectasia: a clinical analysis. J Med Genet 1992; 29: 527–530

132 Johnson DW, Berg JN, Baldwin MA. Mutations in the activin receptor-like kinase 1 gene in hereditary haemorrhagic telangiectasia type 2. Nature Gen 1996; 13: 189–195

133 Plauchu H, de Chadarevian JP, Bedeau A, Robert JM. Age-related clinical profile of herditary hemorrhagic telangiectasia in an epidemiologically recruited population. Am J Med Genet 1989; 32: 291–297

134 Braverman IM, Keh A, Jacobson BS. Ultrastructure and three-dimensional organization of the telangiectases of hereditary hemorrhagic telangiectasia. J Invest Dermat 1990; 95: 422–427

135 Folz BJ, Dünne AA, Wollstein AC, Werner JA. Umfassendes Screening auf okkulte, arterio-venöse Malformationen bei M. Osler-Patienten mit Epistaxis als Indexsymptom. HNO Informationen 2002; 2: 112

136 Siegel MB; Keane WM, Atkins JP, Rosen MR. Control of epistaxis in patients with hereditary hemorrhagic telangiectasia. Otolaryngol Head Neck Surg 1991; 105: 675–679

137 Dobrovic M, Hosch H. Non-contact applications of Nd:YAG laser in nasal surgery. Rhinology 1994; 32: 71–73

138 Kluger PB, Shapshay SM, Hybels RL, Bohigian RK. Neodymium-YAG laser intranasal photocoagulation in hereditary hemorrhagic telangiectasia: an update report. Laryngoscope 1987; 97: 1397–1401

139 Werner JA, Lippert BM, Geisthoff UW, Rudert H. Nd:YAG-Lasertherapie der rezidivierenden Epistaxis bei hereditärer hämorrhagischer Teleaniektasie. Laryngorhinootologie 1997; 76: 495–501

140 Ben-Bassat M, Kaplan I, Levy R. Treatment of hereditary hemorrhagic telangiectasia of the nasal mucosa with the carbon dioxide laser. Br J Plast Surg 1978; 31: 157–158

141 Simpson GT, Shapshay SM, Vaughn CW, Strong MS. Rhinologic surgery with the carbon dioxide laser. Laryngoscope 1982; 92: 412–415

142 Haye R, Austad J. Hereditary haemorrhagic teleangiectasia – argon laser. Rhinology 1991; 29: 5–9

143 Parkin JL, Dixon JA. Argon laser treatment of head and neck vascular lesions. Otolaryngol Head Neck Surg 1985; 93: 211–216

144 Haye R, Austad J. Hereditary haemorrhagic teleangiectasia: ususcessful treatment with the flashlamp-pulsed dye laser. Rhinology 1992; 30: 135–137

145 Harries PG, Brockbank MJ, Shakespeare PG, Carruth JAS. Treatment of hereditary haemorrhagic telangiectasia by the pulsed dye laser. J Laryngol Otol 1997; 111: 1038–1041

146 Hopf JUG, Hopf M, Rohde E, Roggan A, Eichwald H, Scherer H. Die Behandlung der rezidivierenden Epistaxis mit den Diodenlaser. Lasermedizin 2000; 15: 96–106

147 Lennox, Harries M, Lund VJ, Howard DJ. A retrospective study of the role of the argon laser in the management of epistaxis secondary to hereditary haemorrhagic telangiectasia. J Laryngol Otol 1997; 111: 34–37

148 Shapshay SM, Oliver P. Treatment of hereditary hemorrhagic telangiectasia by Nd:YAG laser photocoagulation. Laryngoscope 1984; 94: 1554–1556

149 Illum P, Bjerring P. Hereditary hemorrhagic teleangiectasia treated by laser surgery. Rhinology 1988; 26: 19–24

150 Crockett DM, Healy GB, McGill TJ; Friedman EM. Benign lesions of the nose, oral cavity and oropharynx in children: excision by carbon dioxide laser. Ann Otol Rhonl Lryngol 1985; 94: 489–493

151 Keles N, Deger K. Endonasal endoscopic surgical treatment of paranasal sinus inverted papilloma – first experiences. Rhinology 2001; 39: 156–159

152 Greinwald JH, Burke DK, Bonthius KJ, Baumann NM, Smith RJH. An update on the treatment of hemangiomas in children with interferon alfa-2a. Arch Otolaryngol Head Neck Surg 1999; 125: 21–27

153 Grantzow R. Probleme in der Nd-YAG-Laserbehandlung großer Hämangiome. In: Landthaler M, Hohenleutner U, Voigt T (Hrsg). Benigne Gefäß- und Neubildungen. Berlin: Blackwell, 2002: 99–103

154 Mulliken JB, Glowacki J. Hemangiomas and vascular malformations of infants and children: A classification based on endothelial characteristics. Plast Reconstr Surg 1982; 69: 412–422

155 Hohenleutner U. Möglichkeiten und Grenzen der Lasertherapie. In: Landthaler M, Hohenleutner U, Voigt T (Hrsg). Benigne Gefäß- und Neubildungen. Berlin: Blackwell, 2002: 91–98

156 Kim Y, Stearns G, Davidson TM. Hemangioma of the ethmoid sinus. Otolaryngol Head Neck Surg 2000; 123: 517–519

157 Raboso E, Rosell A, Plaza G, Martinez-Vidal A. Haemangioma of the maxillary sinus. J Laryngol Otol 1997; 111: 638–640

158 Strek P, Modrzejewski M, Kitlinski Z. Lobular capillary hemangioma of the nasal septum. Otolaryngol Pol 1997; 51: 555–557

159 Werner JA, Dünne AA, Folz BJ, Rochels R, Ramaswamy A, Lippert BM. Current concepts in the classification, diagnosis and treatment of hemangiomas and vascular malformations of the head and neck. Eur Arch Otorhinolaryngol 2001; 258: 141–149

160 Werner JA, Bien S, Dünne AA, Rochels R, Seyberth H, Folz BJ, Lippert BM. Fortgeschrittene extrakranielle Hämangiome und vaskuläre Malformationen. Dt Ärzteblatt 2002; 99: 188–193

161 Werner JA, Lippert BM, Gottschlich S, Folz BJ, Fleiner B, Hoeft S, Rudert H. Ultrasound-guided interstitial Nd:YAG laser treatment of voluminous hemangiomas and vascular malformations in 92 patients. Laryngoscope 1998; 108: 463–470

162 Werner JA, Lippert BM, Hoffmann P, Rudert H. Nd:YAG laser therapy of voluminous hemangiomas and vascular malformations. Adv Otorhinolaryngol 1995; 49: 75–80

163 Werner JA, Lippert BM, Godbersen GS, Rudert H. Die Hämangiombehandlung mit dem Neodym:Yttrium-Aluminium-Granat Laser (Nd:YAG-Laser). Laryngorhinootologie 1992; 71: 388–395

164 Denk MJ, Ajkay N, Yuan X, Rosenblum RS, Freda N, Magee, Jr WP. Surgical treatment of nasal hemangiomas. Ann Plast Surg 2002; 48: 489–494, discussion: 494–495

165 McCarthy JG, Borud LJ, Schreiber JS. Hemangiomas of the nasal tip. Plast Reconstr Surg 2002; 109: 31–40

166 Uysal KM, Olgun N, Erbay A, Sarialioglu F. High-dose oral methyl-prednisolone therapy in childhood hemangiomas. Pediatr Hematol Oncol 2001; 18: 335–341

167 Waner M, Suen JY. A classification of congenital vascular malformations of the head and neck. New York: Wiley-Liss, 1999: 1–12

168 Somma AM, Dioguardi D. CO₂-laser surgery in recurrent tumors of the nose. Ann Plast Surg 1982; 9: 172–174

169 Hopf JUG, Hopf M. Funktionell-endoskopische endonasale Laserchirurgie. Tuttlingen: Endo-Press, 2001

170 Levine HL. Lasers in endonasal surgery. Otolaryngol Clin North Am 1997; 30: 451–455

171 Rontal M, Rontal E. Treatment of recurrent carcinoma at the base of the skull with carbon dioxide Laser. Laryngoscope 1983; 93: 1261–1265

172 Feyh J, Gutmann R, Leunig A, Jäger L, Reiser M, Saxton RE, Castro DJ, Kastenbauer E. MRI-guided laser interstitial thermal therapy (LITT) of head and neck tumors: progress with a new method. J Clin Laser Med Surg 1996; 14: 361–366

173 Paiva MB, Blackwell KE, Saxton RE, Calcaterra TC, Ward PH, Soudant J, Castro DJ. Palliative Laser Therapy for recurrent head and neck cancer: a phase II clinical study. Laryngoscope 1998; 108: 1277–1283

174 von Hebra F. Versuch einer auf pathologische Anatomie gegründete Einteilung der Hautkrankheiten. Z der KK Ges d Ärzte 1845; 2: 145

175 Acker DW, Helwig EB. Rhinophyma with carcinoma. Arch Dermatol 1967; 95: 250–254

176 Orenstein A, Haik J, Tamir J, Winkler E, Frand J, Zilinsky I, Kaplan H. Treatment of rhinophyma with Er:YAG laser. Lasers Surg Med 2001; 29: 230–235

177 Har-El G, Shapshay SM, Bohigian RK, Krespi YP, Lucente FE. The treatment of rhinophyma. „Cold" vs laser techniques. Arch Otolaryngol Head Neck Surg 1993; 119: 628–631

178 Wenig BL, Weingarten RT. Excision of rhinophyma with Nd:YAG laser: A new technique. Laryngoscope 1993; 103: 101–103

179 Ali MK, Calleri RH, Mobly DL. Resection of rhinophym with CO₂-laser. Laryngoscope 1987; 7: 1316–1318

180 el-Azhary RA, Roenigk RK, Wang TD. Spectrum of results after treatment of rhinophyma with the carbon dioxide laser. Mayo Clin Proc 1991; 66: 899–905

181 Shapshay SM, Strong MS, Anastasi GW, Vaughan CW. Removal of rhinophyma with the carbon dioxide laser: a preliminary report. Arch Otolaryngol 1980; 106: 257–259

182 Karim Ali M, Streitmann MJ. Excision of rhinophyma with the carbon dioxide laser: a ten-year experience. Ann Otol Rhinol Laryngol 1997; 106: 952–955

183 Sedlmaier B, Fuhrer A, Jovanovic S. New treatment possibilities for skin changes with the CO₂-laser in head and neck surgery. HNO 1997; 45: 625–629

184 Abergel Rp, Dahlman CM. The CO₂-laser approach to the treatment of acne scarring. Cosmetic Dermatol 1995; 8: 33–35

185 Gjuric M, Rettinger G. Comparison of carbon dioxide laser and electro-surgery in the treatment of rhinophyma. Rhinology 1993; 31: 37–39

186 Kaufmann R, Hartmann A, Hibst R. Cutting and skin-ablative properties of pulsed mid-infrared laser surgery. J Dermatol Surg Oncol 1994; 20: 112–118

187 Stucker FJ, Hoasjoe DK, Aarstad RF. Rhinophyma: a new approach to hemostasis. Ann Otol Rhinol Laryngol 1993; 102: 925–929

188 Ell C, Baumgartner R, Gossner L, Häußinger K, Iro H, Jocham D, Szeimies R-M. Photodynamische Therapie. Dt Ärzteblatt 2000; 97: 3337–3343

189 Kulapaditharom B, Boonkitticharoen V. Photodynamic therapy for recurrent nasopharyngeal cancer. J Med Assoc Thai 1999; 82: 1111–1117

190 Tong MC, van Hasselt CA, Woo JK. Preliminary results of photodynamic therapy for recurrent nasolpharyngeal carcinoma. Eur Arch Otorhinolaryngol 1996; 253: 189–192

191 Biel MA. Photodynamic therapy and the treatment of head and neck neoplasia. Laryngoscope 1998; 108: 1259–1268

192 Lofgren LA, Hallgren S, Nilsson E, Westernborn A, Nilsson C, Reizenstein J. Photodynamic therpy for recurrent nasopharyngeal cancer. Arch Otolaryngol Head Neck Surg 1995; 121: 997–1002

193 Lippert BM, Klahr N, Külkens C, Folz BJ, Werner JA. 5-Delta-Aminolävulinsäure induzierte Fluoreszenzdiagnostik bei Karzinomen der oberen Luft- und Speisewege – erste Ergebnisse. In: Lippert BM, Schmidt S, Werner JA (Hrsg). Fluoreszenzdiagnostik und photodynamische Therapie. Aachen: Shaker, 2000: 65–73

194 Feyh J. Photodynamic treatment for cancers of the head and neck. J Photochem Photobiol B 1996; 36: 175–177

195 Kennedy JC, Pottier RH, Pross DC. Photodynamic therapy with endogenous protoporphyrin IX: basic principles and present clinical experience. J Photochem Photobiol B 1990; 6: 143–148

196 Radakovic-Fijan S, Hönigsmann H, Tanew A. Photodynamische Therapie bei Präkanzerosen der Haut (aktinische Keratosen, M. Bowen). In: Szeimies RM, Jocham D, Landthaler M (Hrsg). Klinische Fluoreszenzdiagnostik und Photodynamische Therapie. Berlin: Blackwell, 2002: 191–205

197 Szeimies RM, Abels C, Bäumler W, Karrer S, Landthaler M. Photodynamische Therapie in der Dermatologie. In: Krutmann J, Hönigsmann H (Hrsg). Handbuch der klinischen Photodermatologie. Berlin, Heidelberg: Springer, 1997: 196–233

198 Casas A, Fukuda H, di Venosa G, Batle AM. The influence of the vehicle on the synthesis of porphyrins after topical application of 5-amino-laevulinic acid. Implications in cutaneous photodynamic sensitisation. Br J Dermatol 2000; 143: 564–572

199 Wolf P, Rieger E, Kerl H. Topical photodynamic therapy with endogenous porphyrins after application of 5-aminolevulinic acid. An alternative treatment modality for solar keratoses, superficial squamous cell carcinomas, and basal cell carcinomas? J Am Acad Dermatol 1993; 28: 17–21

200 Heinritz H, Benzel W, Sroka R, Iro H. Photodynamic therapy of superficial skin tumors following local application of delta-aminolaevulinic acid. Adv Otorhinolaryngol 1995; 49: 48–52

201 Lang S, Baumgartner R, Struck R, Leunig A, Gutmann R, Feyh J. Photodynamische Diagnostik und Therapie von Neoplasien der Gesichtshaut nach topischer Applikation von 5-Aminolävulinsäure. Laryngorhinootologie 1995; 74: 85–89

202 Svanberg K, Andersson T, Killander D, Wang I, Stenram U, Andersson-Engels S, Berg R, Johansson J, Svanberg S. Photodynamic therapy of non-melanoma malignant tumors of the skin using topical delta-aminolevulinic acid sensitisation and laser irradiation. Br J Dermatol 1994; 130: 743–751

203 Calzavara-Pinton PG. Repetitive photodynamic therapy with topical delta-aminlaevulinic acid as an appropriate approach to the routine treatment of superficial non-melanoma skin tumours. J Photochem Photobiol B 1995; 29: 53–57

204 Jeffes EW, McCullough JL, Weinstein GD. Photodynamic therapy of actinic keratosis with topical 5-aminolevulinic acid. A pilot doseranging study. Arch Dermatol 1997; 133: 727–732

205 Karrer S, Szeimies RM, Hohenleutner U, Landthaler M. Role of lasers and photodynamic therapy in the treatment of cutaneous malignancy. Am J Clin Dermatol 2001; 2: 229–237

206 Kalka K, Merk H, Mukhtar H. Photodynamic therapy in dermatology. J Am Acad Dermatol 2000; 42: 389–416

4 Laser Use in the Oral Cavity and Oropharynx

W. Bergler

■ Contents

■ Abstract

Good accessibility of the oral cavity and oropharynx has favored the development of numerous laser applications in this region. The CO_2, KTP, and Nd:YAG lasers are most commonly used for cutting mucosa and devitalizing tissue. The most important laser applications in these regions are in tonsillar surgery and soft-palate surgery for sleep-disordered breathing. Besides tonsillectomy, various authors have also described laser tonsillotomies with the goal of preventing intraoperative and postoperative bleeding and reducing postoperative pain. While these positive effects have been documented in several studies, they have not yet been widely confirmed. Laser tonsillectomy is more costly and requires an elaborate safety protocol. Different problems arise in association with laser use on the soft palate, as in laser-assisted uvulopalatoplasty (LAUP). LAUP is a very promising technique owing to the simplicity of the procedure. Unfortunately, published data indicate that LAUP should be used only in the treatment of primary snoring and is not appropriate for sleep apnea. Even with careful patient selection, the potentially severe complications should not be overlooked. Many other possible laser applications have been published including the excision of small tumors, the treatment of leukoplakia, frenectomies, and the fragmentation of salivary stones. Laser application for these indications is just one possible treatment modality offering only marginal advantages over conventional techniques when the added costs are taken into account. Laser use for these indications is basically a matter of individual preference and availability.

■ Characteristics of Lasers Used in the Oral Cavity and Oropharynx

Importance of Laser Surgery in the Oral Cavity and Oropharynx

The carbon dioxide (CO_2), neodymium:yttrium aluminum garnet (Nd:YAG), potassium-titanyl-phosphate (KTP), and argon lasers are most commonly used for soft-tissue surgery in the oral cavity and oropharynx. The lasers are used for cutting and ablation of tissue and the coagulation of tissue surfaces. Depending on the specific indication and the type of laser used, lasers can offer advantages over traditional surgical methods[1, 2]:

- spontaneous occlusion of small transected vessels, providing hemostasis and an almost bloodless field;
- no-touch operating technique;
- precise incisions under microscopic control with little collateral tissue damage;
- no need for sutures. All therapeutic options remain open, such as repeating the laser therapy or resection of an extensive tumor in case of a recurrence.

It is also important, however, to factor in the high costs incurred by laser use (e.g., a dedicated laser operating suite) and the necessary safety measures.

Some cases may not be amenable to a classic en-bloc resection, depending on the extent of the tumor in the oral cavity and oropharynx, and it may be necessary to remove the tumor piecemeal if visualization is poor. The histologic workup can be difficult in some cases and requires close teamwork between the surgeon and pathologist.

Some of the most frequent indications for laser use in the oral cavity and oropharynx are listed below:

- Tongue base reduction
- Tonsillar surgery
- Soft-palate surgery
- Treatment of hemangiomas
- Excision of benign tumors
- Treatment of premalignant lesions
- Excision of malignant tumors
- Frenectomies (of the lip, tongue, or cheek)
- Salivary gland diseases

Properties and Indications of Lasers Used in the Oral Cavity and Oropharynx

CO_2 Laser

The CO_2 laser was first developed by Patel et al. in 1964 [3] and introduced for medical use in the early 1970s [4–6]. The CO_2 laser is a type of gas laser. It emits light at a wavelength of 10.6 µm (10,600 nm) in the invisible, infrared region of the spectrum. This requires the use of a coaxial helium-neon (HeNE) laser aiming beam, whose 0.633-nm wavelength is in the visible (red) region of the spectrum.

Because of its wavelength, the CO_2 laser has strong affinity for water. This accounts for the good absorption of CO_2 laser energy by the oral mucosa, which consists of more than 90 % water. The CO_2 laser has excellent cutting and ablating properties, especially in soft tissue. Its maximum penetration depth in tissue is less than 1 mm. The CO_2 laser beam itself is not reflected or scattered in the mucosa [7]. Absorption of the laser energy by water causes rapid generation of heat, which carbonizes the tissue. The laser can be operated in pulsed mode (superpulse or ultrapulse) or in continuous mode (continuous-wave [CW]). The CW mode is preferred for oral soft-tissue surgery. The CO_2 laser energy is applied to the target tissue using a noncontact technique. One disadvantage compared with the Nd:YAG laser is that the CO_2 laser requires a rigid delivery system.

When applied in the oral cavity and oropharynx, the CO_2 laser is used mainly as a cutting instrument to remove benign and malignant lesions [8–12]. It is also used for intraoral incisional and excisional biopsies and frenectomies.

Nd:YAG Laser

The Nd:YAG laser emits a beam in the invisible, infrared part of the spectrum (similar to the CO_2 laser) at a wavelength of 1064 nm. A coaxial HeNe laser is used to produce a visible aiming beam. YAG, which stands for "yttrium-aluminum-garnet," is the host crystal for the neodymium ion and is distinguished by its relatively high thermal conductivity and good optical quality. The advantage of the

Nd:YAG laser over the CO_2 laser is that the laser energy can be delivered into the oral cavity through a flexible carrier [13] and can be applied through quartz fibers in flexible endoscopes. The Nd:YAG laser can be used interstitially, out of contact, or in contact with the target tissue.

The light emitted by the Nd:YAG laser is weakly absorbed by water, but it has strong affinity for dark and pigmented tissues such as hemoglobin and melanin [14]. Because Nd:YAG laser light is transmitted through water, it penetrates more deeply into tissue than the CO_2 laser beam. It undergoes minimal reflection. Owing to its properties, the Nd:YAG laser is best for treating more deeply situated areas in the oral cavity and oropharynx. Because the Nd:YAG laser energy is strongly absorbed by hemoglobin, it is very effective for coagulation [1]. The laser can be operated in a pulsed or continuous mode.

Argon Laser

The argon laser is a type of ion laser that uses a noble gas as the lasing medium. It emits primarily at 488 nm in the blue part of the visible spectrum and at 514 nm in the green part of the spectrum. As with the Nd:YAG laser, the light can be delivered into the oral cavity through a fiberoptic carrier.

Argon lasers have strong affinity for dark-colored tissue and hemoglobin, such as melanin, hemangiomas, Kaposi sarcoma, and nevi, making them particularly useful for coagulation [15]. The argon laser beam is not reflected from the oral tissues. It undergoes relatively little absorption, transmission, or scattering. Like the Nd:YAG laser, the argon laser can be used in or out of contact with the target tissue.

Unlike the CO_2 and Nd:YAG lasers, the argon laser (blue wavelength) can also polymerize composite resins [16, 17]. This property is used mainly in periodontal therapy, where the laser is used for the photopolymerization and curing of resin materials up to 3 cm thick [18, 19]. The green wavelength is used primarily for intraoral soft-tissue work and hemostasis, particularly in the treatment of vascular and pigmented lesions in the oropharynx and oral cavity. Angiitis can develop as a late reaction in exposed vessels, leading to vascular occlusion. Superficial coagulation with subsequent scarring has not been observed with this laser system.

Erbium:YAG Laser

Like the Nd:YAG laser, the erbium:YAG laser belongs to the category of pulsed solid-state lasers. It emits a beam in the infrared part of the spectrum at a wavelength of 2.94 μm. Because it is strongly absorbed by water, the erbium:YAG laser is useful for cutting and ablation but is not a very effective coagulator [1]. Because of these properties, the erbium:YAG laser is used mainly in dentistry for cutting bone and dental hard tissue [20]. It is not widely used in oral soft-tissue surgery.

Excimer laser

The excimer laser, just as the erbium:YAG laser, has mainly dental applications in the oral cavity and oropharynx. The active medium of the excimer laser is a noble gas combined with a halogen gas, such as xenon–fluoride or argon–fluoride. The composition of the gas determines the wavelength of the laser and is generally in the ultraviolet range [1]. As with the erbium:YAG laser, dental hard tissue can be removed by photoablation. The rate of ablation depends on the mineral content and morphologic structural elements of the dental hard tissue. Tissue affected by caries is ablated at a considerably faster rate than intact dental enamel or dentin [21].

A major drawback of the excimer laser is that its light cannot be transmitted through a flexible carrier. Besides high equipment costs, the energy density at the target can be controlled only by adjusting the focal–object distance, and the beam must be passed through an aperture to screen off areas at the beam periphery [22].

■ Clinical Uses of Lasers in the Oral Cavity and Oropharynx

The following sections deal only with the most frequent clinical indications and applications of lasers in the oral cavity and oropharynx.

Hyperplasia of the Lingual Tonsil

Hyperplastic changes in the region of the base of the tongue may result from chronic recurrent inflammation of the lingual tonsils. However, the differential diagnosis should also include ectopic thyroid tissue and malignant lesions such as lymphoma and squamous cell carcinoma. Hyperplastic changes can lead to swallowing difficulties, globus sensation, or fetid breath odor, and chronic infection can lead to febrile episodes of unknown cause with odynophagia. Laser ablation of the hyperplastic tissue is often recommended in such cases, sometimes after an ineffectual trial of conservative therapy [2].

Owing to its physical properties and hemostatic effect, the CO_2 laser is particularly useful for the reduction of hyperplastic lingual tonsils. The CO_2 laser markedly reduces the risk of collateral deep tissue injury compared with the Nd:YAG laser [23]. As studies by Steiner et al. have shown, laser resection that is confined strictly to lymphatic tissue and does not injure the muscles of the base of the tongue causes less intraoperative bleeding [24]. Laser surgery is associated with significantly less postoperative pain (including neuralgiform pain radiating to the ears) and postoperative edema than more extensive resections, which may be followed by considerably more complications.

Vascular Malformations

See also Chapter 7 (Lasers in Dermatology).

Hemangiomas involving the lips and oral cavity occur predominantly in infants and small children. Approximately 50% of these lesions regress spontaneously, and therefore a wait-and-see approach should be taken initially. If the hemangioma is large and shows a tendency to enlarge, active therapeutic intervention is often required.

Extensive hemangiomas in the oral cavity are frequently related to the mandible, floor of the oral cavity, tongue, and the base of the tongue because of their "cluster-of-grapes" morphology. Their blood supply is derived from multiple branches of the external carotid artery [25]. Interstitial laser therapy with the Nd:YAG laser is of special importance in these cases. It is critical that the target tissue be adequately cooled, however, because the Nd:YAG laser beam can cause uncontrolled thermal damage to the skin and mucosa [26]. Laser probes are inserted into the tumor under sonographic guidance. The hemangiomatous tissue is vaporized by the selective application of a defined wattage. Bulky hemangiomas and vascular malformations are treated with power densities ranging from 500 W/cm^2 (equivalent to 2.5 W of laser power) to 3000 W/cm^2 (equivalent to 15 W of laser power). The size of the hemangioma is progressively reduced in several sittings.

Other Benign Tumors

Benign tumors, which are more common in the oral cavity than the oropharynx, can be easily visualized, enabling the laser to be used in the noncontact mode in an ambulatory setting [23]. The most common benign lesions include papillomas, fibromas, cysts, and ranulas [27]. A lesion can be removed from the oral cavity and oropharynx with two main techniques: excision and vaporization. Of the two, excision is preferred as it permits histologic examination of the specimen and the assessment of adequate margins. Vaporization is effective when the histology of the lesion has already been confirmed. Biological studies have shown that the wound surfaces produced by laser surgery get covered by an eschar consisting of denatured proteins that minimizes postoperative redness and edema. The wound surfaces may be left to heal by granulation without having to use plastic techniques for coverage [28].

The CO$_2$ laser can vaporize tumors that have a solid tissue structure or dense stroma such as fibromas, epidermoid, and dermoid cysts. Deeper vascular lesions should be treated with the KTP or Nd:YAG laser, which have a better coagulating effect than the CO$_2$ laser.

Premalignant Lesions

The ability to vaporize and excise mucosal lesions in the oral cavity and oropharynx with a good hemostatic effect, minimal scarring, and reduced pain and edema gives the CO$_2$ laser a distinct advantage over conventional resection techniques. Several studies have shown that leukoplakia and erythroplakia, which undergo malignant degeneration in 10% of cases, can be effectively ablated with the CO$_2$ laser [23]. It is essential, however, that every lesion be histologically confirmed prior to laser ablation. For deeper lesions extending into the base of the tongue or the soft palate, the laser also permits the resection of muscular tissue without the fascicular contractions in surrounding tissue that occur with electrocautery [2].

Malignant Tumors

See Chapter 6 (Lasers for Malignant Lesions in the Upper Aerodigestive Tract).

Labial and Lingual Frenoplasties

A high labial frenum will often cause a gap to develop between the two maxillary central incisors, called a median diastema. The laser can be used to perform a labial frenoplasty, dividing the constricting bands with minimal trauma and bleeding. A similar technique can be used for short lingual frenula, which may cause speech impediments, promote dental caries, and interfere with denture wearing. The CO$_2$ laser is most commonly used for this procedure.

Many of these laser procedures represent alternatives to established techniques based on the individual preferences of different surgeons. The frequent advantages of laser use, whether substantial or only marginal, are frequently offset by practical constraints relating to time and money, which have prevented the widespread application of laser for some indications.

■ Lasers in the Treatment of Snoring and Sleep Apnea

Despite numerous surgical developments, nasal continuous positive airway pressure (nCPAP) therapy continues to be the gold standard in the treatment of obstructive sleep apnea (OSA). With compliance rates of approximately 70%, both patients and their doctors are seeking alternatives mainly involving surgical techniques. With refinements in imaging procedures and flexible diagnostic endoscopy, it is becoming more feasible to relate the underlying pathology to a specific anatomic region—particularly the velar segment and region of the base of the tongue. Unfortunately, this type of localizing diagnosis has proved accurate only for primary snoring and for certain cases of mild OSA.

The soft palate was identified as a target for surgical correction at a relatively early stage. Ikematsu and Fujita aimed to reduce the hyperplastic velopharyngeal tissue, and this procedure became known as uvulopalatopharyngoplasty (UPPP) [29]. Kamami introduced the CO$_2$ laser into soft-palate surgery [30]. The procedure, known as laser-assisted uvulopalatoplasty (LAUP), is carried out in an outpatient setting under local anesthesia, and thus quickly became popular, even though the results supporting the procedure continue to be very controversial [31]. The growing demand of patients for the treatment of primary snoring is reflected in the numerous publications on the use of this technique, which often do not go beyond anecdotal case reports.

Applications

The relative ease of learning the LAUP technique and the wide availability of lasers, combined with the initial euphoria sparked by enthusiastic publications, often resulted in LAUP being used indiscriminately to treat primary snoring as well as obstructive sleep apnea. The rationale of the procedure is to modify the tissues in a way that eliminates the airway obstruction and snoring noise. Snoring noises are produced by soft-tissue vibrations at constrictions formed mainly by the pharyngeal walls, soft palate, and uvula. The sound is generated one level lower in the region of the epiglottis and base of the tongue. The obstruction is promoted by an increase in tissue pressure, hyperplastic or hypertrophic tissues in the corresponding regions, and a decrease in muscle tonus. The precise location of the obstruction is of key importance and is closely related to the desired endpoint of treatment [32]. A number of localizing techniques are available for determining the site of the lesion. In routine practice, however, it is often too difficult and costly to carry out a complete battery of tests. In over 50 % of cases, the causative lesion of the obstruction and snoring noise is to be found in the velopharyngeal segment [33].

The initial euphoria that LAUP could also treat OSA soon gave way to sobering reality. This may have been due to a failure to achieve the desired result or a higher-than-expected complication rate. Efforts to define criteria for selecting OSA patients for LAUP, based for example on an upper cut-off value of the apnea–hypopnea index (AHI) of 30/h or a maximum body mass index (BMI) of 28 kg/m^2, met with little success. These values are not statistically supported by higher evidence levels; they merely reflect a tendency. It became increasingly clear that, determining the site of the lesion for OSA did not lead to improved success rates. The underlying pathology is believed to be multifactorial [34]. This is reflected in operative treatments and a growing reliance on multilevel procedures, starting from the uvula and soft palate and proceeding to the tonsils, base of the tongue, and the hyoid [35]. Today fewer and fewer surgeons feel that LAUP is appropriate for OSA, regardless of its severity.

Contraindications

There is great diversity of opinion in the literature regarding the severity of sleep-related breathing disorders for which a laser procedure would be indicated. According to Finkelstein et al., neither primary snoring nor OSA is a valid indication for LAUP [36]. Primary snoring is recognized as an indication for LAUP in most publications, and about half of the studies also advocate this procedure for mild OSA. Very few authors still believe that LAUP is appropriate for higher grades of OSA. Based on an analysis of the literature,

we can list the following contraindications for LAUP in primary snoring:
- AHI greater than 20–30/h
- BMI greater than 28 kg/m^2
- Midfacial deformities
- Posterior airway space at the mandibular level smaller than 10 mm
- Severe concomitant medical disease
- Severe neurologic or psychiatric comorbidity

Techniques

The goal of all laser techniques is to resect soft tissues and induce scarring that will increase the stiffness of the velum [37–39]. Nearly all publications describe the use of the CO_2 laser [40, 41]. Some groups prefer the Nd:YAG laser, one group uses the KTP laser, and one group prefers the gallium-aluminum-arsenide laser. Since comparisons are lacking, we cannot present objective advantages and disadvantages.

The surgery basically consists of vaporizing the uvula as needed and reducing the parauvular soft tissues at the free margin of the soft palate. The procedure is extended anteriorly to varying degrees, preserving or dividing the anterior pillars. LAUP differs from UPPP in that it is a brief procedure done under local anesthesia and the tonsils are not involved. The procedure does not require sutures or a hospital stay.

The soft-palate surgery is usually done with the CO_2 laser using a handpiece with a backstop to protect the posterior wall of the pharynx from the laser beam. Three different laser techniques have been described:
- The oldest technique is laser uvulopalatoplasty (LUPP), described by Carenfelt in 1986. It is a radical technique, carried out under general anesthesia, and resembles UPPP. It may include tonsillectomy, and the faucial pillars are sutured following partial resection of the soft palate and uvulectomy (Fig. 4.1) [42].
- The most commonly used technique, the LAUP, was described by Kamani (1990) and is done in the sitting patient under local anesthesia. Vertical incisions are made

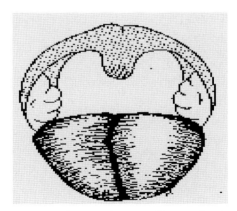

Fig. 4.**1** Schematic diagram of laser uvulopalatoplasty (LUPP), a radical technique. The shaded area is resected [42].

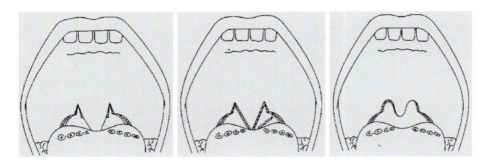

Fig. 4.**2**   Diagrammatic representation of laser-assisted uvulopalatoplasty (LAUP) as a staged procedure [43].

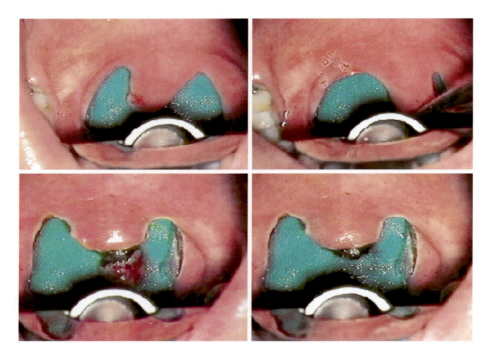

Fig. 4.**3**   LAUP as a muscle-sparing single-stage procedure. The parauvular area to be resected is marked with laser spots, and the mucosal area is resected while sparing the musculature. Finally the tip of the uvula is resected.

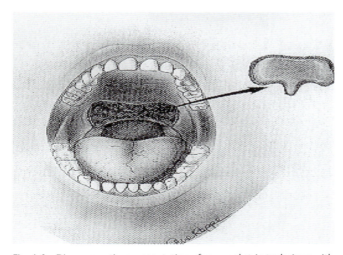

Fig. 4.**4**   Diagrammatic representation of mucosal strip technique with uvulectomy. The mucosa is resected, leaving the musculature [39].

through the anterior and posterior pillars adjacent to the uvula, followed by a complete or partial uvulectomy. LAUP may be done as a single-stage or multistage procedure, depending on the desired extent of the resection (Figs. 4.**2**, 4.**3**) [30, 43].

• A new, less commonly used technique is the mucosal strip technique (MST), first described by Morar in 1995 [39, 44]. It involves resecting only the mucosa of the anterior pillar, leaving the musculature of the velum intact. The uvula and posterior pillar are incised or resected as in LAUP (Fig. 4.**4**).

Evaluating Outcomes

Individual outcome of soft-palate surgery with the laser cannot be accurately predicted. This applies to primary snoring as well as OSA (mild to moderate). It is also difficult to evaluate and analyze results published in the literature due to the different instruments and criteria that have been used to evaluate treatment outcomes. In patients with OSA, polysomnography should be done before and after treatment, accompanied by questionnaires. There are marked differences in what is defined as a successful outcome. Sher et al. recommend that success be defined as a reduction of the AHI to less than 20/h and a reduction of more than 50 % the initial AHI value [32]. Subjective rating is inadequate in OSA patients. Evaluating the outcome of soft-palate laser surgery for primary snoring presents even greater difficulties [45]. Subjective rating of symptoms using a visual analog scale (VAS) by a third party is essential, unless the evaluation is limited to measuring decibel reduction and the duration of snoring phases relative to total sleep. The frequency spectrum of the snoring noise is relevant to the subjective suffering of the bed partner, and alteration of the complex noise pattern by the procedure can have positive effects.

Efficacy of Laser-Assisted Uvulopalatoplasty in Obstructive Sleep Apnea

No controlled randomized studies have been conducted on the efficacy of LAUP in the treatment of OSA. Published series of case reports are of limited value for making a definitive assessment. As in all surgical therapies, the lack of control groups is a problem. Case studies can provide information on a change in respiratory parameters, such as the AHI, when pre- and postoperative polysomnographic records are available [46]. A meta-analysis has shown only minor improvements based on this criterion [40]. Quality-of-life measurements are one of the tools that must be applied to determine whether this reduction of the AHI is clinically significant. However, this type of measurement is absent in almost all studies.

A study by Walker and Gopalsami demonstrated the effect of criterion selection on the evaluation of surgical outcome [47]. These authors found that a 50 % reduction of the AHI is easier to achieve in a patient with severe sleep apnea than in a patient with mild apnea. If an AHI less than 20/h is defined as the success criterion, better success rates will be achieved in mildly apneic patients.

Another problem that calls into question the efficacy of LAUP in OSA is the lack of long-term results over a period of years. The quality of the published data is not sufficient to document efficacy. Studies comparing LAUP and UPPP have been published, but none goes beyond level III in the classification of evidence (where level I represents randomized trials with low alpha and beta errors). Comparisons are also difficult to interpret due to the large diversity in the nonstandardized operating techniques and outcome measures that have been applied.

Efficacy of Laser-Assisted Uvulopalatoplasty for Primary Snoring

The main dilemma is a lack of objective measures for analyzing snoring sounds. As a result, there is no uniform criterion for evaluating response. Walker et al. described a digital method of analyzing snoring noise based on a fast Fourier transform [48]. These authors documented a postoperative change in snoring index and frequency spectrum. LAUP decreased relative loudness at frequencies below 180 Hz, which originate in the velum. With these few exceptions, the severity of snoring is generally rated subjectively by the bed partner. Two long-term studies over periods of up to 8 years and 5 years, respectively, showed improvement of snoring in approximately 90 % of the patients treated [49, 50]. Other studies report a 55 % success rate at 18–24 months [51] and a 43 % success rate up to 24 months [52].

Pain and Laser-Assisted Uvulopalatoplasty

An analysis of publications on postoperative pain symptoms shows that LAUP tends to be more painful than UPPP. Pain assessment also encounters the problem of nonuniform outcome measures and of complex and sometimes unrecognized boundary conditions such as concomitant medications. Ordinarily, the intensity of pain is rated from 1 to 10 on a VAS. A comparative study by Wennmo et al. indicated that LAUP is more painful than UPPP [42]. Shehab and Robin also noted this disadvantage of LAUP compared with UPPP [53]. It is typical of laser procedures in the oral cavity and oropharynx that the greatest pain is experienced on about the third postoperative day. Astor et al. described seven cases in which treatment had to be discontinued due to pain [54]. The implication is that pain medication should be properly adjusted in patients undergoing a laser procedure.

Complications After Laser-Assisted Uvulopalatoplasty

The number and severity of complications after LAUP increase with the extent of the resection. One survey article reported one death in 2900 LAUPs (sepsis on the fourth postoperative day) and three deaths in 9000 UPPPs [55]. One potential danger is the risk of decreased tolerance to nCPAP following the surgery. An oral leak can result from the loss of palatal tissue. The nature and frequency of complications after LAUP are reviewed in Table 4.**1**.

Overall Evaluation of Laser-Assisted Uvulopalatoplasty

The German Society of Otorhinolaryngology–Head and Neck Surgery published its guidelines on OSA and obstructive snoring in 1998 [56]. Three years later, the American Sleep Disorder Association (ASDA) incorporated new study results into its guidelines and issued the following recommendations for the practice of LAUP:
- LAUP is not recommended for the treatment of sleep-related breathing disorders, including OSA (guideline).
- LAUP is not recommended as a substitute for UPPP in the treatment of sleep-related breathing disorders, including OSA (guideline).
- LAUP appears to be comparable to UPPP in the treatment of subjective snoring (guideline).

Table 4.1 Types and incidence (%) of complications after laser-assisted uvulopalatoplasty*

Complications	Incidence (%)
Difficulty swallowing while eating	81
Temporary dysphagia	31
Persistent dysphagia	5–53
Severe dysphagia	1
Anorexia	21
Dry mouth	16–42
Persistent difficulties with drinking	16
Persistent foreign body sensation	10–25
Increased gag reflex	10
Change in swallowing	6
Mild dysphonia	6
Vasovagal episodes	1.8
Temporary voice changes	1.7–17.2
Temporary nasal regurgitation	1.7–10.3
Persistent nasal regurgitation	1–20
Vomiting	1.5
Mild bleeding	1–8
Bleeding sufficient to require treatment	0.4–1.8
Temporary vasovagal insufficiency	0.5–3
Temporary taste disturbance	0.3
Persistent taste disturbance	5
Fibrotic scarring	0.2–30
Oral candidiasis	0.4–2

* Data from a meta-analysis published by Littner et al., 2001 [40].

- Patients who are surgical candidates for LAUP as treatment for snoring should undergo a preoperative examination including polysomnography. The patient should be informed that regular postoperative polysomnography is necessary to detect the possible development of OSA (standard).
- The need for perioperative medication should be assessed (standard).
- Patients should be informed of the risks and complications of LAUP.

LAUP is recommended only for the treatment of primary snoring. It is easier to do than UPPP but has a similar range of potential complications. The preferred candidates for LAUP are patients with small or atrophic tonsils and a hypertrophic uvula.

Laser Use on the Tonsils

Laser Tonsillectomy

Since the introduction of lasers in otolaryngology, reports of laser tonsillectomies with various laser systems have been published. A common goal in these studies is to reduce intraoperative blood loss, postoperative bleeding, and pain through laser use. Because tonsillectomy is one of the most common surgical procedures in otolaryngology, and given the desire to reduce the risks associated with traditional operative procedures, there has been considerable worldwide interest in the results of laser tonsillectomy [57, 58]. Overall tonsillectomy rates range from 13% to 50% of the population in different countries [59].

Martinez and Akin [60] described the use of the CO_2 laser for tonsillectomy in 1987 and Nishimura et al. [61] in 1988. The CO_2 laser is widely used in otolaryngology. In theory, the physical properties of this laser make it an effective tool for laser tonsillectomy. It has a shallow penetration depth in tissue. Theoretically this could reduce thermal damage to the surrounding tissue, with an associated reduction in postoperative morbidity [62]. However, only a few studies have shown clinical confirmation of this theory. Martinez and Akin [60], for example, reported on more than 500 CO_2 laser tonsillectomies carried out at their institution. The patients were not compared with a control group. Without detailing individual results, the authors found that laser use for tonsillectomy reduced intraoperative blood loss and operating time and was followed by less than a 2% incidence of postoperative bleeding. An operating microscope was used to increase the precision of laser application.

Martinez and Akin's results have not been corroborated by other authors [63–65]. Auf et al., Oas and Bartel, and Strunk and Nichols performed tonsillectomies with the KTP-532 laser [66–68]. Auf et al. used the KTP-532 laser because it has a better cutting action than the Nd:YAG laser and a better coagulating effect than the CO_2 laser. Strunk and Nichols and Auf et al. reported a significant reduction of intraoperative bleeding, no difference in operating time, increased postoperative coatings, and delayed healing with the KTP-532 laser tonsillectomy. Strunk and Nichols found no difference in postoperative pain during healing, whereas Auf et al. found that postoperative pain was less on the side treated with the KTP-532 laser on the first and second postoperative days but was significantly worse on the laser side starting on the third postoperative day. Strunk and Nichols found no significant difference in postoperative bleeding between tonsillectomy by the KTP-532 laser and by traditional dissection. In the study by Auf et al., there was a 15% incidence of postoperative bleeding on the laser-treated side, which was adequately managed by conservative treatment. Raine et al. found a 22% incidence of postoperative bleeding in their prospective study of 54 KTP-532 laser tonsillectomies in patients between 16 and 51 years of age [69]. They concluded that KTP-532 laser tonsillectomy compared unfavorably with conventional tonsillectomy in adult patients.

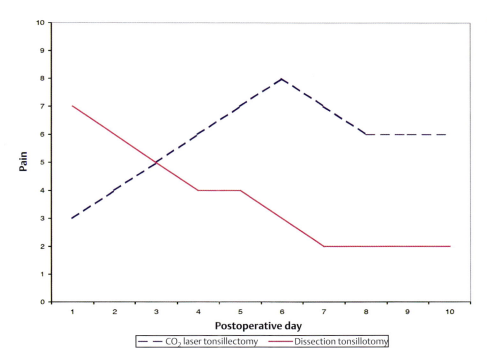

Regardless of the type of laser used and whether or not an operating microscope is used, laser dissection of the tonsil often causes bleeding that obscures the surgical site and cannot be adequately controlled by the laser itself. In this case the surgeon must resort to a conventional method of hemostasis. An increased incidence of postoperative uvular edema has been reported after laser tonsillectomy.

In summary, and based on our own experience, it may be said that laser tonsillectomy is less bloody than a conventional tonsillectomy and allows for greater surgical precision when an operating microscope is used. Patients experience less pain on the first and second postoperative days than after a conventional tonsillectomy, but the pain becomes worse starting on the second or third day after laser tonsillectomy and persists for a longer time (Fig. 4.5). Postoperative wound coatings persist longer after a laser tonsillectomy than a conventional tonsillectomy, and it takes the tonsillar bed longer to reepithelialize. Significant reduction in postoperative bleeding has not been demonstrated.

These factors must be weighed against the special equipment needed before and during laser use, which translates into added time and expense. While a dissection tonsillectomy can be started immediately after insertion of the mouth gag, additional safety aspects must be considered prior to laser tonsillectomy. For example, the orotracheal ventilation tube must be carefully secured outside the operative field, and the tube and posterior pharyngeal wall have to be covered with moist gauze. If an operating microscope is used, the tongue depressor must be accurately placed for optimum exposure of the surgical site and reintroduced as needed. Consequently, a laser tonsillectomy is more technically demanding and is not an operation for beginners. In routine clinical practice, however, tonsillectomies are usually carried out by relatively inexperienced residents.

For the reasons cited above, we must conclude that tonsillectomy with the CO_2 or KTP laser cannot be recommended as a standard method in routine clinical situations. The initial enthusiasm must give way to a more realistic appraisal of the laser's capabilities.

Mucosa-Intact Laser Tonsillar Ablation

In 1996, Volk et al. described a procedure known as mucosa-intact laser tonsillar ablation (MILTA) [62]. They carried out this procedure in five dogs with an 810-nm diode laser, comparing it with conventional tonsillectomy done in four dogs. In MILTA, the tonsillar tissue is lased to denature the lymphoid tissue while leaving the mucosal layer intact. The authors state that the laser energy blanched the superficial mucosa without charring it. In the MILTA group, a reduction of tonsillar tissue was noted on the seventh postoperative day, and complete reduction was achieved by the 45th day. The authors recommend that MILTA be repeated on any residual tonsillar tissue. Postoperative weight loss was less in the MILTA-treated animals compared with the control group. This was interpreted as an indirect sign of reduced postoperative pain. No postoperative bleeding occurred in the MILTA group. The diode laser is a small, portable laser weighing approximately 12 kg with a low maximum power output of 25 W. It is better suited for tonsillar surgery than the Nd:YAG laser, because it has a shallower penetration depth posing less hazard to deeper structures [64].

So far there have been no publications on the clinical use of the theoretically promising technique of tonsillar ablation. Also, the study by Volk et al. did not address the question of whether tonsillar hypertrophy or chronic tonsillitis should be considered a proper indication for MILTA.

Laser Tonsillotomy

Studies have been published on laser tonsillotomy in children with tonsillar hyperplasia who present with symptoms of primary snoring and/or sleep apnea along with eating difficulties [70]. This operation is practiced at various centers in Germany and in the Scandinavian countries [71, 72]. Tonsillotomy has been known for many decades and was long considered to be obsolete [56]. The main criticism was that the tonsillar remnants left by the procedure underwent scarring and caused significant complaints such as severe tonsillitis and abscesses [73]. For this reason, laser tonsillotomy should be strictly limited to patients with hyperplastic tonsils that are easily luxated from the fossa. The patient must have no known history of tonsillitis; if doubt exists in an older child, a tonsillectomy should be done [74]. In patients with chronic tonsillitis, the chronically inflamed tonsillar remnant will behave no differently from the removed tonsillar tissue in the event of a recrudescence. More recent studies on laser tonsillotomy have not found any evidence of increased incidence of tonsillitis or peritonsillar abscess [70].

Tonsillotomy with the CO_2 laser or Nd:YAG laser is done under general endotracheal anesthesia [72]. In principle, KTP or diode lasers could also be used for this procedure. Different laser systems produce different necrotic zones in the tonsillar remnants. Coagulating systems such as the Nd:YAG laser produce a considerably larger necrotic zone than cutting lasers (e.g., the CO_2 laser). With the CO_2 laser, the incisions should be placed through the tonsils such that the margins of the resection are directly in front of the anterior and posterior pillars. With a coagulating laser, they should be placed slightly more medially. The mucosa of the faucial pillars should be completely preserved. Small bleeding sites in the tonsillar tissue are controlled with electrocautery [70].

The vessels at the superior and inferior poles of the tonsil remain intact in a laser tonsillotomy, and therefore the risk of postoperative bleeding is reduced along with postoperative malaise and use of analgesics. The patient is left with functionally competent lymphatic tonsillar tissue [71, 72].

Figure 4.6 illustrates the appearance of the operative site on the first day after CO_2 laser tonsillotomy, and Fig. 4.7 on the eleventh postoperative day.

The cutting and (limited) coagulating properties of the CO_2 laser result in a dry wound bed. This advantage must be weighed against the added time and expense of laser use compared with a monopolar needle and conventional operating technique.

■ Lasers in the Treatment of Salivary Gland Diseases

Sialolithiasis is the most common disease of the major salivary glands, with an incidence of 1.2%. Approximately 80% of salivary stones are located in the submandibular gland and 10% in the parotid gland [75]. The obstruction of salivary outflow typically leads to a glandular swelling at mealtimes. The salivary stasis results in bacterial infection of the gland. Salivary stones are composed of organic material (mucopolysaccharides) and inorganic material (carbonate apatite). Sialolithiasis is believed to be the result of formation of calcium–mucin complexes, from which microliths are formed [76].

In the past, the treatment of sialolithiasis has been almost entirely surgical. Stones located away from the gland, in the distal portion of the excretory duct, can be removed by intraoral incision of the duct. Stones located close to the gland or in the glandular parenchyma have traditionally required excision of the gland [77]. Besides possible complications of impaired wound healing and salivary fistulation, the main risk of excising the gland is damaging important neural structures such as the facial nerve and its branches (parotidectomy) or the lingual nerve (submandibulectomy).

Stone fragmentation by means of laser-induced shockwaves (laser-induced lithotripsy [LIL]) was first used in the treatment of ureteral stones in the early 1980s and has become an established urologic treatment modality during recent years [78, 79].

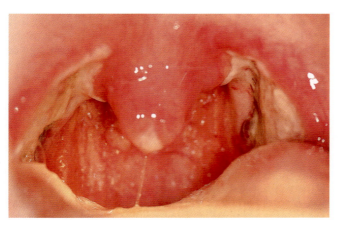

Fig. 4.6 CO_2 laser tonsillotomy: first postoperative day.

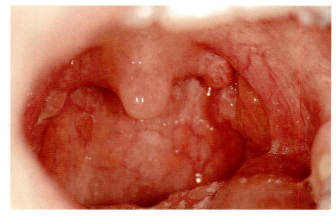

Fig. 4.7 CO_2 laser tonsillotomy: eleventh postoperative day.

The basic physical principle underlying LIL is the phenomenon of photodisruption, also known as "optical breakdown." When laser pulses of sufficiently high energy and short duration are applied to tissue, they form a plasma that causes the sudden volume expansion of fluids and generates a shockwave [80]. The laser fiber is advanced to the stone through an endoscope. The particles of the fragmented stone are either passed spontaneously with the salivary flow or flushed out through the working channel of the endoscope.

In vitro studies of lasers in the CW mode have demonstrated a slight surface ablation of salivary stones that can be attributed to a thermal melting and boring effect. This contrasts with the effect of short-pulse laser systems with pulse lengths of 7 ns to 3 µs, which cause the fragmentation of calculi [77]. With this technique, stones 1 cm in diameter were completely disintegrated within a period of about 10 minutes.

Different laser systems have yielded varying results in the treatment of sialoliths [81]. While the alexandrite laser emitting at 755 nm and the Nd:YAG laser (1064 nm) failed to produce adequate stone fragmentation, Gundlach et al. obtained good results with the excimer laser, achieving complete stone clearance in 91.6% of their patients [77]. The main drawback of the excimer laser is the potential for injury to surrounding tissues such as nerves and blood vessels. Iro et al., on the other hand, reported good results with a dye laser emitting at 595 nm [82]. Their laser had built-in stone-tissue detection based on the optical analysis of the light reflected during the lithotripsy. These authors achieved a stone clearance rate of 46% after one to three treatments.

The laser-induced lithotripsy of salivary stones is well tolerated and can be performed under local anesthesia in an ambulatory setting. Intraglandular abscess formation and transient sialadenitis have been cited as the main complications of LIL [77]. To date, LIL has been performed only in small numbers of otolaryngology patients. The main disadvantages of the method are its higher costs, prolonged operating time, and added personnel requirements.

■ References

1 Rudert H, Werner JA. Lasers in Otorhinolaryngology and Head and Neck Surgery, Adv Oto-Rhino-Laryngol. Basel: Karger 1995
2 Steiner W, Werner JA. Endoskopische Laserchirurgie der oberen Luft- und Atemwege. Schwerpunkt Tumorchirurgie. Stuttgart: Thieme, 1996
3 Matschke RG. Experiences with laser surgery in benign and malignant findings of the oro- and hypopharynx. Adv Otorhinolaryngol 1995; 49: 153–157
4 Polanyi TG. Laser Physics. Otolaryngol Clin N Amer 1983; 16: 753–774
5 Polanyi TG, Bredmesiser HC, Davis TG. A CO_2 laser for surgical research. Med Biol Eng Comput 1970; 8: 541–548
6 Jako FG. Laser surgery of the vocal cord: an experimental study with carbon-dioxide laser on dogs. Laryngoscope 1972; 82: 204–211
7 Pick RM. Using laser in clinical dental practice. JADA 1993; 124: 37–47
8 Iro H, Waldfahrer F, Gewalt K, Zenk J, Altendorf-Hofmann A. Enoral/transoral surgery of malignancies of the oral cavity and the oropharynx. Adv Otorhinolaryngol 1995; 49: 191–195
9 Eckel HE, Thumfart WF. An analysis of recurrences after transoral laser resection of oral carcinoma. Adv Otorhinolaryngol 1995; 49: 196–200
10 Chiesa F, Sala L, Costa L, Iglo K. Excision of oral leukoplakias by CO_2 laser on an outpatient: a useful procedure for prevention and early detection of oral carcinomas. Tumori 1986; 72: 307–312
11 Duncavage JA, Ossoff RH. Use of CO_2 laser for malignant disease of the oral cavity. Lasers Surg Med 1986; 6: 442–444
12 Frame JW. Carbon dioxide laser surgery for benign oral lesions. Br Dent J 1992; 71: 221–228
13 Midgely HC. Nd:YAG contact lasersurgery: a scapel of the future? Otolaryngol Clin N Amer 1990; 23: 99–105
14 Folz BJ, Lippert BM, Gottschlich S, Maass JD, Werner JA. The influence of different dessection techniques on p53 as a possible indicator for local recurrences in carcinomas of the upper aerodigestive tract. Anticancer Res 1999; 19: 2707–2710
15 Ashinoff R. Introduction to lasers. Semin Dermatol 1994; 13: 48–59
16 Blankenau RJ, Kelsey WP, Powell GL, Shearer GO, Barkmeier WW, Cavel WT. Degree of composite resin polymerization with visible light and argon laser. Am Dent J 1991; 4: 40–42
17 Powell GL, Kelsey WP, Blankenau RJ, Barkmeier WW. The use of an argon laser for polymerization of composite resin. J Esthet Dent 1989; 1: 34–37
18 Miserendino TJ. The laser apicoectomy: endodontic application for the CO_2 laser for periapical surgery. Oral Surg 1988; 66: 615–619
19 Morlock BJ, Pippin DJ, Cobb CM, Killoy WJ, Rapley JW. The effect of Nd:YAG laser exposure on root surfaces when used as an adjunct to root planing: an in vitro study. J Periodontol 1992; 7: 637–641
20 Frentzen M. Laser in der Parodontaltherapie: eine kritische Übersicht. Schweiz Monatsschr Zahnmed 1993; 103: 1585–1592
21 Frentzen M, Koort HJ, Kermani O. Bearbeitung von Zahnhartsubstanzen mit einem Excimer-Laser. Dtsch Zahnärztl Z 1989; 44: 431–439
22 Liesenhoff F, Lenz H, Seiler T. Wurzelkanalaufbereitung mit Excimer-Laserstrahlen. Zahnärztl Welt 1989; 98: 1034–1040
23 Rathfoot CJ, Coleman JA. Laser utilization in the oral pharynx. Otolaryngol Clin N Amer 1996; 29: 963–972
24 Steiner W, Werner JA. Lasers in otorhinolaryngology, head and neck surgery. Tuttlingen: Endo-Press, 2000
25 Lindenberger M, Strutz J. Kapitel 21 Laserchirurgie. In: Strutz J, Mann W (Hrsg). Praxis der HNO-Heilkunde, Kopf- u. Halschirurgie. Stuttgart: Thieme, 2000
26 Werner JA, Lippert BM, Hoffmann P, Rudert H. Nd:YAG laser therapy of voluminous hemangiomas and vascular malformations. Adv Otorhinolaryngol 1995; 49: 75–80
27 Crockett DM, Healy GB, McGill TJ, Friedman EM. Benign lesions of the nose, oral cavity, and oropharynx in children: excision by carbon dioxide laser. Ann Otol Rhinol Laryngol 1985; 94: 489–493
28 White JM, Chaudry SI, Kudler JJ, Sekandari N, Schoelch ML, Sil S Jr. Nd:YAG and CO_2 laser therapy of oral mucosal lesions. J Clin Laser Med Surg 1998; 16: 299–304
29 Fujita S, Conway W, Zorick F. Surgical correction of anatomic abnormalities in obstructive sleep apnea syndrom: uvulopalatopharyngoplasty. Otolaryngol Head Neck Surg 1981; 89: 923–934
30 Kamami YV. Laser CO_2 for snoring-preliminary results. Acta Otorhinolaryngol Belg 1990; 44: 451–456
31 Verse T, Pirsig W. Metaanalyse zur laserassistierten Uvulopalatopharyngoplastik. Laryngo-Rhino-Otol 2000; 79: 273–284
32 Sher AE, Schechtman KB, Piccirillo JF. The efficiency of surgical modifications of the upper airway in adults with obstructive sleep apnea syndrome. Sleep 1996; 19: 156–177
33 Shepard JW, Gefter WB, Guilleminault C, Hoffman EA, Hoffstein V, Hudgel DW, Suratt PM, White DP. Evaluation of the upper airway in patients with obstructive sleep apnea. Sleep 1991; 14: 361–371
34 Moore K. Site-specific versus diffuse treatment/presenting severity of OSA. Sleep & Breathing 2001; 4: 145–146
35 Hörmann K, Hirth K, Maurer JT. Operative Therapie schlafbezogener Atmungsstörungen. HNO 1999; 47: 226–235

36 Finkelstein Y, Stein G, Ophir D, Berger R, Berger G. Laser-assisted uvulopalatoplasty for the management of obstructive sleep apnea. Arch Otolaryngol Head Neck Surg 2002; 128: 429–434

37 Kaluskar SK, Kaul GH. Long-term results of KTP/532 laser uvulopalatopharyngoplasty. Rev Laryngol Otol Rhinol (Bord) 2000; 121: 59–62

38 Walker RP, Grigg-Damberger MM, Gopalsami C. Uvulopalatopharyngoplasty versus laser-assisted uvulopalatoplasty for the treatment of obstructive sleep apnea. Laryngoscope 1997; 107: 76–82

39 Skatvedt O. Laser-assisted uvulopalatoplasty. Descritption of technique and pre- and postoperative evaluation of subjective symptoms. Oto-Rhino-Laryngol 1996; 58: 243–247

40 Littner M, Kushida CA, Hartse K, Anderson WMcD, Davila D, Johnson SF, Wise MS, Hirshkowitz M, Woodson BT. Practice parameters for the use of laser-assisted uvulopalatoplasty: an update for 2000. Sleep 2001; 24: 603–619

41 Remacle M, Betsch C, Lawson G, Jamart J, Eloy P. A New Technique for laser-assisted uvulopalatoplasty: decision-tree analysis and results. Laryngoscope 1999; 109: 763–768

42 Wenmo C, Olsson P, Flisberg K, Paulsson B, Luttrup S. Treatment of snoring – with and without carbon dioxide laser. Acta Otolaryngol (Stockh) 1992; 492: 152–155

43 Kamami YV. Section 1: Outpatient treatment of snoring and sleep apnea syndrom with CO_2 Laser: Laser-assisted uvulopalatoplasty. In: Clayman L (Ed). Lasers in Maxillofacial Surgery and Dentistry. 1998: 111–116

44 Morar P, Nandapalan V, Lesser THJ, Swift AC. Mucosal-strip/uvulectomy by the CO_2 laser as a method of treating simple snoring. Clin Otolaryngol 1995; 20: 308–311

45 Pirsig W. There is no rationale for radical UPPP. Somnologie Suppl 1997; 2: 48

46 Seemann RP, DiToppa JC, Holm MA, Hanson J. Does laser-assisted uvulopalatoplasty work? An objective analysis using pre- and postoperative polysomnographie studies. J Otolaryngol 2001; 30: 212–215

47 Walker RP, Gopalsami C. Laser-assisted uvulopalatoplasty; postoperative complications. Laryngoscope 1996; 106: 834–838

48 Walker RP, Gatti WM, Porier N, Davis JS. Objective assessment of snoring before and after laser-assisted uvulopalatoplasty. Laryngoscope 1996; 106: 1372–1377

49 Hagert B, Wahren LK, Wikblad K, Ödkvist L. Patients and cohabitants reports on snoring and daytime sleepiness, 1–8 years after surgical treatment of snoring. Oto-Rhino-Laryngol 1999; 61: 19–24

50 Coleman JA. Laser-assisted uvulopalatoplasty: Long-term results with a treatment for snoring. Ear Nose and Throat J 1998; 77: 22–34

51 Wareing MJ, Callanan VP, Mitchell DB. Laser-assisted uvulopalatoplasty: six and eighteen months results. J Laryngol Otol 1998; 112: 639–641

52 Finkelstein Y, Shapiro-Feinberg M, Stein G, Ophir D. Uvulopalatopharyngoplasty vs laser-assisted uvulopalatoplasty. Anatomical considerations. Arch Otolaryngol Head Neck Surg 1997; 123: 265–276

53 Shebab ZP, Robin PE. Comparison of the effectiveness of uvulopalatopharyngoplasty and laser palatoplasty for snoring. Clin Otolaryngol 1997; 22: 158–161

54 Astor FC, Hanft KL, Benson C, Amaranath A. Analysis of short-term outcome after office based laser-assisted uvulopalatoplasty. Otolaryngol Head Neck Surg 1998; 118: 478–480

55 Carenfelt C, Haraldsson PO. Frequency of complications after uvulopalatopharyngoplasty. Lancet 1993; 341: 437

56 Pirsig W, Hörmann K, Siegert R, Maurer J, Verse T. Obstruktive Schlafapnoe (OSA) und obstruktives Schnarchen. Leitlinien der Deutschen Gesellschaft für Hals-Nasen-Ohren-Heilkunde, Kopf- und Hals-Chirurgie. HNO 1998; 46: 730

57 Feldmann H. 2000 Jahre Geschichte der Tonsillektomie. Laryngol-Rhinol-Otol 1997; 76: 751–760

58 Handler SD, Miller L, Richmond KH, Baranak CC. Post-tonsillectomy hemorrhage: incidence, prevention and management. Laryngoscope 1986; 96: 1243–1247

59 Matzker J, Steinberg A. Tonsillektomie und Leukämie im Erwachsenenalter. Laryngol-Rhinol-Otol 1976; 55: 721–755

60 Martinez SA, Akin DP. Laser tonsillectomy and adenoidectomy. Otolaryngol Clin N Amer 1987; 20: 371–376

61 Nishimura T, Yagisawa M, Suzuki A, Okada T. Laser tonsillectomy. Acta Otolaryngol (Stockh) Suppl 1988; 454: 313–315

62 Volk MS, Wnag Z, Pankratov MM, Perrault DF, Ingrams DR, Shapshay SM. Mucosal intact laser tonsillar ablation. Arch Otolaryngol Head Neck Surg 1996; 122: 1355–1359

63 Scherer H, Fuhrer A, Hopf J, Linnartz M, Philipp C, Wermund K et al. Derzeitiger Stand der Laserchirurgie im Bereich des weichen Gaumens und der angrenzenden Regionen. Laryngol-Rhinol-Otol 1994; 73: 14–20

64 Shah RK, Nemati B, Wang LV, Shapshay SM. Optical-thermal simulation of tonsillar tissue irradiation. Lasers Surg Med 2001; 28: 313–319

65 Maloney RW. Contact Nd:YAG tonsillectomy: effects on weight loss and recovery. Lasers Surg Med 1991; 11: 517–522

66 Auf I, Osborne JE, Sparkes C, Khalil H. Is the KTP laser effective in tonsillectomy? Clin Otolaryngol 1997; 22: 145–146

67 Oas RE, Bartels JP. KTP-532 laser tonsillectomy: a comparison with standard technique. Laryngoscope 1990; 100: 385–388

68 Strunk CL, Nichols ML. A comparison of the KTP-532-Laser tonsillectomy vs traditional dissection/snare tonsillectomy. Otolaryngol Head Neck Surg 1990; 103: 966–971

69 Raine NMN, Whittet HB, Marks NJ, Ryan RM. KTP-532 laser tonsilectomy – a potential day-case procedure? J Laryngol Otol 1995; 109: 515–519

70 Helling K, Abrams J, Bertram WK, Hohner S, Scherer H. Die Lasertonsillotomie bei der Tonsillenhyperplasie des Kleinkindes. HNO 2002; 50: 470–478

71 Hulterantz E, Linder A, Markström A. Tonsillectomy or tonsillotomy? – A randomized study comparing postoperative pain and long-terrm effects. Int J Pediatr Otorhinolaryngol 1999; 51: 171–176

72 Linder A, Markström A, Hulterantz E. Using the carbon dioxide laser for tonsillotomy in children. Int J Pediatr Otorhinolaryngol 1999; 50: 31–36

73 Lenz H. Tonsillektomie mit einem Laserraspatorium – Vorläufige Mitteilung. Laryngol-Rhinol-Otol 1984; 63: 582–584

74 Handrock M. Lasertonsillotomie. HNO 2002; 50: 64

75 Seifert G, Mann W, Kastenbauer E. Sialolithiasis. In: Naumann HH, Helms J, Herberhold C, Kastenbauer E (Hrsg). Oto-Rhino-Laryngologie in Klinik und Praxis. Band 2. Thieme-Verlag, 1992: 729–732

76 Gutmann R, Zigler G, Leunig A. Die endoskopische und extrakorporale Stoßwellen-Lithotripsie von Speichelsteinen. Laryngo-Rhino-Otol 1994; 74: 249–253

77 Gundlach P, Scherer H, Hopf J, Leege N, Müller G, Hirst L, Scholz C. Die endoskopisch kontrollierte Laserlithotripsie von Speichelsteinen. In-vitro-Untersuchungen und erster klinischer Einsatz. HNO 1990; 38: 247–250

78 Dretler SP. Laser photofragmentation of ureteral calculi: analysis of 75 cases. J Endourology 1987; 1: 9–14

79 Königsberger R, Feyh J, Goetz A. Die endoskopisch kontrollierte Laserlithotripsie zur Behandlung der Sialolithiasis. Laryngo-Rhino-Otol 1990; 69: 322–323

80 Helfmann J. Nichtlineare Prozesse. In: Berlin HP, Müller G (Hrsg). Angewandte Lasermedizin. Landsberg, München, Zürich: ecomed Verlagsgesellschaft, 1989

81 Arzoz E, Santiago A, Gorriaran M. Removal of a stone in Stensen's duct with endoscopic laser lithotripsy. Report of a case. J Oral Maxillofac Surg 1994; 52: 1329–1330

82 Iro H, Zenk J, Benzel W. Laser lithotripsy of salivary duct stones. Adv Otorhinolaryngol 1995; 49: 148–152

5 Lasers for Benign Diseases of the Larynx, Hypopharynx, and Trachea

H. E. Eckel

■ Contents

■ Abstract

The use of endoscopic laser surgery for benign lesions of the larynx has led to the modification of numerous operative procedures, which are briefly reviewed in this article. The CO_2 laser meets the criteria for use for most benign laryngeal lesions, particularly in phonosurgery, stenosis surgery, swallowing rehabilitation, and for the resection of most benign laryngeal tumors. Optimum instruments and equipment are even more important in surgical procedures for benign laryngeal lesions than in the surgery of malignant tumors. While the use of surgical lasers in phonosurgery is still somewhat controversial, laser surgery has gained an established place in the treatment of glottic laryngeal stenoses, selected tracheal stenoses, and Zenker diverticula. Today, CO_2 lasers are an indispensable tool for endolaryngeal surgery.

■ Operative Technique: Considerations

Historical Background

Modern endoscopic laryngeal surgery traces its origins to the second half of the nineteenth century. Turck and Czermak of Vienna first used angled mirrors for clinical examination of the larynx in 1857, and two years later Stoerk used these mirrors for endolaryngeal cauterization of the larynx. As a result of these efforts, endolaryngeal surgery became more widely practiced and techniques were advanced by McKenzie, Fränkel, Kirstein, Killian, and Jackson. Thus, the development of endolaryngeal surgery was contemporaneous with, but essentially separate from, that of open laryngeal surgery.

In the U.S., the separation between endolaryngeal surgery and open laryngeal surgery is still evident since while head and neck surgeons in the U.S. are skilled in open laryngeal surgery, they may take a skeptical view toward endoscopic laryngeal surgery, which is the domain of "laryngologists." This "overdivision" into subspecialties helps to explain the long delay in the acceptance of endolaryngeal laser surgery in the U.S.

The decisive breakthrough for endolaryngeal surgery as a universal approach for laryngeal operations occurred when Oskar Kleinsasser of Cologne, Germany, introduced microlaryngoscopy in the early 1960s. This method provides access to most of the mucosal lesions of the larynx and a number of submucous lesions. At the same time, it requires a specialized set of microinstruments that are controlled with both hands, requiring a high degree of manual skills. Moreover, the rich vascular supply of the tissues in the larynx makes it difficult to carry out more extensive procedures, tending to cause troublesome bleeding from the cut tissues, obscuring the operative field and making precision microsurgery difficult or impossible. An early solution to this problem involved using monopolar electrocautery probes in endolaryngeal surgery to improve hemostasis in operations involving the relatively extensive division of submucous tissues (e. g., cordectomy, arytenoidectomy).

In the light of the above situation, the introduction of laser systems into laryngeal surgery marks an important milestone in the development of this operative approach. By coupling a CO_2 laser to the operating microscope and controlling the invisible treatment beam with a micromanipulator, guided by a visible-wavelength coaxial aiming beam, a relatively stationary, noncontact technique was acheived for dividing endolaryngeal tissues while simultaneously coagulating smaller blood vessels. This approach overcame several basic problems in endolaryngeal surgery: the laser beam does not obstruct the surgeon's view of the confined operating field, it provides adequate tissue hemostasis for greater visibility, and it facilitates the surgical dissection.

The obvious advantages of endolaryngeal laser surgery were not generally appreciated at first. A major objection was that laser incisions always caused thermal tissue damage (burns) and therefore did not meet the requirement of clean, atraumatic tissue division with margins that could be histologically evaluated. Over time, technical refinements eliminated most of these objections, and laser use not only made it easier to carry out known surgical procedures but also laid the foundation for developing new therapeutic concepts, especially in the field of oncologic surgery (see Chapter 6). Remarkably, these concepts were not developed in the U.S., where lasers were first used in laryngology [1]. It was left to clinical pioneers in Europe such as Burian and Höfler [2], Rudert and Werner [3, 4], Thumfart [5], and especially Steiner and Ambrosch [6, 7] in the German-speaking world, Motta in Italy [8], Grossenbacher in Switzerland [9], and others to research, describe, apply, and publicize the clinical potential of endolaryngeal laser surgery.

In addition, endoscopic laser surgery has led to a modification of numerous operative procedures for benign lesions of the larynx. These are briefly reviewed in this chapter.

Fundamentals of Endolaryngeal Surgery and Equipment

The necessary ingredients for successful endolaryngeal surgery include:
- a refined operating technique,
- appropriate anesthesia and ventilation,
- a complete instrument set for endolaryngeal surgery.

Other important factors are proper positioning of the patient, preoperative assessment of dental status, adequate mouth protection during the procedure to prevent dental injuries, and a trained, proficient surgeon. Suitable options for anesthesia–ventilation are general endotracheal anesthesia (using a laser-safe ventilation tube!), jet ventilation, or mask ventilation with intermittent apnea [10, 11]. The necessary equipment includes an assortment of laryngoscopes and stands, an operating microscope, microinstruments, the CO_2 laser, monopolar cautery probes, rigid telescopes, and suction. Some procedures also require implants and their corresponding application instruments (collagen, fat, cartilage, dispersed silicone) and photographic or video equipment [12].

The essential problems in any minimally invasive procedure, regardless of whether it is in the abdominal cavity, knee joint, or larynx, are obtaining an adequate view of the operative field and the ability to use the necessary instruments at the surgical site. In laryngeal surgery, operating laryngoscopes are employed for this purpose. Since no laryngoscope can satisfy all requirements, the laryngeal surgeon should have an assortment of different models on hand. The most important are listed below:

- Kleinsasser laryngoscopes (sizes A–C, DN, J, JL)
- Bivalved laryngoscopes in various sizes (Rudert, Steiner, Weerda)
- Lindholm laryngoscope—when this is inserted into the vallecula epiglottica, it affords an excellent view of supraglottic structures (ideally, of the whole larynx)
- Diverticuloscope (Holinger-Benjamin) for endoscopic cricopharyngeal myotomy
- Pediatric laryngoscopes (various models)

Optimum instrumentation is just as important in the treatment of benign laryngeal lesions as it is in the surgery of malignant tumors. It may be even more so, inasmuch as tumor surgery is basically a destructive process while the surgery of benign laryngeal lesions is often a tailoring procedure. The goal in this type of surgery is not just to remove abnormalities but rather to modify and adapt (tailor) anatomic changes to allow for optimum functional rehabilitation of the voice, swallowing, and respiration. This can be achieved, as in phonosurgery, only by means of precise, noncharring laser tissue cutting without collateral thermal tissue damage, requiring the use of optimum instruments and equipment.

Laser Systems Used in the Endoscopic Surgery of Benign Laryngeal and Tracheal Lesions

The CO_2 laser is the undisputed workhorse of laser surgery in laryngology. Owing to its frequent use in tumor surgery, nowadays it is available in the ENT departments of most larger hospitals. The CO_2 laser meets the requirements for use for most benign laryngeal lesions, particularly in phonosurgery, stenosis surgery, swallowing rehabilitation, and in the resection of most benign laryngeal tumors [3, 13–17].

Besides the laser unit itself, accessories are available for the optimum delivery of laser energy to the operative site. These include devices for optimum focusing of the surgical beam (e. g., AccuSpot, Lumenis) [18], which focus the beam to an extremely small spot for precision cutting. Scanner systems (e. g., Surgitouch, Lumenis) [16] are also available for making a precise linear incision or for coagulating predefined mucosal areas while preserving the underlying tissue (e. g., in the treatment of laryngeal papillomatosis). A scanner system consists of a robotic guidance mechanism that tracks the CO_2 laser beam over a rectangular, round, or elliptical mucosal area selected by the operator on the micromanipulator of the laser head. Following a prede-

fined algorithm, the robotic mechanism scans the laser beam over the targeted area in a cruciform pattern at a preset speed and constant power output. This ensures that equal power densities and exposure times are delivered to all subareas of the selected scan area. The rapid movement of the laser beam leads to rapid heat dispersion in the tissue. Meanwhile the surface of the selected mucosal area is vaporized completely and uniformly while the underlying anatomic structures are largely preserved. This mode of laser use is suitable for the selective, superficial removal of mucosal lesions in cases where histologic examination is not required and the main aim is to achieve uniform tissue ablation with the least possible collateral injury. An example is the removal of papillomas or patchy areas of leukoplakia, which can be histologically confirmed prior to actual laser ablation. The result of this procedure is a superficial mucosal wound with no thermal alteration of the underlying tissue. This type of wound undergoes rapid secondary epithelialization and can heal to an excellent functional result. Scanners based on a similar working principle are also available for producing straight or curved incisions, as in a cricopharyngeal myotomy for a Zenker diverticulum (Accublade, Lumenis).

For the selection of suitable laser parameters (pulse shape and duration, power output, etc.), the reader is referred to selected publications [see references 19–22] and to Chapters 1, 2, and 6 of this volume.

In the treatment of laryngeal hemangiomas, especially when large, the neodymium:yttrium aluminum garnet (Nd:YAG) laser has the advantage of a greater penetration depth in tissue, producing deeper coagulation of the hemangioma [23, 24]. However, circumscribed hemangiomas can be successfully excised locally with the CO_2 laser. Argon lasers can also be used to treat vascular neoplasms owing to the absorption of the light by red blood pigment.

A special laser treatment modality is photodynamic therapy (tissue lasing following the selective uptake of a photosensitizing agent) [25–28]. The efficacy of photodynamic therapy has been documented for a number of benign, preneoplastic, and neoplastic mucosal lesions. On the other hand, the costs of the procedure and concerns about unpredictable mucosal scarring still limit its application in the treatment of benign lesions of the larynx and trachea.

Alternatives to Surgical Laser Use

Surgical lasers, particularly the CO_2 laser, can be used in various ways for the treatment of benign laryngeal and tracheal lesions:

- Tissue ablation (precise cutting with minimal coagulation for the resection of abnormal tissue)
- Coagulation (of blood vessels or very vascular neoplasms)
- Vaporization (of tissues, as for papilloma removal)
- Induction of photochemical processes (in photodynamic therapy)

Alternative techniques are available for all of these applications and will be briefly described below.

Tissue Ablation

Tissue ablation can be accomplished with sharp cutting instruments (knives, scissors)—the essential tools for selective tissue ablation in every surgical discipline. Special small knives and microscissors are available for traditional tissue ablation in the larynx and trachea [29], but these instruments require expert manual skills and rigorous practice. They are designed to have a long shaft that must be passed down the operating laryngoscope, making them less effective than the scalpels and scissors used in open operations. At the same time, the division of tissues with cutting instruments always involves capillaries and small arterial or venous vessels, leading to diffuse bleeding at the surgical site. Although the blood loss in the larynx is not quantitatively significant in itself, the bleeding nevertheless obscures the operative field and makes it difficult to assess the progress of the operation. This type of bleeding is particularly troublesome in the situation of maximum-precision microsurgery. Not infrequently, it prevents the surgical precision that is desired from a functional standpoint and prolongs the operating time. The bleeding, and the associated obstacles created during the surgery, can result in functional failures and persistent, undesired anatomic changes (scars, synechiae).

On the other hand, "cold" instruments offer the significant advantage of precise cutting with no thermal damage to surrounding tissues. This makes it easier for the pathologist to evaluate the margins of the excised tissues and eliminates the deleterious effects of collateral thermal damage on wound healing [30, 31]. Moreover, the use of cutting microinstruments in laryngeal surgery does not require the elaborate technical precautions necessitated by laser use.

In summary, there is no question that the ability of cold instruments to remove small lesions confined to the mucosa, especially in phonosurgery, is the equal of surgical lasers and is even superior to lasers in some situations. The CO_2 laser should be used for the phonosurgical ablation of mucosal lesions only by a highly skilled surgeon and only in settings where optimum technical facilities are available (Accuspot micromanipulator, precisely adjusted laser system, proficiency in laser use) [32–35].

Besides conventional instruments, powered instruments (microdebriders, shavers) for use in laryngeal and tracheal surgery have been described recently [36–38]. These instruments have been widely used in paranasal sinus surgery. Basically, they consist of a motorized blade rotating in a sheath with suction at the tip. Tissue is excised superficially by the rotating blade and simultaneously aspirated out of the sheath. Those advocating this type of instrument for endolaryngeal surgery (especially papilloma removal) have noted that shaver systems require less time for tissue ablation and do not generate a smoke plume. This argument is worth mentioning because human papillomavirus (HPV) DNA has been identified in the plume produced during the CO_2 laser vaporization of respiratory tract papillomas [39, 40]. Its clinical significance is uncertain however.

The difficult healing of "tissue burns" caused by endolaryngeal laser surgery has been cited as another argument for the use of microdebriders [41]. One fact should be emphasized at this point: surgical lasers cause burns in the larynx and trachea only if the surgeon is using an outdated device or is not well versed in modern laser surgery. In other words, burns following laser surgery are the fault of the operator, not of the method. Modern, fully equipped CO_2 laser systems enable the surgeon to divide tissue with absolute precision with a focused beam, without causing clinically significant thermal damage to normal surrounding tissue. Thus, the concern voiced by many authors that lasers cause "burns" is based on observations either from the early days of laser surgery or of improper laser use. When all facts are considered, the argument of thermal tissue damage and its implications for wound healing can no longer be taken seriously.

Moreover, it is unclear whether motorized instruments used on the very fine structures of the vocal cord mucosa pose an equal or even greater risk of inadvertent tissue damage than present-day laser technology. Let us consider an analogy with middle ear surgery: CO_2 lasers have gained an established place in stapes surgery, and today no ear surgeon would think of using shaver systems on the auditory ossicles. At the same time, microdebriders are probably an effective supplement to the surgical armamentarium for the rapid removal of larger neoplasms that do not require further histologic evaluation.

Coagulation

Besides surgical lasers (CO_2, Nd:YAG), electrocautery probes are commonly used to coagulate blood vessels and tissues having a rich blood supply. Before the advent of surgical lasers, electrocautery probes were widely used in endolaryngeal surgery [29, 42, 43]. They were used for cutting (e. g., arytenoidectomy) and tissue ablation (suction–coagulation during papilloma removal) and for the selective cauterization of small blood vessels. Today, classic electrosurgery is more of an adjunct to endolaryngeal laser surgery than a competing modality. It is no longer considered an acceptable tool for most procedures because it causes far more extensive thermal damage and cauterization of specimen margins than the CO_2 laser and cannot be manipulated as precisely as the laser beam.

When used as an adjunct to the CO_2 laser, electrosurgery is indispensable in all major endolaryngeal procedures because the CO_2 laser can only coagulate blood vessels up to a certain size. It is unable to coagulate large bleeders, such as those encountered in an arytenoidectomy or endolaryngeal partial laryngectomy, even when applied in the continuous mode with a defocused beam. In these cases the electrocautery probe is an essential adjunct to the laser for obtaining surgical hemostasis.

Electrosurgery as a stand-alone method has undergone technical refinements in recent years, and these improvements have eliminated some of the inherent disadvantages of electrosurgical procedures. For example, thermal tissue damage can be substantially reduced by irrigating the surgical site with water [44]. Good clinical results have been achieved by applying a continuous stream of noble gas to the tissue to be coagulated (argon beamer, argon plasma coagulation) [45–47]. This technique permits optimum electrocoagulation of the tissue while preventing carbonization. It has become an accepted alternative to laser surgery, particularly in operations on the nose and paranasal sinuses. So far there has been very little clinical experience with argon plasma coagulation in laryngeal surgery. But it is entirely conceivable that the method could be effective in treating vascular lesions located away from the vocal cords.

Vaporization

Aside from the argon plasma coagulation systems described above, basically there is no alternative to the CO_2 laser for tissue vaporization.

Photodynamic Therapy

Laser systems have ideal technical properties for inducing the desired photochemical reactions in tissue. Photodynamic therapy would not be possible without lasers. The question is which laser system is the most suitable. This question, just as that of choosing the best photosensitizing agent, is a topic of current research [48] and is beyond the scope of this chapter.

Anesthesia, Perioperative Care, and Adjunctive Medical Therapy

Laser surgery can be done under general endotracheal anesthesia and using jet ventilation [10, 11]. Endotracheal intubation is generally preferred in operations where there is likely to be heavy bleeding (tumor resections, arytenoidectomies, laryngeal papillomatosis). Special laser-safe tubes can be used to protect against tube combustion and airway fires, but they are expensive. Jet ventilation is preferred in operations for airway stenosis and in many phonosurgical procedures, as it provides a better view of the glottis and subglottis.

Even extensive endolaryngeal procedures can almost always be done without a prior tracheotomy when surgical lasers are used [49–51]. The present author has achieved good results with the routine i.v. administration of 250 mg methylprednisolone before endolaryngeal procedures. Antibiotic prophylaxis (e.g., 3 g ampicillin–sulbactam or 600 mg clindamycin i.v.) is also given for more extensive procedures, especially those involving the exposure of laryngeal cartilages. Patients generally require postoperative monitoring in an intensive care unit (ICU) following laser surgery for airway stenosis. At this time the patient should be awake and extubated. For all other procedures, ICU monitoring is generally unnecessary from a surgical standpoint.

Surgical Endoscopy

Diagnostic laryngoscopy is indicated for all laryngeal diseases in which the larynx cannot be examined in the conscious patient (children) or in which mirror laryngoscopy, telescopic laryngoscopy, or flexible endoscopy has revealed findings in the larynx, hypopharynx, or trachea that require further investigation. Suspension laryngoscopy provides ideal access for many diagnostic and therapeutic procedures in the trachea, in which the laryngoscope can serve as a "sheath" for the introduction of tracheoscopes and operating instruments (Figs. 5.**1**, 5.**2**). Besides inspection of the mucosal surface with the operating microscope and introduction of rigid endoscopes, this technique allows selective excisional biopsies, even enabling the surgeon to take large samples if required. In additional, visual inspection can be supplemented by tactile examination (e.g., to assess the mobility of an ankylosed arytenoid cartilage).

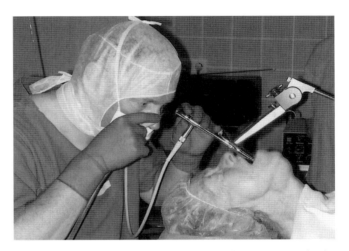

Fig. 5.**1** Suspension laryngoscopy for tracheal access. A rigid telescope is passed into the trachea through the laryngoscope. Tracheal secretions are simultaneously aspirated.

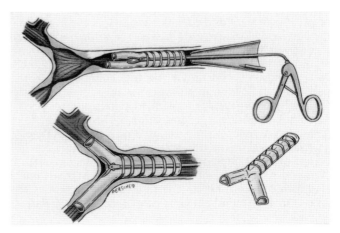

Fig. 5.**2** Endoscopic tracheal surgery through the laryngoscope using jet ventilation. A rigid tracheoscope is introduced through the laryngoscope, allowing dilatation and stenting of a neoplastic tracheal stenosis.

Currently, the CO_2 laser can be used for excisional biopsies, completely resecting smaller mucosal lesions of indeterminate nature in a procedure that is both diagnostic and therapeutic.

■ Phonosurgery

Phonosurgery is the term applied to all surgical measures aimed at improving the voice (in a broad sense, it also includes voice rehabilitation after laryngectomy).

Classification

Based on a proposal by the European Laryngological Society (ELS), phonosurgical procedures can be grouped into four classes [52]:
- Vocal fold surgery: surgical procedures carried out directly on the vocal cords (generally endolaryngeal) with the goal of improving the vibrational properties of the vocal cords or glottic closure.
- Laryngeal framework surgery: procedures done on the cartilaginous skeleton of the larynx or the laryngeal musculature to correct the position, shape, or tension of the vocal cords.
- Neuromuscular surgery: procedures done on the nerves of the larynx with the goal of restoring or improving the mobility and/or tension of the vocal cords.
- Reconstructive surgery addressing partial or total laryngeal defects: procedures done to restore or improve the voice after surgically induced loss of function.

This chapter deals with the predominant use of lasers in phonosurgery: vocal cord surgery. Other works should be consulted for details of laryngeal framework procedures and neuromuscular surgery.

Preoperative Diagnosis

In otologic surgery, one or more preoperative tests are done to provide a functional description of the affected ear. The preoperative audiogram describes the existing functional impairment and provides a baseline for evaluating the outcome of the tympanoplasty. The same basic principles should be applied in phonosurgery. These cases also require a preoperative functional description, although there is no universal measuring tool comparable to the pure-tone audiogram in otology. The author feels that the minimal workup before a planned phonosurgical procedure should include an examination of the larynx by telescopic laryngoscopy and stroboscopy, a perceptual voice analysis (based on the HBR scale), and generally a determination of vocal pitch and loudness range and maximum phonation time. Videoendoscopic documentation and a digital voice recording provide an ideal baseline for evaluating the treatment outcome, although these resources will not be available at every center.

Laser Surgery of the Vocal Cords

Laser surgery on the vocal cords may be done for a number of conditions such as epithelial changes (vocal nodules, leukoplakia, hyperkeratosis, acanthosis, dysplasia, etc.), exudative changes in the Reinke space (vocal cord polyps, Reinke edema), granulomas (contact granuloma, intubation granuloma), scarring, and subepithelial lesions (cysts) [16, 53–57]. The use of the CO_2 laser in particular is highly controversial for these indications [31, 33, 57, 58]. While the advocates of laser surgery state that lasers using non-contact technique are ideal for making precise, atraumatic, bloodless mucosal incisions, the proponents of "cold instruments" claim that laser incisions always cause poorly healing burns followed by unpredictable scarring, often with adverse functional consequences. It is likely that both views are correct,

With a modern CO_2 laser operated by a well-trained surgeon using optimum equipment and state-of-the-art peripheral devices (AccuSpot), the laser can indeed cut tissues atraumatically and without charring [15, 16, 18, 20, 30]. Under these ideal conditions, CO_2 lasers are excellent instruments for use in phonosurgery, although operating time can be considerably prolonged in some cases. The use of less optimal lasers by inadequately trained surgeons can cause significant thermal damage to the mucosa far beyond that caused by microsurgical incisions with conventional instruments. Thus, vocal cord surgery with or without a CO_2 laser (i. e., using hot or cold instruments) is less a matter of deciding in favor of one technique or the other than a matter of the availability of equipment and the surgeon's training and proficiency. Moreover, the use of a laser system does not compel the surgeon to use the laser exclusively. The laser surgeon is free to use the instrument (hot or cold) that is best for any given situation.

Several common surgical lesions of the vocal cords are discussed briefly in the sections below.

Idiopathic Granulomas (Contact Granulomas)

The etiology of contact granulomas is not yet fully understood. The disease affects males almost exclusively. The typical configuration of the male larynx, where there is a relatively small angle between the thyroid laminae, is believed to contribute to the more frequent occurrence of contact granulomas in males. The causal mechanism may be repeated microtrauma to the mucosa on the medial side of the arytenoid cartilage during phonation. The microtrauma, whose repetitive nature keeps the mucosal wound from healing once it has developed, apparently incites the formation of granulation tissue. Gastroesophageal reflux into the pharynx has also been cited as a possible etiologic factor [59–61].

Telescopic laryngoscopy generally reveals a typical granuloma located on the medial side of an arytenoid cartilage (Fig. 5.3). In any given case, it is often unclear whether the dysphonia is related to the granuloma or whether it is a sign of abnormal functional processes in the larynx, which

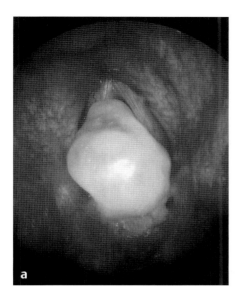

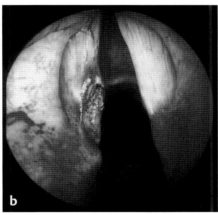

Fig. 5.**3** Large contact granuloma on the left vocal cord. **a** Microlaryngoscopic view. **b** Appearance after laser ablation.

in turn may contribute to the granuloma formation. Granulomas should be surgically removed to establish the diagnosis. This can be done in ideal fashion with the CO_2 laser (using jet ventilation), because the laser allows precise ablation with good hemostasis without damaging the cartilaginous tissue. Medical treatment with proton pump inhibitors is often recommended in the literature to prevent a recurrence, but the author has not had encouraging results with these agents. While this conclusion is not based on a systematic analysis, it is the author's impression that this therapy does not reduce the number of recurrences compared with patients who have not received proton pump inhibitors. Also, the phenotype and psychological profile of patients with contact granuloma do not appear to support reflux disease as the cause of the lesions. The disease is particularly common in patients with a very correct, conscientious personality type who are not overweight, generally do not smoke, and do not drink excessively. In contrast, vocal cord granulomas occur very rarely in patients with a known history of severe reflux disease. Thus, once the lesions have been removed by laser abla-

tion, the patient often undergoes counseling until the condition resolves spontaneously, often after a period of years.

Intubation Granulomas

Intubation granulomas resemble contact granulomas in their gross and microscopic features, but they may be bilateral and also occur in women and children. Removal follows the principles outlined above with the lesions much less likely to recur than in contact granulomas.

Vocal Nodules

Functional voice disorders and vocal overuse often lead to circumscribed epithelial thickening of the free edges of the vocal cords, usually located at the junction of the anterior and middle thirds and situated at opposite sites on both cords. All vocal nodules do not require surgical removal. They should be removed only if they obstruct complete glottic closure. Whether the nodules are resected (very sparingly, always preserving the underlying vocal ligament) with microinstrumentation or a meticulous laser technique (single pulse, low power density) depends less on theoretical considerations than on the personal experience of the surgeon [34, 35].

Reinke Edema

Fluid accumulation in Reinke's space beneath the surface of the vocal cords increases the volume and mass of the vibrating portions of the cords, lowering the pitch of the voice in affected individuals [62, 63]. Many patients accept this low-pitched voice as a personality trait. Surgery should be withheld in these cases unless the edema is hampering respiration or there are concomitant mucosal changes suspicious for malignancy (leukoplakia, etc.). But if the edema is causing a subjective deterioration of voice quality, decreased voice performance, or a fluctuating voice quality, it should be surgically corrected.

In all cases the vocal effects of surgical ablation should be discussed with the patient preoperatively, giving particular attention to the anticipated (irreversible) increase in vocal pitch, the transient worsening of dysphonia, and the fact that surgical procedures for Reinke edema generally do not completely restore the voice [64]. The patient should be informed that the surgical treatment and the subsequent period of voice rest are only part of the overall treatment plan, which should include functional voice therapy and long-term vocal hygiene which involves avoiding vocal misuse and smoking.

The operation begins by making a mucosal incision lateral to the free edge of the vocal cord, near the floor of Morgagni's pouch, extending the full length of the cord. The incision can be made with a microsurgical instrument or a surgical laser. The CO_2 laser can also provide point coagulation of thickened blood vessels in the mucosa. Next the gelatinous edema is suctioned from Reinke's space without causing further damage to the mucosa. The mucosal flaps are then reapproximated, resecting (with a laser or cold instrument) the mucosa made redundant by the decreased volume. Ideally, the mucosal flaps should be apposed edge to edge. The free edges of the vocal cords should be protected from injury and should be covered with intact epithelium at the end of the operation. In this way both sides can be treated in one sitting. If there is very extensive edema with scarring, it can be difficult or impossible to carry out the technique as described. If there is epithelial tearing or the vocal ligament is exposed at the free edge on one side, it is better to defer operating on the second side to avoid the risk of synechia formation. These cases require a two-stage procedure in which the second side is treated after the first side has healed.

Vocal Cord Polyps

Vocal cord polyps, as Reinke edema, are exudative lesions of Reinke's space but are more circumscribed than the edema. They can be removed with microscissors or with a CO_2 laser beam in the single-pulse mode (Fig. 5.**4 a–d**) [65].

Vocal Cord Cysts

Typical subepithelial vocal cord cysts should be exposed by careful incision of the mucosa, isolated by blunt dissection, and removed in one piece without opening the cyst wall to reduce the risk of recurrence (similar to middle ear cholesteatomas) (Fig. 5.5 **a, b**). The author prefers to use the Kleinsasser microinstrument set (Karl Storz) or Bouchayer set (Micro-France, Xomed) for this purpose, and not the laser.

Surgical Voice Rehabilitation

Surgical lasers are occasionally used to create a speech fistula in patients who have undergone a total laryngectomy [66]. The author does not feel that this procedure offers any special advantages over established methods of prosthetic voice restoration, and these options will not be described here.

■ Surgery to Improve Swallowing

Difficulty in swallowing (dysphagia) is a relatively common presenting complaint in the practice of otolaryngolo-

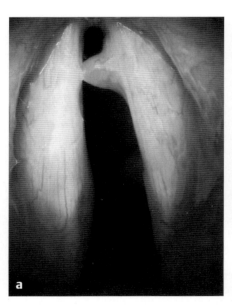
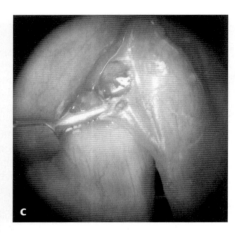
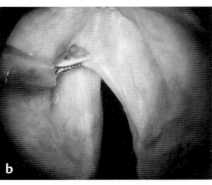
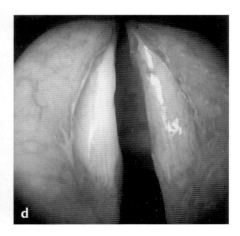

Fig. 5.**4** Polyp on the right vocal cord. **a** Microlaryngoscopic view. **b** The mucosa is grasped with a Bouchayer forceps. **c** The mucosa is incised with the CO_2 laser in single-pulse mode, using the AccuSpot system for bloodless cutting without charring. **d** Appearance at the end of the operation.

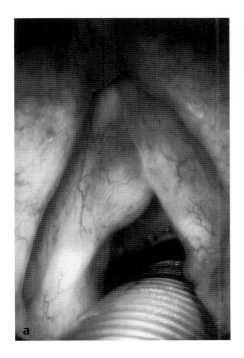 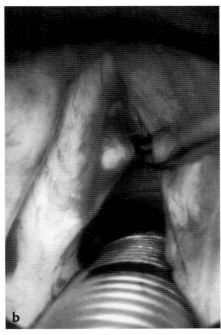

Fig. 5.**5** Large subepithelial cyst of the left vocal cord. **a** Microlaryngoscopic view. **b** The cyst is exposed by microsurgical (not laser) incision of the mucosa and removed in toto.

gy. It is reasonable to expect that, with the growing percentage of older individuals in the overall population, the numbers will increase in the future.

Classification

Dysphagia may present with any one of three main symptoms:
- Obstruction (impairment of bolus transport)
- Aspiration (inhalation of food particles or saliva)
- Globus sensation (vague feeling of fullness in the throat, often perceived subjectively as "difficult swallowing" although solid foods and fluids are still swallowed normally)

Surgical treatment is an option only for obstruction or aspiration-related dysphagia. No sound rationale exists for the operative treatment of globus sensation.

Obstruction

Swallowing of food may be obstructed by mass lesions in the oral cavity, oropharynx, hypopharynx, or esophagus or by disturbances of neuromuscular regulation, especially absent or delayed opening of the upper esophageal sphincter (cricopharyngeus muscle) during swallowing. Pharyngeal masses leading to dysphagia may be due to hyperplasia of the lymphatic Waldeyer ring (hyperplasia of the tonsils or lymphatic tissue at the base of the tongue) or benign and malignant tumors of the oral cavity, pharynx, and esophagus. The treatment of benign tumors is covered later and the treatment of malignant tumors is discussed in Chapter 6.

Obstruction of the foodway by tonsillar hyperplasia can be treated medically (for acute inflammation) or surgically

(tonsillectomy) (see Chapter 4). In children, laser tonsillotomy may be appropriate if the goal is to reduce the volume of the tonsils while preserving tonsillar remnants for immunologic reasons [67].

The treatment of Zenker diverticulum has become an established domain of laser surgery during recent years. These diverticula develop as a result of deficient or delayed relaxation of the cricopharyngeus muscle [68] during swallowing. Until a few years ago, open cricopharyngeus myotomy combined with diverticulectomy through a left transcervical approach was the standard surgical treatment for Zenker diverticula [69–71]. Although endoscopic myotomy (division of the posterior part of the annular cricopharyngeus muscle) was described as early as 1917, the endoscopic approach was abandoned later due to excessive complications. Van Overbeek, in particular, showed that endoscopic crico-pharyngeal myotomy could be undertaken with a high degree of precision using the CO_2 laser (Fig. 5.**6 a–e**) [71]. According to the literature, the complications and results of endoscopic myotomies appear to be comparable to or better than those achieved with open surgery [72–76]. In any case, endoscopic myotomy obviates the need for an external neck incision and practically eliminates the risk of recurrent nerve paralysis. Generally the myotomy can be done without difficulty when a special diverticuloscope (Dohlman type) is used. There is disagreement as to whether patients should be fed through a temporary nasogastric tube (placed preoperatively and carefully protected during laser use) or by temporary parenteral nutrition. Opinions also vary as to the timing of the initial feeding after endoscopic myotomy. An interval of 2–7 days is most commonly recommended. In all cases, oral contrast examination with a water-soluble medium (Gastrografin) should be done before the resumption of oral intake to exclude paravasation into the upper mediastinum.

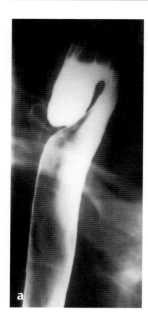

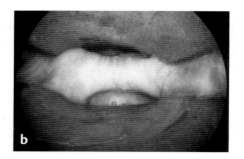

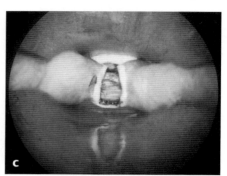

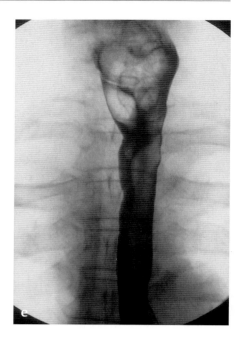

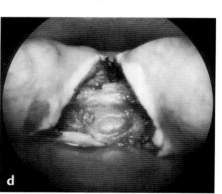

Fig. 5.**6** A typical Zenker diverticulum. **a** Preoperative contrast radiograph of the esophagus. **b** Diverticuloscope demonstrates the common wall between the diverticular sac and esophagus. **c** Laser incision of the common wall in the midline. **d** Complete cricopharyngeal myotomy. **e** No swallowing difficulties 3 months after endoscopic laser myotomy.

Although endoscopic myotomy is technically straightforward, it should be emphasized that this procedure is by no means without risks. Contrary to van Overbeek's belief that the anterior wall of the diverticular sac is always fused to the posterior wall of the esophagus by inflammatory adhesions, minimizing the risk of opening the mediastinum during endoscopic myotomy, in the author's experience in the open surgery of Zenker diverticula such adhesions are rarely if ever present. In any case, they do not offer adequate protection against opening the mediastinum. It should be assumed, rather, that any complete cricopharyngeal myotomy will open the upper mediastinum. This underscores the urgent need for preoperative antibiotic prophylaxis. Local mucosal antisepsis in the region of the hypopharynx and diverticular sac may also help lower the risk of infection.

Mild wound pain, leukocytosis, and temperature elevation are common after the operation, especially during the first night [72]. These findings alone do not indicate significant mediastinitis. But if the temperature remains elevated beyond the first day or does not respond promptly to antipyretic agents, and if the patient has res-

piration-dependent back pain, local warmth in the neck region, or other manifestations of a septic systemic process, appropriate imaging studies should be done at once to assess the need for surgical intervention (opening the upper mediastinum through a left cervical incision, oversewing an esophageal perforation, local irrigation) (Fig. 5.7). Thus, endoscopic surgery for Zenker diverticula is relatively easy to do but is not risk free. The surgeon should take note of the potential risks and should be prepared to manage them.

Aspiration

Aspiration may result from loss of substance, especially in the larynx (e. g., after a supraglottic partial laryngectomy), or it may have a neurogenic cause (e. g., lesions of the superior laryngeal nerve or vagus nerve). These forms of dysphagia are not amenable to correction by laser surgery [70].

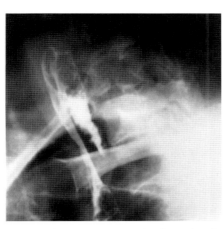

Fig. 5.**7**   Contrast extravasation from the pharynx after endoscopic myotomy, with incipient mediastinitis—treated surgically by mediastinal drainage through a lateral neck incision.

Cricopharyngeus Motility Disorders without Diverticula

Delayed relaxation of the cricopharyngeus muscle during swallowing can occasionally lead to dysphagia, which often is accompanied by secondary aspiration. A diverticulum is not (yet) demonstrable in all cases. The disorder is more common in older individuals. Video cinematography is generally necessary to make a diagnosis. Unlike a conventional oral contrast examination, the temporal resolution of this technique is high enough to demonstrate the underlying functional disorder. As for Zenker diverticula, the recommended treatment is endoscopic myotomy [77]. The author has no personal experience with the endoscopic treatment of this disorder and would prefer an open-neck myotomy (to avoid the risk of opening the pharynx and possibly causing mediastinitis).

Surgical Alternatives to Laser Use (Stapler, Botulinum Toxin, Open Myotomy)

A number of alternatives to laser surgery are available for the treatment of Zenker diverticulum and cricopharyngeal dysfunction. Endoscopic myotomy with a stapler has been recommended from a surgical and laryngologic standpoint in recent years [69, 78, 79]. The device is an automatic stapler of the type commonly used in open abdominal surgery. A special stapler has beed developed for the treatment of Zenker diverticula and can be introduced and operated through a diverticuloscope. It divides the common wall between the diverticular sac and esophagus, simultaneously closing the wound surfaces on both sides with staples. This technique is supposed to prevent leakage into the mediastinum. Because of the way the stapler is designed, a part of the wound always remains open at the lowest point of the incision [80]. The author has no personal basis for judging whether this method actually offers advantages over endolaryngeal laser surgery. The results in the literature are comparable to those of endolaryngeal laser surgery, and there is no published evidence showing definite advantages.

Open myotomy is always available as an alternative to endoscopic myotomy in cases where it is important to avoid opening the pharynx. The surgery is done through a left transcervical approach, like the classic operation for treating a Zenker diverticulum. Following meticulous division of the cricopharyngeus muscle, the pharynx is closed. There is virtually no risk of infection under these conditions (with proper attention to surgical asepsis). The procedure can thus provide an alternative to endoscopic myotomy and the classic open operation for Zenker diverticula in all patients considered to be at increased risk for mediastinitis (patients with multiple morbidities, older patients). To the author's knowledge, however, no comparative studies on this technique have been published.

An elegant, minimally invasive treatment option is to temporarily paralyze the cricopharyngeus muscle by the localized injection of botulinum toxin [81]. The advantage of this method is that it is practically free of complications when carried out correctly. The disadvantage is that its effect lasts only a few months, at which time the treatment may have to be repeated (generally necessitating brief general anesthesia). Thus botulinum toxin injection is not a permanent treatment option. It does, however, provide an ideal test method in equivocal cases to determine whether the proposed surgical division of the cricopharyngeus muscle will improve the patient's symptoms. If the symptoms improve following transient paralysis of the muscle with botulinum toxin and then worsen again after the effect has subsided, the patient can be scheduled for a definitive cricopharyngeal myotomy.

■ Laser Treatment of Airway Stenosis

The larynx forms the narrowest part of the central respiratory tract [82]. As a result, anatomic changes can easily lead to clinically significant airway narrowing [83]. The relative narrowness of the respiratory tract at this level is based on the physiologic function of the larynx as a safety valve between the upper respiratory and alimentary tracts. Because of its dual functions in preventing aspiration and producing speech, the larynx must be able to close the airway temporarily when needed. Disturbances of this physiologic process can lead to permanent narrowing of the airway lumen. Inflammatory swelling, scarring, and tumor masses can also narrow or obstruct the airway.

Classification

The symptoms of central airway stenosis depend on the location and type of the stenosis and the degree of airway narrowing. The main etiologic factors are summarized in Table 5.**1**. Several etiologic categories of airway stenosis are described below.

Malformations

The most common laryngeal malformation causing respiratory obstruction is laryngomalacia. Based on a congenital

Table 5.**1**   Classification of laryngeal stenosis

Time course	Acute
	Subacute
	Chronic
	Recurrent
Location of the stenosis	Supraglottis (accompanying feature: dysphagia)
	Glottis (accompanying feature: dysphonia)
	Subglottis
	Laryngotracheal junction
Degree of airway narrowing	Mild (no clinical manifestations)
	Moderate (with clinical signs of obstruction but not life-threatening)
	Severe (pronounced airway obstruction with risk of respiratory decompensation)
	Asphyxia
Anatomic form of the stenosis	Bilateral recurrent nerve paralysis or arytenoid cartilage fixation
	Mucosal scar (web)
	Postchondritic scar
	Extraluminal compression
	Intraluminal tumor growth
	Floppy wall leading to stenosis (malacia)
	Mixed forms
Etiology	
Malformations	Laryngeal malformations
	Laryngomalacia
Inflammatory	Diphtheria (croup)
	Epiglottis
	Bacterial tracheitis
	Viral laryngotracheitis (pseudocroup)
	Tuberculosis, sarcoidosis
Traumatic	Laryngeal fractures, soft-tissue injuries
	Insect stings
	Intubation trauma (arytenoid cartilage fixation)
Immunologic	Allergic mucosal swelling
	Rheumatoid arthritis
	Polychondritis
	Wegener granulomatosis
	Amyloidosis
Neurogenic	Recurrent or vagus nerve paralysis
	Iatrogenic
	Traumatic
	Inflammatory
	Compression or vascular disease
	CNS or skull base tumors
	Neck tumors
	Mediastinal tumors
	Papilloma
	Hemangioma
	Lipoma
	Many other rare tumors
	Laryngeal carcinoma
	Sarcoma
	Malignant lymphoma
	Secondary tumor invasion
	Laryngoceles
	Intubation-related (postchondritic stenosis)
	Intubation-related (arytenoid cartilage fixation)
	After tracheotomy
	Malacias

flaccidity of the entire epiglottis, it allows the epiglottis to prolapse over the larynx during inspiration, producing a stridorous noise on forced inspiration. In the great majority of cases, the symptoms resolve completely with further growth as the cartilaginous part of the epiglottis becomes stiff enough to prevent inspiratory prolapse. Only a few cases require an endoscopic procedure to improve respira-

tion. Less common congenital malformations are synechiae of the ligamentous glottis, laryngeal clefts, and subglottic hemangiomas [2, 53]. Laryngeal atresia is an extremely rare anomaly that generally leads to immediate postpartum death from asphyxiation after the umbilical cord has been cut. With improvements in prenatal diagnosis, however, it is reasonable to expect that more of these children will be saved by intrauterine or intrapartum surgery.

Inflammatory Stenosis

Inflammatory laryngeal stenosis is very rare in adults (exceptions: epiglottitis and glottic stenosis due to severe Reinke edema) but is a frequent and dreaded condition in children [84, 85]. Acute infections of the larynx and trachea are particularly ominous in children due to the small size of their airways [83]. Swelling of the mucosa or a buildup of tracheal secretions can cause considerably greater obstruction of the anatomically smaller airways than that in adult patients. Acute obstructive airway inflammations in children are a heterogeneous group of infectious diseases with a common presentation marked by a typical barking cough (croup), inspiratory stridor, hoarseness, and airway obstruction [86]. Generally these cases are managed by endoscopy, endolaryngeal intubation or tracheotomy, specific high-dose antibiotic therapy, or intensive care of the affected child. Further surgical measures are not required.

Traumatic Laryngeal Stenosis

Blunt and sharp trauma to the neck can cause acute laryngeal stenosis. Emergency intubation can be difficult in these cases, and tracheotomy is occasionally required. Particularly severe injuries are seen after suicidal hanging or gunshot injuries to the larynx (avulsing the trachea from the larynx). The most common laryngeal injuries today, which generally resolve spontaneously, are caused by intubation [87, 88]. Emergency intubation under unfavorable conditions can cause permanent trauma-related changes in the larynx, especially arytenoid cartilage fixation (see Fig. 5.3). In this condition the arytenoid cartilage is fixed in the cricoarytenoid joint, causing vocal cord immobility [89]. Some of these cases are clinically indistinguishable from recurrent nerve paralysis, but the correct diagnosis is suggested by the history, passive mobility of the arytenoid cartilage during microlaryngoscopic examination under anesthesia, and by electromyography to record summation action potentials from the muscle groups supplied by the inferior laryngeal nerve [90, 91]. Table 5.**2** gives the frequency of various etiologic factors in recurrent nerve paralysis and arytenoid cartilage fixation.

Neurogenic Laryngeal Stenosis

Paralysis of the vagus nerve or, more commonly, of the inferior laryngeal nerve most frequently occurs after surgical procedures in the neck (especially on the thyroid gland) and upper mediastinum (see Table 5.**2**) [92]. It may also be caused by malignant tumors invading the larynx, hypopharynx, esophagus, thyroid, or tracheobronchial tree

Table 5.**2**   Etiologic factors in 218 consecutive patients with bilateral vocal cord fixation in a paramedian or median position and consequent airway stenosis requiring surgery*

Etiologic factor	Bilateral recurrent nerve paralysis		Bilateral arytenoid cartilage fixation		Total	
	n	%	n	%	n	%
Iatrogenic (postsurgical)	154	82.8	1	3.1	155	71.1
Revision thyroid surgery	141	75.8	0		141	91.0
Primary thyroid surgery	4	2.2	0		4	2.6
Esophageal surgery	4	2.2	0		4	2.6
Other surgery	5	2.7	1	100	6	3.8
Long-term intubation (>24 hours)	0		22	68.8	22	10.1
Malignant tumors	16	8.6	0		16	7.3
Esophageal carcinoma	9	56.2	0		9	56.2
Bronchial carcinoma	4	25.0	0		4	25.0
Others	3	18.8	0		3	18.8
Short-term intubation	5	2.7	3	9.4	8	3.7
Neurogenic	7	3.8	0		7	3.2
Wegener granulomatosis	0		3	9.4	3	1.4
Rheumatoid arthritis	0		2	6.2	2	0.9
Suicidal caustic ingestion	0		1	3.1	1	0.5
Others or unknown	4	2.2	0		4	1.8
Total	186	100	32	100	218	100

*   Department of Otorhinolaryngology, Cologne University Hospital, 1991–2000 (after [89]).

and other malignant neoplasms in the lower neck or upper mediastinum [51]. Neurogenic laryngeal stenosis may also develop during the course of viral inflammations or as a result of central nervous system processes (cerebral or skull-base tumors, injuries, surgical procedures on the lateral skull base) [89]. The preoperative recognition of concomitant superior laryngeal nerve paralysis on one side is important because it is a contraindication for surgical measures (especially arytenoidectomy) that could result in increased aspiration.

Cicatricial Stenosis

Stenosis due to scarring most commonly results from intubation or surgical procedures on the larynx and trachea (partial laryngectomy, tracheotomy, surgery of laryngeal papillomas). The most dreaded lesions are subglottic stenosis and laryngotracheal junction stenosis secondary to previous cricoid chondritis. These severe stenoses consistently warrant complex surgical procedures for airway restoration.

Cicatricial stenoses develop gradually over time and therefore they often remain undetected in hospitalized patients following prolonged intubation. A slowly progressive central airway obstruction develops only after the patient has been released. Less commonly, a cicatricial stenosis at the laryngotracheal junction may develop in the setting of Wegener granulomatosis with the secondary development of vasculitis. Generally the disease begins with a prolonged inflammatory process involving the upper respiratory tract, especially the nose and paranasal sinuses, but the larynx is also commonly involved. This leads to a granulating,

nonresolving inflammation of the subglottic larynx often culminating in scarring and stenosis.

Malacic Tracheal Stenosis

Prolonged external pressure on the trachea or the cartilaginous framework of the subglottic larynx, as well as prior inflammatory reactions, can lead to softening of the cartilaginous framework, resulting in malacic stenosis of the airway. Similar instability may develop following surgical procedures on the trachea. Collapse of the malacic airway is most likely to occur during inspiration, but increased expiratory resistance may also be found. Typically the degree of stenosis increases with the forcefulness of inspiration. While respiration is only mildly impaired during shallow breathing, the airway compromise becomes worse with increasing exertion, and complete obstruction can occur in extreme cases. In many patients, malacic stenosis is reliably detected by imaging procedures and is often missed during rigid endoscopy, since the malacic portions of the trachea does not prolapse in response to respiratory pressure changes during this examination. The most reliable diagnostic procedure is flexible tracheoscopy in the conscious, spontaneously breathing patient.

Tumor-Related Stenosis

Most stenoses of the central airways develop as a result of nonneoplastic disease. Occasionally, however, benign and malignant tumors can produce this type of stenosis. While there is often no difficulty in diagnosing the cause since the underlying disease is usually known, these stenoses are often difficult to treat unless the tumor can be treated surgically or radiotherapeutically with curative intent (e. g., primary laryngeal carcinoma). Higher-grade strictures of the central airways caused by tumors and metastases can lead to life-threatening airway obstruction. If the underlying disease is not amenable to curative treatment (e. g., an advanced thyroid or esophageal malignancy that has invaded the larynx), the airway should be recanalized to prevent death from asphyxia. Often this requires an interdisciplinary approach, tailored to the individual case, to spare the patient an agonizing death by asphyxiation [4, 15, 39, 71].

Primary tumors of the trachea are very rare, and malignant tracheal tumors are believed to be slightly more common than benign tumors. The most frequent histologic entities are adenoid cystic carcinoma, squamous cell carcinoma, mucoepidermoid tumors, and carcinoids. Besides rare mesenchymal malignancies (malignant lymphoma, sarcoma, malignant melanoma), distant metastases from tumors in other organs are occasionally found in the trachea (hypernephroma, breast carcinoma, malignant melanoma) [15]. Primary tracheal tumors are a less common cause of malignant tracheal stenosis than tumors invading the trachea secondarily from the esophagus, thyroid, larynx, or bronchial tree. The symptoms of primary tracheal tumors are nonspecific: persistent cough and an eventual inspiratory stridor, often mistaken initially for asthma. The correct diagnosis is not made until the patient manifests dyspnea due to progressive tracheal narrowing, hemoptysis, or persistent hoarseness due to infiltration of the recurrent nerve. In cases where the trachea is involved secondarily by solid tumors from adjacent organs, the underlying disease is generally known and it is not difficult to interpret the symptoms.

Indications for Surgical Treatment

Surgical correction is not appropriate for every central airway stenosis. The need for surgery depends in part on whether the stenosis is acute or chronic, the resulting adaptation of the respiratory muscles to the increased central airway resistance (conditioning), and especially the degree to which the respiratory compromise restricts normal levels of physical activity. Studies by the author indicate that an inspiratory resistance of more than 2.5 kPa × s/L is a good empirical cut-off point for selecting patients who require surgical correction. Ultimately, however, the decision to operate will depend on the level of physical exertion at which the patient can still compensate for the stenosis through increased respiration [93, 94].

Preoperative Diagnosis

Electrophysiologic Testing

Bilateral recurrent nerve palsy is reversible in principle, but its treatment is irreversible (in the case of surgical glottis expansion) or invasive (in the case of tracheotomy). This unusual set of circumstances calls for a particularly rigorous approach to diagnosis. On the one hand, it is important to select cases in which adequate functional restoration of

vocal cord mobility will not be achieved so that respiration can be normalized by an endoscopic procedure to widen the glottis. This should be done as soon as possible after the onset of damage to spare the patient a tracheotomy if at all possible. On the other hand, it is important to withhold definitive glottic expansion in cases where vocal cord mobility would be expected to recover adequately without further surgery. At present, electrophysiologic testing offers the only means of satisfying these requirements in a large number of cases with an acceptable degree of confidence [90, 91].

Respiratory Function Testing

The flow–volume curve is the simplest and most rewarding function test for diagnosing a central airway obstruction. Glottic stenosis alter the flow–volume curve by causing increased airway resistance, turbulence (at high flow rates), and a decrease in luminal cross section. Unlike an anatomically fixed cicatricial stenosis of the subglottis or trachea, the airway stenosis associated with bilateral recurrent nerve paralysis is characterized by a passive abduction of the vocal cords during expiration and adduction (medialization) of the cords through a suction effect (Bernoulli) during inspiration. This produces a characteristic curve with extreme inspiratory flattening, often accompanied by an essentially normal expiratory pattern [94].

Therapeutic Options

Supraglottic Stenosis

Supraglottic stenosis of the larynx is rare. It occasionally develops as a sequel to caustic injuries of the larynx and pharynx or as a result of surgical procedures, especially supraglottic partial laryngectomy. Laser surgery has repeatedly been used in an attempt to divide circumferential scar-tissue bands, but personal experience indicates that the results are hardly ever permanent. Generally this type of stenosis is repaired in an open operation either by resecting the stenosis and restoring the circumferential continuity of the larynx or by creating an epiglottic advancement flap to reconstruct the supraglottic airway [95].

Glottic Airway Stenosis

Bilateral Recurrent Nerve Paralysis

Acute bilateral recurrent nerve paralysis generally presents at once as a severe inspiratory airway obstruction, which is often stridorous. Occasionally a tracheotomy may be necessary if the patient can no longer tolerate the increased inspiratory resistance. It must be decided on a case-by-case basis whether immediate surgery should be done to expand the larynx as an alternative to tracheotomy, although it is usually still too early to make an accurate prognostic assessment in patients whose paralysis is of very recent onset [90]. Occasionally the prognosis of recurrent nerve paralysis can be based on the clinical situation, as in the case of a thyroidectomy for thyroid carcinoma in which a recurrent nerve had to be deliberately sacrificed. It is rarely possible, however, to make such a confident prognosis based on clinical status alone. Electromyography is useful for making a prognostic assessment, although this cannot be done with certainty in patients with neurapraxic paralysis [90, 91, 96]. A confident prognosis can be made only by waiting and watching for the return of normal vocal cord mobility over a period of 6–9 (up to 12) months. It should be noted that in cases with bilateral paralysis, the prognosis may be quite different for each of the affected sides. It is not unusual for the paralysis on one side to regress over time while that on the opposite side persists indefinitely.

Once the acute respiratory compromise caused by bilateral recurrent nerve paralysis of recent onset has been overcome by adaptation of the respiratory muscles, most patients can breathe well at rest and during mild physical exertion. The indication for glottis-expanding surgery in these cases is based on (i) a lack of exercise tolerance and (ii) the potential risk to the patient from sporadic respiratory inflammations (flu-like infections) that may cause swelling of the already-tight glottis. With few exceptions, we feel that glottis-expanding surgery is indicated for bilateral recurrent nerve paralysis to restore at least partially the patient's exercise tolerance and reduce the risk of asphyxiation due to respiratory infections. As long as the degree of respiratory compromise is acceptable to the patient at rest and during mild exercise, it is reasonable to wait for approximately 9 months after the onset of paralysis to watch for spontaneous recovery of nerve function.

While extralaryngeal surgical procedures (lateral fixation with its numerous variants) were once the standard treatment for bilateral vocal cord paralysis [97, 98], endoscopic techniques have advanced considerably since the popularization of endolaryngeal arytenoidectomy by Kleinsasser [42, 43] and especially since the advent of endolaryngeal laser surgery. Today, endoscopic procedures have largely replaced open laryngeal surgery in the treatment of this disorder. A number of endolaryngeal procedures for expanding the glottis have been described in recent years as a treatment for bilateral recurrent nerve paralysis [49, 99–108]. Some of these techniques expand the airway by resecting tissues bordering the glottis, while others are designed to relieve tension on the glottis and especially on the conus elasticus. Typical resection techniques are arytenoidectomy and cordectomy.

Typical relaxation techniques are the muscular tenotomy [109] and especially the posterior cordotomy [106–108, 110]. The goal in the latter technique is complete division of the vocal cord at its attachment to the vocal process of the arytenoid cartilage, supplemented by complete division of the conus elasticus as far as the cricoid cartilage. The effect of the cordotomy is to shift the ligamentous portions of the vocal cords anteriorly. This produces a triangular widening of the glottic aperture anterior to the arytenoid cartilage. While this does not restore normal respiration, most patients notice a marked improvement of respiration by about 2 months after the procedure, when epithelialization is complete. Generally the rule still applies that enlarging the airway results in deterioration of voice function. All opera-

tions that expand the glottis create static changes in laryngeal anatomy that compromise the ability of the larynx to expand for respiration and also close the glottis for swallowing. This means that a trade-off must be accepted between these conflicting requirements [49].

The distinguishing features of the various surgical procedures are summarized below:
- *Arytenoidectomy* [42, 43, 99, 111] is very effective for expanding the airway if the surgeon can completely remove the arytenoid cartilage and completely divide the conus elasticus as far as the cricoid cartilage. Even a partial arytenoidectomy is believed to provide satisfactory airway enlargement. A temporary tracheotomy is generally unnecessary when arytenoidectomy is carried out with a CO_2 laser. But the drawbacks of this technique include frequent transient aspiration and the risk of cricoid chondritis in patients who have had previous radiation to the neck. Arytenoidectomy is contraindicated in these patients and also in patients who would be jeopardized by transient aspiration [49, 112].
- *Cordectomy* [51, 101] is as effective as arytenoidectomy for airway restoration. There is no risk of aspiration with this procedure, but there may be a greater adverse effect on voice quality than after arytenoidectomy.
- *Posterior cordectomy* [106–108, 110], in which the vocal cord is divided in the area of the vocal process of the arytenoid cartilage combined with division of the conus elasticus, is considered by many laryngologists to be the best compromise between expanding the airway and preserving voice quality. It can be done bilaterally, but the present author has found that the unilateral procedure provides adequate airway enlargement (Fig. 5.**8 a–d**).
- *Temporary lateral fixation* [105] of the vocal cord as described by Lichtenberger is a potentially reversible procedure for airway expansion. Once nerve function has recovered, the endoscopically performed lateral fixation of the vocal cord can be released.

As a rule, modern endoscopic laser operations to expand the glottis are considered to be reliable techniques for airway restoration. Generally they can be performed without a temporary tracheotomy, making them easier for patients to tolerate [49].

To summarize, a variety of surgical techniques are available for expanding the glottis in patients with bilateral recurrent nerve paralysis. Varying degrees of glottic enlargement can be achieved. It should be noted that while expanding the airway results in improved breathing, it often leads to a weak, breathy voice because more air escapes through the enlarged glottis during phonation. This weakening of the voice can be objectively documented by a decrease in maximum phonation time [49]. Thus, despite the many advances in laryngeal surgery, it is still true that enlarging the glottic aperture leads to a deterioration of vocal performance, and that both of these qualities are inversely proportional to each other. These relations should be discussed with the patient preoperatively in order to weigh the physical activity needs of the patient against anticipated voice deterioration and strive for a compromise that is best for the individual situation—although the phonatory

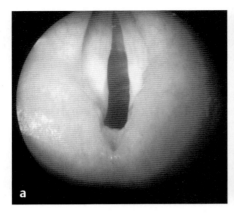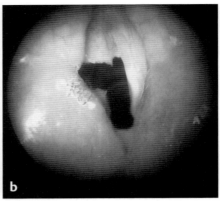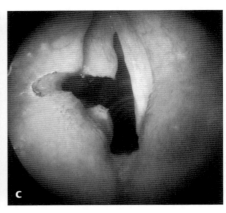

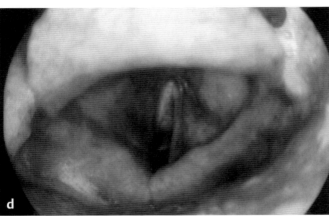

Fig. 5.**8** Posterior cordectomy on the left side for bilateral recurrent nerve paralysis. **a** Microlaryngoscopic view into the larynx before the operation. **b** The vocal cord is divided at the vocal process. **c** The conus elasticus is completely divided out to the superior border of the cricoid cartilage. **d** Healed site 6 months after surgery.

outcome of a glottis-expanding operation can never be predicted with complete accuracy.

Arytenoid Cartilage Fixation

Bilateral recurrent nerve paralysis needs to be differentiated mainly from bilateral arytenoid cartilage fixation (rare cases may also involve paralysis on one side and cartilage fixation on the other) [89]. Ankylosis of the arytenoid cartilage or fibrosis of the connective tissue capsule of the cricoarytenoid joint most commonly develops as a result of previous intubation. As a result, often it is not possible to distinguish between cartilage fixation (ankylosis) and paralysis based on the history alone. In any case, arytenoid cartilage fixation or posttraumatic fibrosis of the joint capsule should be considered in every patient who presents with limited vocal cord motion and a prior history of intubation. Mechanical restriction of joint motion can be differentiated from paralysis by means of laryngeal electromyography [91] and also by testing the passive mobility of the arytenoid cartilage during microlaryngoscopic examination of the larynx under general anesthesia.

It is important to distinguish between paralysis and ankylosis because when ankylosis is present, often there is no alternative to an arytenoidectomy for glottic expansion, and occasionally this must be done in a tracheotomized patient. In contrast, a glottis-enlarging procedure for bilateral recurrent nerve paralysis can generally be done in

the intubated patient without a prior tracheotomy [89, 113, 114].

Other Glottic Airway Stenoses

Besides paralysis or arytenoid cartilage fixation, glottic stenoses are occasionally caused by congenital malformations (webs), synechiae (postoperative or postinflammatory), and of course by inflammations and tumors. Synechiae can be divided by laser surgery. In patients with synechiae of the anterior commissure, the surgery should include stent insertion and, if necessary, a free mucosal graft, but even then the vocal results are usually unsatisfactory.

Subglottic and Tracheal Stenoses

Cicatricial stenoses involving the subglottic larynx and cervical trachea (laryngotracheal junction) are among the most difficult central airway stenoses to rehabilitate. They continue to pose a therapeutic challenge that cannot always be adequately resolved. Cicatricial stenoses of the subglottic larynx are much more common than congenital stenoses in this region. They usually develop as a result of endolaryngeal intubation (especially prolonged intubation) and occasionally result from tracheotomies and other surgical procedures in the neck.

The subglottic larynx is a site of predilection owing to the special anatomy of this region [82, 83, 115, 116]. The airway lumen is considerably narrower at this level than in the cervical trachea, and so endolaryngeal tubes are more likely to exert pressure on the subglottic mucosa leading to circulatory compromise and eventual necrosis. The resulting mucosal ulcerations are consistently contaminated with bacteria because the tracheal secretions are never sterile when an endotracheal tube is in place. This often leads to bacterial infection of the cartilaginous tissue. Since cartilage, as a bradytrophic tissue, is particularly susceptible to bacterial inflammation, the frequent outcome is inflammatory destruction of the affected cartilage tissue, scarring, and cicatricial stenosis.

Thin-walled scar-tissue webs in the subglottic larynx or trachea are rare. But when they are found and the adjacent cartilaginous framework of the larynx and trachea is intact, a stellate incision of the web can significantly expand the airway lumen and provide adequate correction of the stenosis [3, 117]. This procedure, however, is appropriate only for thin webs no more than 2–3 mm thick [118].

Most stenoses of the subglottic larynx, laryngotracheal junction, and cervical trachea are caused by postchondritic scarring after a previous cartilage inflammation. The cartilaginous skeleton of the airway is consistently absent in these cases. The lesions consist of thick, circular or crescent-shaped scars that feel rigid when probed with a suction tip. Laser ablation or incision of the scars is occasionally successful in the short term but does not offer a permanent solution. This treatment may even incite additional chondritis which worsens the situation. Consequently, lasers should not be used on this type of stenosis.

The treatment of choice is a continuity-restoring resection of the stenotic airway segment followed by an end-to-end anastomosis or a laryngotracheoplasty in which costal cartilage is implanted into the anterior and/or posterior wall of the larynx and trachea [119–123]. Complete or partial tracheal allograft reconstruction may be considered in particularly severe cases and in patients with long segmental stenoses [124, 125]. Tracheoplasties and allograft reconstructions generally require the temporary placement of a tracheal stent (Dumont stent, Montgomery stent, etc.). To eliminate troublesome granulation tissue at the ends of the stent or after stent removal, the CO_2 laser can be used for precise, atraumatic tissue ablation in the subglottic larynx and trachea.

Laser surgery has no particular role in the treatment of tracheomalacia.

Airway Stenosis Due to Malignant Disease

Malignant diseases (laryngeal or tracheal carcinoma, esophageal carcinoma invading the cervical trachea, central bronchial carcinoma, locally advanced thyroid carcinoma, malignant tumors of the upper mediastinum) can occasionally lead to malignant central airway stenosis. This type of stenosis may be caused by extrinsic airway compression, tumor invasion of the tracheal wall with subsequent malacia, or intraluminal tumor growth in the trachea and larynx [126]. Tumor infiltration of the recurrent nerve with subsequent vocal cord paralysis in a paramedian position can also lead to functional airway stenosis [51]. In all of these situations, endolaryngeal surgery with the CO_2 laser (or occasionally the Nd:YAG laser for larger tumor masses) provides an excellent tool for airway recanalization. The laser-enlarged airway can be maintained in the intermediate term by implanting stents in the carina, thoracic trachea, and cervical trachea as far as the laryngotracheal junction (see Fig. 5.2). The cranial end of these stents should not reach the subglottic vocal cord appendages, as this would lead to granulation tissue formation with poor tolerance of the stents. If airway restriction recurs at the ends of the stents due to tumor growth, this can be remedied either by ablating the tumor tissue with the laser or by inserting additional stents (into the stent already present) [127].

On the whole, malignant airway stenoses pose a special challenge to the attending otolaryngologist, bronchologist, and anesthesiologist, but most of these lesions can be successfully managed by the use of surgical lasers and other modern endoscopic techniques.

Medical Therapy in Conjunction With Operative Treatment of Airway Stenosis

In the laser surgery and open operative treatment of airway stenoses, medical therapy should generally be provided in addition to the surgical procedure itself. The medical options are outlined below.

In all procedures in which the cartilaginous structures of the larynx and/or trachea are exposed, preoperative antibiotic prophylaxis is indicated to prevent wound infection. A bactericidal antibiotic should be administered approximately 30 minutes before the start of the operation. The agents of choice are first- or second-generation cephalosporins, a combination of penicillins and penicillinase inhibitors, or clindamycin.

The efficacy of steroids is a controversial issue. High steroid doses (e.g., 250 mg methylprednisolone) during the immediate postoperative period have a number of beneficial effects, most notably the prevention of surgery-related tissue swelling and a reduction of surgical trauma [128]. Occasionally steroids are given for a prolonged period after stenosis surgery to prevent new connective tissue formation and undesired new scarring. It is the present author's opinion, however, that this therapy is of dubious benefit. Delaying or reducing new connective tissue formation ultimately means a delay in wound healing. The author himself does not routinely prescribe steroids during the initial days after the surgical correction of airway stenoses.

Recently, several reports have been published on the local application of mitomycin C for the prevention and treatment of undesired scarring of the larynx and trachea [129, 130]. Mitomycin C is an antibiotic first isolated from *Streptomyces caespitosus* in 1958. It inhibits DNA synthesis due to alkylation and is a potent inhibitor of connective tissue formation. Mitomycin C is an effective antineoplastic cytostatic drug that is used systemically and locally for the treatment of carcinoma at various sites. High local concentrations and low plasma levels are achieved following local application. Mitomycin C is widely used in ophthalmology for modifying wound healing processes after glaucoma operations and dacryocystorhinostomies. It is used particularly for the prevention of restenosis.

In laryngology, the use of this agent has been described following endoscopic laser treatment of airway stenosis and after open operations. Neurosurgical cotton soaked with 1 mL of a solution of 0.4 mg mitomycin C/mL is applied topically to the wound and left in place for about 5 minutes. Several authors recommend irrigating the wound with saline solution after this treatment. Some studies indicate promising results in the prevention of restenosis and also in preventing the recurrence of ablated contact granulomas [129, 130].

■ Laser Surgery of Benign Tumors of the Larynx and Trachea

Benign tumors of the larynx and trachea are much rarer than malignant tumors, especially laryngeal carcinoma. The tumors are classified into various groups based on their tissues of origin: epithelial tumors, neurogenic tumors, fibrocystic tumors, histiocytic tumors, tumors of cartilage and bone (due to frequent ossification of the cartilaginous laryngeal skeleton), myogenic tumors, tumors of fatty tissue, tumors of the vascular system, and lymphoreticular tumors. Besides true tumors, pseudotumors are also occasionally found in the larynx including laryngoceles, circumscribed laryngeal amyloidosis, and sarcoidosis [131–133].

Diagnosis

Except for papillomatosis and vascular tumors, generally these lesions cannot be identified by their clinical manifestations alone. Diagnostic imaging of benign tumors can supply information on the nature of the tumor mass, as in the case of lipomas and tumors of cartilaginous tissue.

Generally the etiology of these laryngeal masses is unknown, and the primary application of endoscopic laser surgery is to provide a biopsy sample for diagnosis. The CO_2 laser can be used during a microlaryngoscopic examination to take selective biopsies not only from the mucosa lining the inner larynx but also from the subepithelial tissues. Benign tumors of the laryngeal cartilage are the only lesions that may require exposure of the tumor for confirming the benign/malignant nature of the lesion.

Principles of Pathomorphologic Classification and Treatment

A complete and detailed classification of benign laryngeal tumors is beyond the scope of this chapter. The reader may

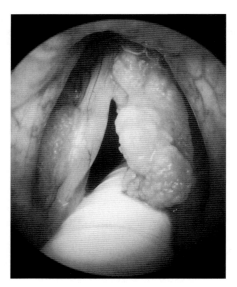

Fig 5.**9**   Typical extensive papillomatosis of the larynx.

find this information in works by Kleinsasser, Michaels, and Friedmann and Ferlito [134–136]. Some of the more common benign laryngeal tumors are discussed below.

Papillomas

Papillomas are benign tumors of the mucosa of the larynx and occasionally affect other parts of the upper respiratory tract (nose, pharynx, trachea, bronchial tree). The tumors result from HPV viral infection of the mucosa [137, 138]. Affected individuals most likely have an immune defect that allows the infection to cause papilloma formation.

Besides the (rare) solitary papillomas, which are classified as premalignant lesions and develop exclusively in adults, a condition known as recurrent laryngeal papillomatosis may be seen in both children and adults (Fig. 5.9) [45, 139, 140]. This disease is characterized by a more or less high recurrence rate and the presence of multifocal, often disseminated papillomas that occur predominantly in the larynx.

The disease is not amenable to surgical treatment (ablation of the papillomas). Nevertheless, papillomas in affected patients should be removed at intervals to relieve the functional compromise caused by the lesions. Extensive papillomatosis can cause life-threatening airway obstruction, especially in children, and it often necessitates repeated interventions for papilloma removal. Nowadays these procedures are generally carried out with a CO_2 laser, which removes the papillomas by a combination of ablation and vaporization [2, 141]. Histologic analysis of representative portions of the lesions is always advised, since recurrent laryngeal papillomatosis can occasionally undergo malignant transformation [142].

In cases with extensive involvement of the laryngeal mucosa, papilloma resections (to obtain tissue samples) are frequently combined with laser vaporization. An evacuator with a microfilter system should be routinely used to trap viral particles from the laser plume. Experimental studies have shown that the smoke plume from a surgical laser may contain viruses capable of reproducing. It is still uncertain whether this experimental finding is actually relevant to the safety of operating room personnel. In any case, there have been no reports of an increased incidence of papillomas in operating room personnel who work in areas where the laser surgery of papillomas is practiced. It may be that very few people have the immune defect that predisposes to papillomatosis following a viral infection.

Alternative surgical procedures such as the use of a monopolar electrocautery probe, photodynamic therapy [25, 143, 144], argon plasma coagulation [46], and shaver systems [38] have repeatedly been described in the literature. However, these techniques have not significantly altered the importance of the CO_2 laser in the treatment of laryngeal papillomatosis.

The treatment goal is superficial removal of the papillomas while preserving the submucous tissue. To prevent webs and synechiae, especially in the anterior commissure, it is often necessary to leave some papillomas in the larynx initially and resect them later in a second stage [3]. It is essential to avoid the creation of opposing open wounds in the anterior commissure, which often lead to anterior webbing with significant, intractable dysphonia [145]. In cases of extensive, rapidly recurrent papillomatosis, especially in children, the airways should be endoscopically inspected and the papillomas removed in procedures that are initially scheduled at frequent intervals. The goal of this close-interval endoscopic surveillance is to remove the papillomas promptly without jeopardizing the airway so that the procedures can be carried out without a tracheotomy [141]. Even with a meticulous operating technique, complete papilloma removal cannot prevent the lesions from recurring. As a result, radical tumor clearance is not only unnecessary but can even be hazardous if it leads to functional compromise (e. g., due to laryngeal scarring) [146, 147]. Even the photodynamic therapy of laryngeal papillomatosis cannot always produce a complete remission. It is also more costly than conventional endoscopic laser surgery.

Given the unsatisfactory results of surgical treatment for laryngeal papillomatosis, a number of adjuvant therapies have been employed. Besides physical removal of the papillomas (by conventional surgical excision, cryosurgery, electrocautery, ultrasound, laser surgery, photodynamic therapy, ablation with shaver systems), there are also medical regimens designed either to modulate the body's immune response (interferon) or inhibit the growth of the papillomas (with antimetabolites, hormones, podophyllin, antibiotics, or virostatics) [148]. Local interferon therapy is reportedly effective, causes fewer complications than systemic therapy, and is practiced at several large hospitals [149, 150].

Recently, encouraging reports have been published on the use of the new virostatic drug cidofovir (Vistide) [151–154]. This drug is currently used at the Cologne University Hospital in adult patients who have had multiple unsuccessful surgical interventions for papillomatosis confined

to the supraglottis, glottis, or subglottis. Cidofovir is ordinarily used in ophthalmology for the treatment of cytomegalovirus retinitis in immunosuppressed patients, where it is administered by i. v. infusion. The first off-label use of cidofovir for papillomatosis was described in 1994, when the drug was injected locally into laryngeal papillomas by Snoeck et al. [152]. We follow the regimen described by Bielamowicz et al. [154], using a concentration of 6.25 mg/mL for intralesional laryngeal injections. A maximum dose of 37.5 mg is given per injection in 6 mL of saline. The therapy is administered during microlaryngoscopy, injecting the solution directly into the papillomas with a butterfly needle until the surrounding mucosa blanches. This procedure is repeated at 4–6-week intervals until papillomas are no longer visible by telescopic laryngoscopy. On average, six injections are required to achieve complete remission of disease. The papillomas are not surgically removed during the treatment, but one representative sample is taken for histologic examination during each microlaryngoscopic procedure. No side effects have been seen with this therapy, but cidofovir should not be used in patients with known renal disease, in pregnant or lactating patients, or in patients who intend to become pregnant.

Lipomas

Laryngeal lipomas most commonly develop in the ventricular folds, aryepiglottic folds, and piriform sinuses [155]. They present clinically as laryngeal masses beneath intact, healthy-appearing mucosa. The typical signal pattern seen with magnetic resonance imaging will generally establish the diagnosis. Lipomas, even when extensive, are generally resectable by endoscopic laser surgery [156].

Hemangiomas

Subglottic hemangiomas are a potential cause of airway stenosis in newborns. They typically present with increasing inspiratory stridor during the first months of life. Endoscopy generally shows a pad-like thickening and bluish discoloration of the subglottic larynx, usually affecting the anterior or lateral walls and often spreading to involve the laryngotracheal junction.

Hemangiomas may be associated with other vascular malformations in the scalp. Often they regress spontaneously over time. In some children airway obstruction must be relieved by creating a temporary tracheotomy or performing endoscopic laser coagulation (which may have to be repeated). The CO_2 laser is best for this purpose, applied during intermittent apnea. When children are treated, the procedure requires close collaboration with the anesthesiologist and with an experienced pediatric ICU (for postoperative surveillance).

Lesions in adults consist mainly of cavernous hemangiomas located in the ventricular folds, aryepiglottic folds, and piriform sinuses (Fig. 5.**10 a, b**). Treatment consists of excising the papillomas (generally with a microlaryngoscopic CO_2 laser) or coagulating the lesions with a Nd:YAG laser [4, 23, 157, 158].

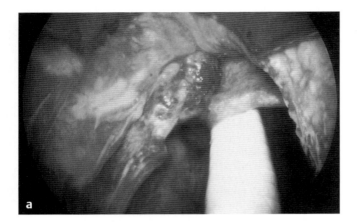

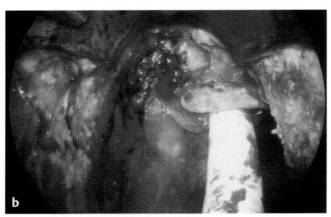

Fig. 5.**10** Cavernous hemangioma of the glossoepiglottic valeculla and aryepiglottic fold on the left side. **a** Microlaryngoscopic view. **b** Appearance after complete removal by CO_2 laser surgery.

Pseudotumors

Laryngoceles and retention cysts of the larynx can occasionally present as tumor-like masses in the larynx. Following endoscopic evaluation of the mass during microlaryngoscopy, treatment consists of laser resection of the cysts or sacs, which occur predominantly in the area of the ventricular folds [133]. Great care is taken to preserve the vocal cord mucosa during the procedure. Subtotal removal of the affected ventricular fold, combined with broad exposure of the ventricle, is generally necessary with laryngoceles to prevent a recurrence.

Endolaryngeal versus Extralaryngeal Approach to the Larynx

In the great majority of cases, the surgical resection of benign laryngeal tumors is the only reasonable therapeutic option in cases where treatment is warranted. Different principles are followed than in the surgical treatment of malignant laryngeal tumors. Functional considerations are assigned a much higher priority than in malignant tumor surgery. If doubt exists, it may be prudent to leave some of the tumor behind and resect it in a later sitting if this will

better preserve the functional integrity of the larynx (for swallowing and phonation).

The great majority of all benign laryngeal tumors are located in the mucosa or submucous space of the larynx, making them easily accessible to endoscopic inspection [159]. Another advantage is that the endoscopic approach does not require a skin incision, division of the thyroid cartilage, or tracheotomy and therefore does not cause additional morbidity [160]. For these reasons, open operations on the larynx are now considered obsolete unless surgery is required for the cartilaginous structures of the larynx, if the position of the larynx is to be altered, or if there are special problems that prevent adequate endoscopic visualization of the anatomic structures.

■ Complications of Endoscopic Laser Surgery

A number of authors have described complications of endoscopic laser surgery in the larynx, trachea, and hypopharynx [30, 161–164]. These mostly involve the combustion of ventilation tube materials and anesthetic gas mixtures during surgical laser use in the larynx [165]. The surgeon should consider the possibility of these complications in every laser operation and take appropriate precautions. Combustion of tube materials can be avoided by the use of laser-safe tubes. Ignition of anesthetic gas mixtures during procedures using jet ventilation can be prevented by ventilating the patient with room air (rather than pure oxygen) and by operating in intermittent apnea. On the whole, such incidents can be safely avoided nowadays by the selection of suitable materials, operating methods, and analgesic techniques. Reports of airway fires in the current literature must be viewed more as a result of poorly trained operating room personnel than as inherent risks of laser surgery.

Possible laser-associated complications are less important in endolaryngeal surgery than complications caused by the microlaryngoscope itself. In a study by the author, 75 % of 339 consecutive microlaryngoscopy patients were found to have small mucosal lesions of the lips, oral cavity, and oropharynx. These lesions caused significant complaints for some time but resolved without sequelae in a few days. Dental injuries occur in approximately 6 % of all patients, but they affect only patients who already have significant carious damage to the teeth, preexisting loose teeth, periodontal disease, or a fixed denture. Patients with healthy dentitions did not sustain dental injuries in this study. The nature of the denture injuries ranged from simple loosening and enamel fractures to chipped teeth and complete dental displacement. No laser-associated complications were observed [166, 167].

Microlaryngoscopic procedures may be followed by transient functional impairment of the hypoglossal nerve and lingual nerve. By and large, this type of complication cannot be completely avoided in microlaryngoscopic surgery, but the range of complications is definitely more limited than in open laryngeal surgery. In summary, laser surgery of benign lesions of the larynx, pharynx, and trachea can be considered a minimally invasive surgical approach with a very low risk of complications.

■ Acknowledgments

The author expresses thanks to the following individuals: Prof. Dr. med. E. Stennert, Director of the Department of Otorhinolaryngology, Cologne University; Dr. med. Christian Sittel (Department of Otorhinolaryngology, Homburg University); Dr. M. Damm, Dr. med. Ursula Schröder, Dr. O. Guntinas-Lichius, Dr. Gero Quante, Dr. M. Streppel, Dr. med. Claus Wittekind, and Dr. med. Jens Peter Klussmann of the Department of Otorhinolaryngology, Cologne University; Dr. med. S. Berendes and Dr. H. Knopf of the Department of Anesthesiology, Cologne University; Dr. med. Markus Jungehülsing of the Department of Otorhinolaryngology, Potsdam Medical Center; speech therapists Ute Mlynczak, Manuela Motzko, and Marie Lotter, Ms. Marion Schmidt (photo lab), Ms. Gabriele Heske (secretary), Ms. Sabine Ricke (laryngeal lab), Dr. H. Klünter (data processing), all of the Department of Otorhinolaryngology, Cologne University, and Ms. Ursula Sima, Department of Otorhinolaryngology at Klagenfurt Hospital, for their support in the preparation of this article; Dr. med. K. Lackner, Director of the Department of Diagnostic Radiology, Cologne University Medial Center, for supplying the radiographic films that were used; Dr. med. K. Wassermann, Third Medical Hospital, Cologne University, for providing Fig. 5.2 and for many years of intense clinical and scientific collaboration.

■ References

1 Strong MS, Jako GJ. Laser surgery in the larynx. Early clinical experience with continuous CO_2-laser. Ann Otol Rhinol Laryngol 1972; 81: 791–798

2 Hofler H. Ergebnisse der CO_2-Laserbehandlng von Larynxmalignomen. Wien Klin Wochenschr 1983; 95: 545–547

3 Rudert H. Laser-Chirurgie in der HNO-Heilkunde. Laryngol Rhinol Otol (Stuttg) 1988; 67: 261–268

4 Werner JA, Rudert H. Der Einsatz des Nd:YAG-Lasers in der Hals-, Nasen-, Ohrenheilkunde. HNO 1992; 40: 248–258

5 Thumfart WF, Eckel HE. Endolaryngeale Laserchirurgie zur Behandlung von Kehlkopfkarzinomen. Das aktuelle Kölner Konzept. HNO 1990; 38: 174–178

6 Steiner W, Jaumann MP, Pesch HJ. Endoskopische Laserchirurgie im Larynx. Ther Umsch 1980: 37: 1103–1109

7 Ambrosch P, Kron M, Steiner W. Carbon dioxide laser microsurgery for early supraglottic carcinoma. Ann Otol Rhinol Laryngol 1998; 107: 680–688

8 Motta G, Villari G, Motta G Jr., Ripa G, Salerno G. The CO_2-laser in the laryngeal microsurgery. Acta Otolaryngol Suppl 1986; 433: 1–30

9 Grossenbacher R. Erste Erfahrungen mit der endolaryngealen CO_2-Laser-Chirurgie beim umschriebenen Kehlkopfkarzinom. Fortschr Med 1983; 101: 1030–1032

10 Jeckstrom W, Wawersik J, Werner JA. Narkosetechnik bei laserchirurgischen Eingriffen im Kehlkopfbereich. HNO 1992; 40: 28–32

11 Lanzenberger-Schragl E, Donner A, Grasl MC, Zimpfer M, Aloy A. Superimposed high-frequency jet ventilation for laryngeal and tracheal surgery. Arch Otolaryngol Head Neck Surg 2000; 126: 40–44

12 Rudert H. Instrumentarium für die CO_2-Laser-Chirurgie. HNO 1989; 37: 76–77

13 Ayache D, Wagner I, Denoyelle F, Garabedian EN. Use of the carbon dioxide laser for tracheobronchial pathology in children. Eur Arch Otorhinolaryngol 2000; 257: 287–289

14 Lippert BM, Werner JA, Rudert H. Tissue effects of CO_2-laser and Nd:YAG laser. Adv Otorhinolaryngol 1995; 49: 1–4

15 Ossoff RH, Coleman JA, Courey MS, Duncavage JA, Werkhaven JA, Reinisch L. Clinical applications of lasers in otolaryngology – head and neck surgery. Lasers Surg Med 1994; 15: 217–248

16 Remacle M, Lawson G, Watelet JB. Carbon dioxide laser microsurgery of benign vocal fold lesions: indications, techniques, and results in 251 patients. Ann Otol Rhinol Laryngol 1999; 108: 156–164

17 Robinson PM, Weir AM. Excision of benign laryngeal lesions: comparison of carbon dioxide laser with conventional surgery. J Laryngol Otol 1987; 101: 1254–1257

18 Ossoff RH, Werkhaven JA, Raif J, Abraham M. Advanced microspot microslad for the CO_2-laser. Otolaryngol Head Neck Surg 1991; 105: 411–414

19 Converse GM, Ries WR, Reinisch L. Comparison of wound healing using the CO_2-laser at 10.6 microm and 9.55 microm. Laryngoscope 2001; 111: 1231–1236

20 Garrett CG, Reinisch L. New-generation pulsed carbon dioxide laser: comparative effects on vocal fold wound healing. Ann Otol Rhinol Laryngol 2002; 111: 471–476

21 Schunke M, Kruss C, Mecke H, Werner JA. Charachteristic features of wound healing in laser-induced incisions. Adv Otorhinolaryngol 1995; 49: 8–14

22 Werner JA, Lippert BM, Heissenberg MC, Rudert H. Laser delivery systems and laser instruments in otorhinolaryngology. Adv Otorhinolaryngol 1995; 49: 27–30

23 Werner JA, Lippert BM, Godbersen GS, Rudert H. Die Hämangiombehandlung mit dem Neodym:Yttrium-Aluminium-Granat-Laser (Nd:YAG-Laser). Laryngorhinootologie 1992; 71: 388–395

24 Cholewa D, Waldschmidt J. Laser treatment of hemangiomas of the larynx and trachea. Lasers Surg Med 1998; 23: 221–232

25 Feyh J, Kastenbauer E. Die Behandlung der Larynxpapillomatose mit Hilfe der photodynamischen Lasertherapie. Laryngorhinootologie 1992; 71: 190–192

26 Maier A, Tomaselli F, Matzi V et al. Comparison of 5-aminolaevulinic acid and porphyrin photosensitization for photodynamic therapy of malignant bronchial stenosis: a clinical pilot study. Lasers Surg Med 2002; 30: 12–17

27 Savary JF, Monnier P, Fontolliet C et al. Photodynamic therapy for early squamous cell carcinomas of the esophagus, bronchi, and mouth with m-tetra (hydroxyphenyl) chlorin. Arch Otolaryngol Head Neck Surg 1997; 123: 162–168

28 Savary JF, Grosjean P, Monnier P et al. Photodynamic therapy of early squamous cell carcinomas of the esophagus: a review of 31 cases. Endoscopy 1998; 30: 258–265

29 Kleinsasser O. Mikrolaryngoskopie und endolaryngeale Mikrochirurgie. Stuttgart: Schattauer, 1991

30 Ossoff RH, Werkhaven JA, Dere H. Soft-tissue complications of laser surgery for recurrent respiratory papillomatosis. Laryngoscope 1991; 101: 1162–1166

31 Shapshay SM, Rebeiz EE, Bohigian RK, Hybels RL. Benign lesions of the larynx: should the laser be used? Laryngoscope 1990; 100: 953–957

32 Hochman II, Zeitels SM. Phonomicrosurgical management of vocal fold polyps: the subepithelial microflap resection technique. J Voice 2000; 14: 112–118

33 Zeitels SM. Laser versus cold instruments for microlaryngoscopic surgery. Laryngoscope 1996; 106: 545–552

34 Zeitels SM, Casiano RR, Gardner GM, Hogikyan ND, Koufman JA, Rosen CA. Management of common voice problems: Committee report. Otolaryngol Head Neck Surg 2002; 126: 333–348

35 Friedrich G. Grundprinzipien für die Indikationsstellung zur Phonochirurgie. Laryngorhinootologie 1995; 74: 663–665

36 El Bitar MA, Zalzal GH. Powered instrumentation in the treatment of recurrent respiratory papillomatosis: an alternative to the carbon dioxide laser. Arch Otolaryngol Head Neck Surg 2002; 128: 425–428

37 Flint PW. Powered surgical instruments for laryngeal surgery. Otolaryngol Head Neck Surg 2000; 122: 263–266

38 Myer CM, III, Willging JP, McMurray S, Cotton RT. Use of a laryngeal micro resector system. Laryngoscope 1999; 109: 1165–1166

39 Kashima HK, Kessis T, Mounts P, Shah K. Polymerase chain reaction identification of human papillomavirus DNA in CO_2-laser plume from recurrent of respiratory papillomatosis. Otolaryngol Head Neck Surg 1991; 104: 191–195

40 Abramson AL, DiLorenzo TP, Steinberg BM. Is papillomavirus detectable in the plume of laser-treated laryngeal papilloma? Arch Otolaryngol Head Neck Surg 1990; 116: 604–607

41 Fried MP. Complications of CO_2-laser surgery of the larynx. Laryngoscope 1983; 93: 275–278

42 Kleinsasser O, Nolte E. Endolaryngeale Arytaenoidektomie und submuköse partielle Chordektomie bei bilateralen Stimmlippenlähmungen. Laryngol Rhinol Otol (Stuttg) 1981; 60: 397–401

43 Kleinsasser O. Endolaryngeale Arytaenoidektomie und submuköse Hemichordektomie zur Erweiterung der Glottis bei bilateraler Abduktorenparese. Monatsschr Ohrenheilkd Laryngorhinol 1968; 102: 443–446

44 Eckel HE, Dollinger K, Feaux dL, Reidenbach HD, Thumfart WF. An electrohydrohermosation system for application in endolaryngeal and enoral surgery: a technical report. Eur Surg Res 1992; 24: 302–308

45 Bergler WF, Gotte K. Current advances in the basic research and clinical management of juvenile-onset recurrent respiratory papillomatosis. Eur Arch Otorhinolaryngol 2000; 257: 263–269

46 Bergler W, Farin G, Fischer K, Hörmann K. Die Argon-Plasma-Chirurgie (APC) im oberen Aerodigestivtrakt. Erste Resultate. HNO 1998; 46: 672–677

47 Bergler W, Sadick H, Gotte K, Riedel F, Hörmann K. Topical estrogens combined with argon plasma coagulation in the management of epistaxis in hereditary hemorrhagic telangiectasia. Ann Otol Rhinol Laryngol 2002; 111: 222–228

48 Heinritz H, Waldfahrer F, Benzel W, Sroka R, Iro H. Meta-tetrahydroxyphenylchlorin: a new photosensitizer for photodynamic therapy of head and neck tumors. Adv Otorhinolaryngol 1995; 49: 44–47

49 Eckel HE, Thumfart M, Wassermann K, Vössing M, Thumfart WF. Cordectomy versus arytenoidectomy in the management of bilateral vocal cord paralysis. Ann Otol Rhinol Laryngol 1994; 103: 852–857

50 Eckel HE. Endoscopic laser resection of supraglottic carcinoma. Otolaryngol Head Neck Surg 1997; 117: 681–687

51 Wassermann K, Mathen F, Eckel HE. Concurrent glottic and tracheal stenoses: restoration of airway continuity in end-stage malignant disease. Ann Otol Rhinol Laryngol 2001; 110: 349–355

52 Friedrich G, de Jong FI, Mahieu HF, Benninger MS, Isshiki N. Laryngeal framework surgery: a proposal for classification and nomenclature by the Phonosurgery Committee of the European Laryngological Society. Eur Arch Otorhinolaryngol 2001; 258: 389–396

53 Hochman I, Sataloff RT, Hillman RE, Zeitels SM. Ectasias and varices of the vocal fold: clearing the striking zone. Ann Otol Rhinol Laryngol 1999; 108: 10–16

54 Damm M, Jungehülsing M, Sittel C, Eckel HE. Ackerman-Tumoren des Larynx – Ergebnisse mit der CO_2-Laser-Chirurgie. Laryngorhinootologie 2000; 79: 565–572

55 Damm M, Eckel HE, Schneider D, Arnold G. CO_2-laser surgery for verrucous carcinoma of the larynx. Lasers Surg Med 1997; 21: 117–123

56 Damm M, Sittel C, Streppel M, Eckel HE. Transoral CO_2-laser for surgical management of glottic carcinoma in situ. Laryngoscope 2000; 110: 1215–1221

57 Hörmann K, Baker-Schreyer A, Keilmann A, Biermann G. Functional results after CO_2-laser surgery compared with conventional phonosurgery. J Laryngol Otol 1999; 113: 140–144

58 Keilmann A, Biermann G, Hörmann K. CO_2-Laser versus konventionelle Mikrolaryngoskopie bei gutartigen Veränderungen der Stimmlippe. Laryngorhinootologie 1997; 76: 484–489

59 Habermann W, Eherer A, Lindbichler F, Raith J, Friedrich G. Ex juvantibus approach for chronic posterior laryngitis: results of short-term pantoprazole therapy. J Laryngol Otol 1999; 113: 734–739

60 Issing WJ, Gross M, Tauber S. Manifestationen von gastroösophagealem Reflux im HNO-Bereich. Laryngorhinootologie 2001; 80: 464–469

61 Ylitalo R, Ramel S. Extraesophageal reflux in patients with contact granuloma: a prospective controlled study. Ann Otol Rhinol Laryngol 2002; 111: 441–446

62 Zeitels SM, Hillman RE, Bunting GW. Vaughn T. Reinke's edema: phonatory mechanisms and management strategies. Ann Otol Rhinol Laryngol 1997; 106: 533–543

63 Marcotullio D, Magliulo G, Pezone T. Reinke's edema and risk factors: clinical and histopathologic aspects. Am J Otolaryngol 2002; 23: 81–84

64 Murry T, Abitbol J, Hersan R. Quantitative assessment of voice quality following laser surgery for Reinke's edema. J Voice 1999; 13: 257–264

65 Remacle M, Degols JC, Delos M. Exudative lesions of Reinke's space. An anatomopathological correlation. Acta Otorhinolaryngol Belg 1996; 50: 253–264

66 Gross M, Hess M. Sekundäre ambulante Stimmprothesen-Implantation mit Argon-Laser in Lokalanästhesie. Laryngorhinootologie 1994; 73: 496–499

67 Helling K, Abrams J, Bertram WK, Hohner S, Scherer H. Die Lasertonsillotomie bei der Tonsillenhyperplasie des Kleinkindes. HNO 2002; 50: 470–478

68 Schulze SL, Rhee JS, Kulpa JI, Danielson SK, Toohill RJ, Jaradeh SS. Morphology of the cricopharyngeal muscle in Zenker and control specimens. Ann Otol Rhinol Laryngol 2002; 111: 573–578

69 Busaba NY, Ishoo E, Kieff D. Open Zenker's diverticulectomy using stapling techniques. Ann Otol Rhinol Laryngol 2001; 110: 498–501

70 EY W, Denecke-Singer U, Ey M, Guastella C, Onder N. Chirurgische Behandlung der Dysphagien im Bereich des pharyngoösophagealen Überganges. Arch Otorhinolaryngol Suppl 1990; 1: 107–156

71 van Overbeek JJ. Meditation on the pathogenesis of hypopharyngeal (Zenker's) diverticulum and a report of endoscopic treatment in 545 patients. Ann Otol Rhinol Laryngol 1994; 103: 178–185

72 Lippert BM, Werner JA. Ergebnisse und operative Erfahrungen bei der Schwellendurchtrennung des Hypopharynx-(Zenker-)-Divertikels mit dem CO_2-Laser. HNO 1995; 43: 605–610

73 Lippert BM, Folz BJ, Gottschlich S, Werner JA. Microendoscopic treatment of the hypopharyngeal diverticulum with the CO_2-laser. Lasers Surg Med 1997; 20: 394–401

74 Lippert BM, Folz BJ, Rudert HH, Werner JA. Management of Zenker's diverticulum and postlaryngectomy pseudodiverticulum with the CO_2-laser. Otolaryngol Head Neck Surg 1999; 121: 809–814

75 Zbaren P, Schar P, Tschopp L, Becker M, Hausler R. Surgical treatment of Zenker's diverticulum: transcutaneous diverticulectomy versus microendoscopic myotomy of the cricopharyngeal muscle with CO_2-laser. Otolaryngol Head Neck Surg 1999; 121: 482–487

76 Mattinger C, Hörmann K. Endoscopic diverticulotomy of Zenker's diverticulum: management and complications. Dysphagia 2002; 17: 34–39

77 Lacau SG, Zhang KX, Perie S, Copin H, Butler-Browne GS, Barbet JP. Improvement of dysphagia following cricopharyngeal myotomy in an group of elderly patients. Histochemical and biochemical assessment of the cricopharyngeal muscle. Ann Otol Rhinol Laryngol 1995; 104: 603–609

78 Smith SR, Genden EM, Urken ML. Endoscopic stapling technique for the treatment of Zenker diverticulum vs standard open-neck technique: a direct comparison and charge analysis. Arch Otolaryngol Head Neck Surg 2002; 128: 141–144

79 Thaler ER, Weber RS, Goldberg AN, Weinstein GS. Feasibility and outcome of endoscopic staple-assisted esophagodiverticulostomy for Zenker's diverticulum. Laryngoscope 2002; 111: 1506–1508

80 Richtsmeier WJ, Monzon JR. Postendoscopic Zenker esophagodiverticulostomy leaks associated with a specific stapler cartridge. Arch Otolaryngol Head Neck Surg 2002; 128: 137–140

81 Schneider I, Thumfart WF, Pototschnig C, Eckel HE. Treatment of dysfunction of the cricopharyngeal muscle with botulinum A

toxin: introduction of a new, noninvasive method. Ann Otol Rhinol Laryngol 1994; 103: 31–35

82 Eckel HE, Sittel C. Morphometrische Untersuchungen der Glottisebene als Grundlage kehlkopferweiternder mikrolaryngoskopischer Operationsverfahren bei beidseitiger Rekurrenslähmung. Laryngorhinootologie 1994; 73: 417–422

83 Eckel HE, Koebke J, Sittel C, Sprinzl GM, Pototschnig C, Stennert E. Morphology of the human larynx during the first five years of life studied on whole organ serial sections. Ann Otol Rhinol Laryngol 1999; 108: 232–238

84 Eckel HE, Widemann B, Damm M, Roth B. Airway endoscopy in the diagnoses and treatment of bacterial tracheitis in children. Int J Pediatr Otorhinolaryngol 1993; 27: 147–157

85 Damm M, Eckel HE, Jungehülsing M, Roth B. Management of acute inflammatory childhood stridor. Otolaryngol Head Neck Surg 1999; 121: 633–638

86 Damm M, Eckel HE, Roth B, Schneider D, Streppel M. Interdisziplinares Therapiekonzept bei schweren bakteriellen Infektionen des zentralen Respirationstraktes im Kindesalter. Laryngorhinootologie 1996; 75: 293–300

87 Grzonka MA, Kleinsasser O. Intubationsschaden im Kehlkopf. Erscheinungsformen, Anmerkungen zur Pathogenese, Behandlung und Prävention. Laryngorhinootologie 1996; 75: 70–76

88 Rudert H. Über seltene intubationsbedingte innere Kehlkopftraumen. Rekurrensparesen, Distorsionen und Luxationen der Cricoarytaenoidgelenke. HNO 1984; 32: 393–398

89 Eckel HE, Wittekind C, Klussmann JP, Schroder U, Sittel C. Management of bilateral Arytenoid cartilage fixation (ACF) versus recurrent laryngeal verne paralysis (RLNP). Ann Otol Rhinol Laryngol 2003; 112: 103–108

90 Eckel HE, Sittel C. Beidseitige Rekurrenslähmungen. HNO 2001; 49: 166–179

91 Sittel C, Stennert E. Thumfart WF, Dapunt U, Eckel HE. Prognostic value of laryngeal electromyography in vocal fold paralysis. Arch Otolaryngol Head Neck Surg 2001; 127: 155–160

92 Jung H. Schlager B. Rekurrensparesen nach Strumektomien. Laryngorhinootologie 2000; 79: 297–303

93 Wassermann K, Koch A, Warschkow A, Mathen F, Muller-Ehmsen J, Eckel HE. Measuring in situ central airway resistance in patients with laryngotracheal stenosis. Laryngoscope 1999; 109: 1516–1520

94 Wassermann K, Eckel HE. Funktionsdiagnostik zentraler Atemwegsstenosen. HNO 1999; 47: 947–956

95 Schroder U, Eckel HE, Jungehülsing M, Thumfart W. Indikation, Technik und Ergebnisse der rekontruktiven Kehlkopfteilresektion nach Sedlacek-Kambic-Tucker. HNO 1997; 45: 915–922

96 Thumfart WF, Pototschnig C, Zorowka P, Eckel HE. Electrophysiologic investigation of lower cranial nerve diseases by means of magnetically stimulated neuromyography of the larynx. Ann Otol Rhinol Laryngol 1992; 101: 629–634

97 Langnickel R. Langzeitergebnisse nach endolaryngealer Latero-Vertikalverlagerung einer Stimmlippe bei doppelseitiger Postikuslähmung. Laryngol Rhinol Otol (Stuttg) 1982; 61: 254–257

98 Schobel H. Glottiserweiterung bei beidseitiger Stimmlippenlähmung. Ein Überblick über die verschiedenen Operationsverfahren und ein Erfahrungsbericht über eine persönliche Operationstechnik „Die funktionelle Lateralfixation". HNO 1986; 34: 485–495

99 Ossoff RH, Duncavage JA, Shapshay SM, Krespi YP, Sisson Sr GA. Endoscopic laser arytenidectomy revisted. Ann Otol Rhinol Laryngol 1990; 99: 764–771

100 Rudert H. Laser surgical techniques for the treatment of glottic stenoses. Adv Otorhinolaryngol 1995; 49: 176–178

101 Eckel HE. Die laserchirurgische mikrolaryngoskopische Glottiserweiterung zur Behandlung der beidseitigen Rekurrensparese. Operationstechnik und Ergebnisse. Laryngorhinootologie 1991; 70: 17–20

102 Eckel HE, Vössing M. Endolaryngeale Operationsverfahren zur Glottiserweiterung bei beidseitiger Rekurrenslähmung. Laryngorhinootologie 1996; 75: 215–222

103 Bigenzahn W, Hoefler H. Minimally invasive laser surgery for the treatment of bilateral vocal cord paralysis. Laryngoscope 1996; 106: 791–793

104 Remacle M, Lawson G, Mayne A, Jamart J. Subtotal carbon dioxide laser arytenoidectomy by endoscopic approach for treatment of bilateral cord immobility in adduction. Ann Otol Rhinol Laryngol 1996; 105: 438–445

105 Lichtenberger G. Reversible immediate and definitive lateralization of paralyzed vocal cords. Eur Arch Otorhinolaryngol 1999; 256: 407–411

106 Reker U, Rudert H. Die modifizierte posteriore Chordektomie nach Dennis und Kashima bei der Behandlung beidseitiger Rekurrensparesen. Laryngorhinootologie 1998; 77: 213–218

107 Dennis DP, Kashima H. Carbon dioxide laser posterior cordectomy for treatment of bilateral vocal cord paralysis. Ann Otol Rhinol Laryngol 1989; 98: 930–934

108 Herberhold C, Huck P. Posterior cordotomy by CO_2-laser surgery for bilateral vocal cord paralysis: Kashima's technique and modified technique. Adv Otorhinolaryngol 1995; 49: 174–175

109 Rontal M, Rontal E. Use of laryngeal muscular tenotomy for bilateral midline vocal cord fixation. Ann Otol Rhinol Laryngol 1994; 103: 583–589

110 Kashima HK: Bilateral vocal fold motion impairment: pathophysiology and management by transverse cordotomy. Ann Otol Rhinol Laryngol 1991; 100: 717–721

111 Szmeja Z, Wojtowicz JG. Laser arytenoidectomy in the treatment of bilateral vocal cord paralysis. Eur Arch Otorhinolaryngol 1999; 256: 388–389

112 Sprinzl GM, Eckel HE, Ernst S, Motamedi K. Cricoid cartilage necrosis after arytenoidectomy in a previously irradiated larynx. Arch Otolaryngol Head Neck Surg 1999; 125: 1154–1157

113 Carrat X, Verhulst J, Duroux S, Pescio P, Devars F, Traissac L. Postintubation interarytenoid adhesion. Ann Otol Rhinol Laryngol 2000; 109: 736–740

114 Lichtenberger G. Endoscopic microsurgical management of scars in the posterior commissure and interarytenoid region resulting in vocal cord pseudoparalysis. Eur Arch Otorhinolaryngol 1999; 256: 412–414

115 Sprinzl GM, Eckel HE, Sittel C. Pototschnig C, Koebke J. Morphometric measurements of the cartilaginous larynx: An anatomic correlate of laryngeal surgery. Head Neck 1999; 21: 743–750

116 Eckel HE, Sittel C. Morphometry of the larynx in horizontal sections. Am J Otolaryngol 1995; 16: 40–48

117 Ossoff RH, Tucker Jr GF, Duncavage JA, Toohill RJ. Efficacy of bronchoscopic carbon dioxide laser surgery for benign strictures of the trachea. Laryngoscope 1985; 95: 1220–1223

118 Cotton RT, Tewfik TL. Laryngeal stenosis following carbon dioxide laser in subglottic hemangioma. Report of three cases. Ann Otol Rhinol Laryngol 1985; 94: 494–497

119 Vollrath M, von der HH Freihorst J. Die Chirurgie der erworbenen laryngotrachealen Stenosen im Kindesalter. Erfahrungen und Ergebnisse von 1988–1998. Teil II: Die cricotracheale Resektion. HNO 1999; 47: 611–622

120 Schultz-Coulon HJ, Laubert A. Laryngotrachealplastik im frühen Kindesalter. HNO 1988; 36: 1–12

121 Deitmer T. Offene chirurgische Therapie bei kindlichen laryngo-trachealen Stenosen. Laryngorhinootologie 2001; 80: 90–95

122 Monnier P, Lang F, Savary M. Traitement des stenoses sousglottiques de l'enfant par resection crico-tracheale. Ann Otolaryngol Chir Cervicofac 2001; 118: 299–305

123 Monnier P, Lang F, Savary M. Partial cricotracheal resection for severe pediatric subglottic stenosis: update of the Lausanne experience. Ann Otol Rhinol Laryngol 1998; 107: 961–968

124 Jacobs J, Quintessenza JA, Andrews T et al. Tracheal allograft reconstruction: the total North American and worldwide pediatric experiences. Ann Thorac Surg 1999; 68: 1043–1051

125 Herberhold C. Tracheal-Rekonstruktion mit konserviertem Homograft. Laryngorhinootologie 2001; 80: 57–60

126 Wassermann K, Mathen F, Eckel HE. Malignant laryngotracheal obstruction: A way to treat serial stenoses of the upper airways. Ann Thorac Surg 2000; 70: 1197–1201

127 Wassermann K, Eckel HE, Michel O, Muller RP. Emergency stenting of malignant obstruction of the upper airways: long-term follow-up with two types of silicone prostheses. J Thorac Cardiovasc Surg 1996; 112: 859–866

128 Nagelschmidt M, Fu ZX, Saad S, Dimmeler S, Neugebauer E. Preoperative high dose methylprednisolone improves pa-

tients outcome after abdominal surgery. Eur J Surg 1999; 165: 971–978

129 Rahbar R, Jones DT, Nuss RC et al. The role of mitomycin in the prevention and treatment of scar formation in the pediatric aerodigestive tract: friend or foe? Arch Otolaryngol Head Neck Surg 2002; 128: 401–406

130 Rahbar R, Shapshay SM, Healy GB. Mitomycin: effects on laryngeal and tracheal stenosis, benefits, and complications. Ann Otol Rhinol Laryngol 2001; 110: 1–6

131 Godbersen GS, Leh, JF, Hansmann ML, Rudert H, Linke RP. Organ-limited laryngeal amyloid deposits: clinical morphological, and immunohistochemical results of five cases. Ann Otol Rhinol Laryngol 1992; 101: 770–775

132 Myssiorek D, Persky M. Laser endoscopic treatment of laryngoceles and laryngeal cysts. Otolaryngol Head Neck Surg 1989; 100: 538–541

133 Piquet JJ, Darras JA, Burny A, Ton VJ, Verplanken M. Le traitement endoscopique au laser des kystes du larynx et des laryngoceles. Ann Otolaryngol Chir Cervicofac 1984; 101: 283–285

134 Kleinsasser O. Tumoren des Larynx und des Hypopharynx. Stuttgart: 1987

135 Michaels L. Pathology of the larynx. Berlin, Heidelberg; Springer, 1984

136 Friedmann I, Ferlito A. Granulomas and neoplasms of the larynx. Edinburgh: Churchill Livingstone, 1988

137 Pou AM, Rimell FL, Fordan JA et al. Adult respiratory papillomatosis: human papillomavirus type and viral coinfections as predictors of prognosis. Ann Otol Rhinol Laryngol 1995; 104: 758–762

138 Kimberlin DW, Malis DJ. Juvenile onset recurrent respiratory papillomatoses: possibilities for successful antiviral therapy. Antiviral Res 2000; 45: 83–93

139 Doyle DJ, Gianoli GJ, Espinola T, Miller RH. Recurrent respiratory papillomatosis: juvenile versus adult forms. Laryngoscope 1994; 104: 523–527

140 Armstrong LR, Preston EJ, Reichert M et al. Incidence and prevalence of recurrent respiratory papillomatosis among children in Atlanta and Seattle. Clin Infect Dis 2000; 31: 107–109

141 Hill DS, Akhtar S, Corroll A, Croft CB. Quality of life issues in recurrent respiratory papillomatosis. Clin Otolaryngol 2000; 25: 153–160

142 Rehberg E, Kleinsasser O. Malignant transformation in non-irradiated juvenile laryngeal papillomatosis. Eur Arch Otorhinolaryngol 1999; 256: 450–454

143 Franco, Jr RA, Zeitels SM, Farinelli WA, Anderson RR, 585 nm pulsed dye laser treatment of glottal papillomatosis. Ann Otol Rhinol Laryngol 2002; 111: 486–492

144 McMillan K, Shapshay SM, McGilligan JA, Wang Z, Rebeiz EE. A 585-nanometer pulsed dye laser reatment of laryngeal papillomas: preliminary report. Laryngoscope 1998; 108: 968–972

145 Desloge RB, Zeitels SM. Endolaryngeal microsurgery at the anterior glottal commissure: controversies and observations. Ann Otol Rhinol Laryngol 2000; 109: 385–392

146 Wetmore SJ, Key JM, Suen JY. Complications of laser surgery for laryngeal papillomatosis. Laryngoscope 1985; 95: 798–801

147 Uloza V. The course of laryngeal papillomatosis treated by endolaryngeal microsurgery. Eur Arch Otorhinolaryngol 2000; 257: 498–501

148 Dedo HH, Jackler RK. Laryngeal papilloma: results of treatment with the CO_2-laser and podophyllum. Ann Otol Rhinol Laryngol 1982; 91: 425–430

149 Walther EK, Herberhold C. Behandlung der laryngotrachealen Papillomatose mit kombinierter Anwendung von Laserchirurgie und intraläsionaler Applikation von Alpha-Interferon (Roferon). Laryngorhinootologie 1993; 72: 485–491

150 Benjamin BN, Gatenby PA, Kitchen R, Harrison H, Cameron K, Basten A. Alpha-interferon (Wellferon) as an adjunct to standard surgical therapy in the management of recurrent respiratory papillomatosis. Ann Otol Rhinol Laryngol 1988; 97: 376–-380

151 Snoeck R, Bossens M, Parent D et al. Phase II double-blind, placebo-controlled study of the safety and efficacy of cidofovir topical gel for the treatment of patients with human papillomavirus infection. Clin Infect Dis 2001; 33: 597–602

152 Snoeck R, Wellens W, Desloovere C et al. Treatment of severe laryngeal papillomatosis with intralesional injections of cidofovir [(S)-1-(3-hydroxy-2-phosphonylmethoxypropyl)cytosine]. J Med Virol 1998; 54: 219–225

153 van Valckenborgh I, Wellens W, de Boeck K, Snoeck R, de Clerq E, Feenstra L. Systemic cidofovir in papillomatosis. Clin Infect Dis 2001; 32: E62–E64

154 Bielamowicz S, Villagomez V, Stager SV, Wilson WR. Intralesional cidofovir therapy for laryngeal papilloma in an adult cohort. Laryngoscope 2002; 112: 696–699

155 Eckel HE, Jungehülsing M. Lipoma of the hypopharynx: preoperative diagnosis and transoral resection. J Laryngol Otol 1994; 108: 174–177

156 Jungehülsing M, Fischbach R, Pototschnig C, Eckel HE, Damm M. Rare benign tumors: laryngeal and hypopharyngeal lipomata. Ann Otol Rhinol Laryngol 2000; 109: 301–305

157 Werner JA, Lippert BM, Hoffmann P, Rudert H. Nd:YAG laser therapy of voluminous hemangiomas and vascular malformations. Adv Otorhinolaryngol 1995; 49: 75–80

158 Yellin SA, LaBruna A, Anand VK. Nd:YAG laser treatment for laryngeal and hypopharyngeal hemangiomas: a new technique. Ann Otol Rhinol Laryngol 1996; 105: 510–515

159 Glanz H. Pathomorphologische Aspekte zur transoralen Resektion von Hypopharynxkarzinomen mit Erhalt des Kehlkopfes. Selektion von Patienten – Therapieergebnisse. Laryngorhinootologie 1999; 78: 654–662

160 Steiner W. Endoskopische Chirurgie in den oberen Atemwegen. Laryngol Rhinol Otol (Stuttg) 1984; 63: 198–202

161 Meyers A. Complications of CO_2-laser surgery of the larynx. Ann Otol Rhinol Laryngol 1981; 90: 132–134

162 Dejonckere PH, Franceschi D, Scholtes JL. Extensive granuloma pyogenicum as a complication of endolaryngeal argon laser surgery. Lasers Surg Med 1985; 5: 41–45

163 Eckel HE, Thumfart WF. Synechieprophylaxe und -therapie nach Laserresektion von Kehlkopftumoren. Laryngol Rhinol Otol (Stuttg) 1988; 67: 116–117

164 Ilgner J, Falter F, Westhofen M. Long-term follow-up after laser induced endotracheal fire. J Laryngol Otol 2002; 116: 213–215

165 Santos P, Ayuso A, Luis M, Martinez G, Sala X. Airway ignition during CO_2-laser laryngeal surgery and high frequency jet ventilation. Eur J Anaesthesiol 2000; 17: 204–207

166 Klussmann JP, Knoedgen R, Eckel HE. Easy and safe dental protection in rigid endoscopy. Laryngoscope: (in press)

167 Klussmann JP, Knoedgen R, Wittekind C, Damm M, Eckel HE. Complications of suspension laryngoscopy. Ann Otol Rhinol Laryngol 2002; 11: 972–976

6 Lasers for Malignant Lesions in the Upper Aerodigestive Tract

P. Ambrosch

■ Contents

■ Abstract

Transoral laser microsurgery has developed in recent years into an operating method combining a minimally invasive approach with the special advantages of the laser: surgical precision, ease of control, optimum tissue effect, and non-contact technique. This chapter describes the principles of laser use in the microsurgical resection of carcinomas of the oral cavity, oropharynx, hypopharynx, and larynx. The oncologic and functional results of laser microsurgery are compared with the results of competitive standard procedures. Laser microsurgery is widely acknowledged to have advantages in the treatment of early glottic carcinoma. The role of laser surgery in the treatment of glottic carcinoma causing impaired mobility or fixation of the vocal cords has not yet been definitively assessed. Based on results published to date, primary laser therapy can achieve local tumor clearance with a functional residual larynx in approximately 70 % of cases. Laser microsurgery is of comparable efficacy to classic partial laryngectomy in the treatment of recurrent laryngeal carcinoma following primary radiotherapy and leads to fewer complications. In patients with early or moderately advanced supraglottic carcinoma, laser microsurgery is comparable to classic partial laryngectomy in terms of local control and survival. With regard to organ preservation, laser microsurgery is comparable to classic partial laryngectomy but superior to radiotherapy. Microsurgery can preserve functionally important structures, allowing for early swallowing rehabilitation while avoiding tracheotomy. Cancers of the hypopharynx can also be treated by laser surgery with good preservation of anatomy and function and good oncologic results. Laser microsurgery provides a therapeutic alternative to standard therapies and newer protocols aimed at organ preservation (neoadjuvant chemotherapy and radiotherapy, simultaneous chemotherapy and radiotherapy). For cancers of the oral cavity and oropharynx, approaching the lesion by the endoral or transoral route greatly reduces morbidity by eliminating the need for a pharyngotomy, mandibulotomy or mandibulectomy, and tracheotomy. Even large defects in the oral cavity and oropharynx do not require plastic surgical repair. This will not necessarily have adverse effects on postoperative swallowing and phonation.

■ Introduction

The treatment of malignant tumors of the upper aerodigestive tract has long posed a great challenge to head and neck surgeons due to the complex anatomy and functions of this region. Tumors were generally resected through a transcervical approach that exposes the affected region. The introduction of microlaryngoscopy was a great step forward in the treatment of early glottic carcinoma, providing a minimally invasive endoscopic approach and the opportunity to utilize the advantages of the operating microscope. Microlaryngoscopy was an essential prelude to the subsequent development of laser microsurgery.

When surgical laser use was introduced during the early 1970s, surgeons mainly used the CO_2 laser as a new kind of scalpel. The laser was held in a handpiece and used for open surgery. Later, however, it became increasingly clear that the real benefit of lasers lay in endoscopic and microscopic applications. During recent years, transoral laser microsurgery has developed into an operating method that combines a minimally invasive approach with the special advantages of the laser: surgical precision, ease of control, optimum tissue effect, and noncontact technique. This permits an organ- and function-conserving mode of tumor surgery whose current importance is reflected in its expanding range of indications compared with competitive, established therapeutic procedures.

This article explores the principles of laser microsurgery in the resection of carcinomas of the oral cavity, oropharynx, hypopharynx, and larynx. The oncologic and functional results of this surgery are compared with those of standard therapeutic procedures. The original results in this article are drawn from cases treated since 1986 at the Department of Otorhinolaryngology at the University of Göttingen (director: Prof. Dr. W. Steiner).

■ Methods

Instrumentation

CO_2 Laser

A CO_2 laser coupled to an operating microscope is used for tumor surgery in the oral cavity, pharynx, and larynx. The tissue effects of the laser beam depend on its specific properties and the characteristics of the treated tissue. Surgical laser use basically involves the conversion of light energy into thermal energy, the energy transformation in the tissue depending mainly on absorption, scattering, and heat conduction. With the CO_2 laser, all the laser energy is converted into heat when the beam strikes the tissue. With a wavelength of 10,600 nm, the CO_2 laser light is strongly absorbed by water. Since biological tissue has a very high water content, the superficial tissue layer absorbs virtually all of the laser light, resulting in an extremely shallow penetration depth and almost no scattering. This means that the conversion of laser energy to thermal energy takes place within a very small tissue volume. It takes just a few milliseconds for the CO_2 laser to heat tissue water to the boiling point, causing an intense evaporation which entrains nonfluid tissue elements. The thermal effect spreads to adjacent layers via heat conduction in the tissue, although the thermal effect zone measures only a fraction of a millimeter. The heat is sufficient to seal small blood vessels at the periphery of the beam. These tissue effects explain both the good cutting properties of the CO_2 laser and its relatively weak coagulating effect. The diameter of the CO_2 laser beam can be adjusted to produce either of two effects: tissue ablation with a spot size of 1–4 mm or tissue cutting with a spot size of 0.2–1 mm.

A key technical advance in recent years has been the development of CO_2 lasers emitting pulsed energy in the microsecond range, which can be focused to a diameter of 250 µm with a micromanipulator. This extremely small spot size allows very precise energy application, and the short pulse duration allows the tissue to cool between pulses by thermal relaxation and diffusion. The resulting tissue incision is almost free of charring. This development is of interest not only in the prevention of thermal damage to the vocal ligament in phonosurgery but also in the surgical treatment of early glottic carcinoma. For tumor surgery, it is generally sufficient to use a micromanipulator with a spot size of 0.2–0.5 mm. It is desirable to connect a video camera to the microscope so the assistants, anesthesiologist, and scrub nurse can follow the procedure.

Laryngoscopes

The laryngoscopes designed by Kleinsasser have been modified and adapted for the specific requirements of laser surgery. Manufacturers offer a range of laryngoscopes with built-in or removable side arms for smoke evacuation, a matted finish, and assorted working lengths and diameters. We have achieved the best results with a medium-sized closed laryngoscope, used mainly for the endolarynx; an extended-length, closed, small-caliber laryngoscope for the more difficult endolarynx and for exposing the anterior commissure, interarytenoid region, and subglottis; and an adjustable laryngopharyngoscope (bivalved laryngoscope), available in two lengths, for exposing the tongue base, vallecula, supraglottis, and hypopharynx. The laryngoscopes are supported on an adjustable round stand, specially designed for laser microsurgery, which is attached to the operating table. The stand has a large working radius that can also accommodate laryngoscopes introduced from the side.

Microinstrumentation

Necessary microinstruments include assorted grasping forceps, insulated suction tube for both aspiration and monopolar cautery, small coagulation forceps, clip-applying forceps, and protectors for protecting and retracting tissue.

Anesthesia

Intravenous, balanced, or inhalation anesthesia can be used for endoscopic operations in the oral cavity, pharynx, and larynx. The selection of agents is determined by the condition of the patient, the pharmacologic properties of the agents, and the personal preference of the anesthesiologist.

Intubation is the safest and most effective method of establishing a clear airway and permits optimum monitoring of ventilation and gas concentrations. For laser microsurgery of carcinomas of the upper aerodigestive tract, we prefer to use the smallest endotracheal tube that can maintain adequate ventilation. We adjust the tube placement as needed during the operation (e.g., to expose the posterior commissure of the larynx). If moving the tube does not permit adequate visualization, parts of the operation can be done in intermittent apnea. In this technique the patient is initially ventilated with 100% inspiratory oxygen for 1–2 minutes. The surgeon then removes the tube, continues the operation in apnea, and reintroduces the tube between apneic phases through the laryngoscope. This technique requires optimum monitoring and good teamwork between the surgeon and anesthesiologist to prevent hypoxia. It can be used whenever jet ventilation is unavailable or contraindicated.

Lasers can be used with special endotracheal tubes like the Laser Shield II (Xomed-Treace), an aluminum and Teflon-coated silicone tube, or the Laser Flex (Mallinckrodt), a spiral metallic tube with two cuffs. For years we have used the MLT Tube (Mallinckrodt) made of polyvinyl chloride (PVC), preferring the tube with a 6-mm inside diameter for most applications. The tube cuff is filled with saline solution and covered with moist pledgets in the area of the subglottis. The tube shaft can be wrapped with Merocel Laser Guard (silver foil coated with water-soaked foam) to protect it from an accidental laser strike. We also use a bare MLT Tube to improve vision in confined anatomic spaces. Studies by Braun [1] indicate that a continuous, perpendicular laser beam with a spot size of 0.5 mm can perforate the tube wall in 30 seconds at 5 W, in 11 seconds at 10 W, and in 2 seconds at 35 W. In clinical use, the tube will withstand accidental laser exposure at a tangential angle for a considerable period. We have had positive experience with this tube, but the technique described cannot be generally recommended due to concerns regarding laser safety.

When jet ventilation is diligently done with modern equipment and when due attention is given to contraindications, it is a safe ventilation technique [2] that can even be used in laryngeal cancer surgery [3]. In the clinical use of jet ventilation, it is important to maintain a free return flow of gas from the bronchial system. The patient should be relaxed. Pulse oximetry is an essential monitoring tool. The injector probe is mounted in the laryngoscope and positioned in front of the glottis. Insufficient attention to gas outflow can lead to typical jet-ventilation–associated complications such as pneumothorax, mediastinal emphysema, gastric distension, regurgitation, and aspiration of gastric contents. One disadvantage of jet ventilation is that the air flow causes movements of the true and false vocal cords, which can hamper precise surgery. Jet ventilation should not be used in patients with severe glottic or subglottic stenosis (e. g., from an obstructing tumor) that can interfere with gas outflow. It is also contraindicated in other obstructive and restrictive ventilation problems, severe cardiovascular disease, and by prolonged operating time and anticipated intraoperative bleeding.

Surgical Principles

The goal of laser microsurgery is no different from that of conventional tumor resections: to remove the tumor completely with clear surgical margins. The main advantages of transoral laser surgery over standard procedures lie in its methodology.

Basically laser surgery is guided by intraoperative findings, i. e., the surgeon traces the tumor and makes operative decisions based on the tumor extent. With larger tumors, the depth of infiltration can be evaluated by resecting the tumor piecemeal. The limits of the resection are defined by the tumor extent visible under the operating microscope and can be adapted to individual circumstances. Healthy tissue can be spared to the extent necessary to preserve the organ and its function. Patient morbidity is much lower than in conventional tumor surgery because a tracheotomy is rarely necessary and swallowing is quickly reestablished after the operation [4].

The procedure for a transoral laser resection is fundamentally different from, say, a classic partial laryngectomy. In a supracricoid partial laryngectomy, for example, a standard resection is carried out to achieve reproducible functional results. The surgeon determines whether a standard resection is possible during preoperative microlaryngoscopy. If more extensive disease is found at operation, it may be necessary to convert a planned partial resection to a total laryngectomy. The ability to preserve almost any structure and tissue with laser microsurgery also carries some risks, as the following two examples show: In patients with glottic carcinoma, the mobility of the vocal cords is restricted due to invasion of the thyroarytenoid muscle. Laser microsurgery makes it possible to preserve portions of the muscle, but this poses a risk of recurrence that is entirely unnecessary, since a muscular remnant is not useful for postoperative voice rehabilitation. The other example is the resection of preepiglottic fatty tissue in patients with supraglottic cancer. Parts of this tissue can be spared, but it carries a risk of leaving behind tumor remnants that cannot be seen with the operating microscope. Complete resection of the preepiglottic fat will remove any tumor cell aggregates that may be present while only slightly delaying the rehabilitation of swallowing.

Histopathologic Examination of Surgical Specimens

A major objection to laser tumor excision was the inability to adequately evaluate the margins of laser-resected specimens. The lasers available in the 1970s produced a charred zone approximately 250 µm wide, which hampered histologic evaluation of the specimen margins. The tissue effects of lasers available today have been substantially improved by more precise focusing. The zone of charring and necrosis seen in histologic specimens depends on the beam parameters (power, focusing, continuous or pulsed mode of operation). We have found that this charred zone measures approximately 25 µm with an underlying edematous zone no larger than 50 µm. Thermal tissue alteration by the laser does not affect the assessability of even small specimens [5].

The resection of oropharyngeal cancers must include a sufficiently wide tissue margin around the tumor (approximately 5–10 mm), since fingers of submucous cancer may extend peripherally from the grossly visible tumor borders ("reticular" type of infiltration) [6]. A less generous margin is generally considered adequate around vocal cord and supraglottic tumors (approximately 1–3 mm). Smaller tumors can be encompassed and removed in one piece. All the margins of a small specimen can be histologically examined. We follow the principle described by Mohs for skin tumors and its modification by Davidson [6, 7] for mucosal tumors of the upper aerodigestive tract, which involves sectioning and examining all surgical margins parallel to the tumor margins.

More extensive or unfavorably situated cancers of the oral cavity, pharynx, and larynx should be removed in a piecemeal, mosaic pattern. In this technique the surgeon should carefully label all the specimens. It is particularly important to label the basal surface of specimens from deeper sites that do not have epithelium to aid orientation. The specimens are cut into slices by the pathologist, embedded, and sectioned perpendicular to the surface. The pathologist evaluates the depth of tumor infiltration, the tumor grade, basal clearance, and margins. The surgeon must be able to reassemble the mosaic from the histologic findings for pT staging. In laser microsurgery as in conventional surgery, all of the margins of larger tumors cannot be completely evaluated at the histologic level. If one surgical margin is found to be positive for tumor cell aggregates by histopathology, the reexcision of further tissue is indicated. This can be done at any time, since the wound bed is left open and is not resurfaced by a flap procedure.

The histologic processing of a specimen excised from the vocal cord is carried out using the method described by Kleinsasser and Glanz [8]. With cancers involving the anterior commissure, the perichondrium about the vocal cord attachment should be dissected from the cartilage with a round knife to protect it from thermal damage and preserve it for histologic examination. With deeply infiltrating and transglottic laryngeal cancers, the perichondrium of the thyroid cartilage should also be resected. Tumor removal with an adequate margin of normal tissue cannot be demonstrated in all histologic sections for tumors infiltrating the perichondrium. It is the surgeon's responsibility in these cases to decide whether the resection should be considered complete. If necessary, portions of the thyroid and/or cricoid cartilage can be included in the resection.

Special Aspects of Pretherapeutic Diagnosis of the Primary Tumor

Laryngeal Carcinoma

Accurate staging of glottic carcinoma and supraglottic carcinoma must include an assessment of vocal cord mobility. This requires inspection by magnifying or flexible laryngoscopy as well as stroboscopic inspection for early glottic cancers. The tumor extent is determined at microlaryngoscopy. Angled rigid scopes are useful for evaluating the subglottis.

A cytologic smear taken from the endolarynx under topical anesthesia is helpful in the benign/malignant differentiation of a proliferative lesion, particularly since this technique does not alter the gross appearance of the lesion. However, smear cytology is rewarding only if cancer cells are detected. Otherwise, with an early lesion, all grossly visible tumor should be removed using excisional biopsy technique.

Multiple biopsies should not be taken from a glottic cancer to confirm the diagnosis. Inflammatory reactions and granulations in biopsied or partially resected vocal cord lesions can make it extremely difficult to distinguish between tumor and uninvolved tissue so that precise laser microsurgical resection can be carried out. Unfortunately, this often results in needless sacrifice of functionally useful ligamentous and muscular structures due to difficulties in evaluating the tissue.

For a cancer that has caused fixation or impaired mobility of the vocal cords or an anterior commissure carcinoma with supra- and/or subglottic extension, computed tomography (CT) should be performed to exclude cartilage invasion and extralaryngeal disease. Supraglottic cancers should be staged with either CT or magnetic resonance imaging (MRI) for detecting any infiltration of the pre- and paraglottic space and cartilage invasion. MRI is particularly useful for detecting submucous tumor spread and invasion of the preepiglottic fat. Imaging studies should always be done prior to diagnostic microlaryngoscopy and biopsy.

Carcinoma of the Oral Cavity

Preoperative diagnosis in oral carcinoma includes the assessment of tongue mobility (involvement of the intrinsic muscles or hypoglossal nerve) and the clinical evaluation of submucous tumor spread and the invasion of surrounding structures (mandible, faucial pillars, tonsils). Tumors within the body of the tongue and oral floor are best delineated by contrast-enhanced CT or MRI. Both studies can demonstrate tumor size, tumor spread across the midline, extension to the tongue base, and invasion of the masticatory muscles and parapharyngeal space. The advantages of MRI consist of arbitrary plane selection and high soft-tissue contrast, which more clearly define the spread of tongue cancer across the midline and extension to the oral floor. CT is better for demonstrating osteolytic foci that indicate bone destruction; this is particularly common with floor of the mouth cancers which have infiltrated the mandible.

Pharyngeal Carcinoma

The preoperative workup of carcinoma of the soft palate and tonsil includes defining the visible and submucous extent of disease by inspection, palpation, and endoscopy of neighboring regions. For carcinoma of the tongue base, the flexible endoscopic examination is supplemented by bimanual palpation since small and predominantly submucous cancers may be overlooked at endoscopy. With hypopharyngeal carcinoma, it is important during preoperative endoscopy to test the mobility of the vocal cords and arytenoid cartilage since mobile vocal cords mean that a function-conserving tumor resection by laser microsurgery can be performed in most cases. It should also be determined during diagnostic microlaryngoscopy whether the apex of the piriform sinus, cervical esophagus, and larynx are involved by tumor.

Imaging studies are essential in patients with oropharyngeal and hypopharyngeal cancers. They are the only means of diagnosing the often clinically undetectable presence of submucous tumor spread into the lateral cervical soft tissues, larynx, and paraesophageal tissues. Sagittal MRI may afford a particularly high-contrast view of tongue base carcinomas in relation to the surrounding lingual muscles and preepiglottic fat.

■ Laser Microsurgery of Glottic Carcinoma

Since microlaryngoscopic laser surgery was introduced in head and neck surgery [9], the range of indications for endoscopic surgery, initially limited to the resection of vocal cord microcarcinomas and the palliative debulking of large tumors obstructing the airway, has significantly expanded. Today laser surgery is a widely accepted alternative to traditional endoscopic resection techniques with cold cutting instruments [10], open partial laryngectomies, and radiotherapy, especially in the treatment of early glottic cancers. A tumor confined *to the middle third* of the vocal cord with normal cord mobility (T1a) has become a widely recognized indication for resection by laser microsurgery. The tumor can be removed without placing the lines of resection through the lesion. For some years now, supraglottic laryngeal cancers have also been recognized as an indication for glottis-preserving partial laryngectomy using laser microsurgery [11]. Given these recent developments, it is necessary to consider the role of transoral laser microsurgery in cases where this technique competes with or replaces conventional partial laryngectomy, primary radiotherapy, or total laryngectomy.

T1 and T2a Glottic Carcinoma

There is no generally accepted definition for an "early" glottic carcinoma. While some authors believe that this definition includes premalignant changes (severe dysplasia), others classify T1 tumors as early glottic carcinomas, and some even include T2 lesions in this category. We define early glottic cancer as carcinoma in situ and carcinoma involving one (T1a) or both (T1b) vocal folds, as well as unilateral or bilateral glottic carcinoma involving the supra- and/or subglottis with preservation of vocal cord mobility (T2a).

Operative Technique

Small midcordal tumors can be resected en bloc (Fig. 6.**1**). More extensive vocal cord lesions are removed piecemeal with a clear margin of approximately 1–3 mm (Figs. 6.**2**–6.**4**). We try to maintain narrow margins and preserve as much healthy tissue as possible to improve the prospects for postoperative voice recovery. A positive margin in the histopathologic specimen means that additional tissue should be resected by laser microsurgery to exclude and if necessary remove any residual tumor. Morbidity associated with transoral laser microsurgery of early glottic carcinoma is low. A tracheotomy is never required and complications are rare, enabling the surgery to be performed on an outpatient basis.

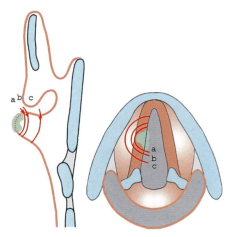

Fig. 6.**1** Lines of resection for an early glottic carcinoma confined to the middle third of the vocal cord. **a** Inadequate safety margin: the line of resection is touching the tumor border. **b** Resection with a narrow margin of healthy tissue. **c** Resection with a wide margin (diagram from [4]).

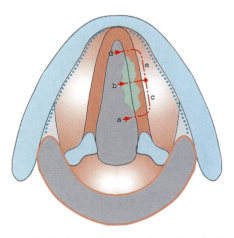

Fig. 6.**2** Technique for two-part resection of a glottic carcinoma (diagram from [4]).

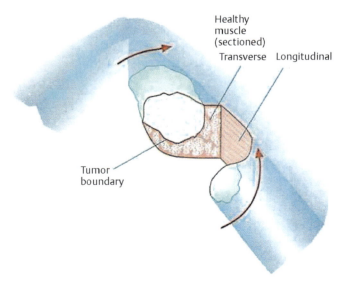

Healthy muscle (sectioned)

Transverse   Longitudinal

Tumor boundary

Fig. 6.**3** Section through a T1 glottic carcinoma. The cut surface shows the tumor and healthy muscle tissue (diagram from [4]).

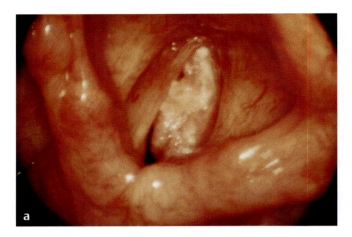

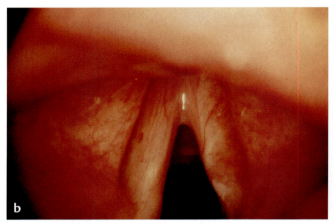

Fig. 6.**4** Carcinoma of the right vocal cord (T1). **a** Preoperative appearance. **b** Appearance one year after tumor resection by laser microsurgery.

Classification of Endolaryngeal Cordectomy

Various proposals have been made in recent years for standardizing laser microsurgical resections of the vocal cords [12, 13]. In 2000, Remacle et al. [14] published a classification proposed by the European Laryngological Society. This classification distinguishes eight types of endoscopic cordectomies based on the extent of the resection. Classifications of this kind appear to be justified from the standpoint of comparing treatment results, and it remains to be seen whether this classification system will be adopted by surgeons who practice cordectomies.

Results of Laser Microsurgery

A number of authors in recent years have reported good oncologic and functional results with laser microsurgery in the treatment of Tis–T2a glottic carcinomas. The 5-year local control rate for these tumors ranged from 80% to 94%. It was possible to preserve the larynx in more than 92% of cases (Table 6.1).

Table 6.1 Results of laser microsurgery of early glottic carcinoma

Author	Number of patients	Local control	Larynx preservation	Indication
Shapshay et al. 1990 [15]	20	90%	–	T1a
Eckel and Thumfart 1992 [16]	24	92%	100%	T1a
Steiner 1993 [17]	159	94%	99%	Tis–T2a
Czigner et al. 1994 [18]	55	85%	92%	Tis–T2
Rudert and Werner 1995 [19]	114	91%	100%	Tis–T2
Lindholm & Elner 1995 [20]	47	91%	100%	T1a
Thumfart et al. 1996 [21]	97	88%	95%	T1a, T1b
Motta et al. 1997 [22]	321	82%	94%	T1a, T1b
Peretti et al. 1997 [23]	140	80%	96%	Tis–T2
Mahieu et al. 2000 [24]	127	92%	99%	T1a
Ambrosch et al. 2001 [25]	248	92%	99%	T1a
	35	80%	94%	T1b
	109	84%	96%	T2a
Peretti et al. 2001 [26]	88	91%	94%	Tis, T1
Gallo et al. 2002 [27]	117	94%	–	T1b
	22	91%	–	T1b
	17	100%	100%	Tis

Among our own patients, the Kaplan–Meier 5-year local control rate for pT1a lesions (n = 248) was 92%. The control rate was 80% for pT1b carcinomas (n = 35) and 84% for pT2a carcinomas (n = 109). The secondary laryngectomy rates were 1.2% for pT1a lesions, 5.7% for pT1b lesions, and 3.7% for pT2a lesions. The Kaplan–Meier 5-year rate for definitive local control ("ultimate local control rate") was 99% in patients with pT1a tumors, 97% in patients with pT1b tumors, and 98% in patients with pT2a tumors [25].

Treatment of Recurrent Tumors

A key advantage of laser microsurgery for glottic carcinoma is that it leaves open all treatment options in patients found to have a local recurrence or a second primary tumor in the head and neck region, including laser reexcision, open partial laryngectomy, and radiation therapy [17, 25, 28]. The majority of local recurrences in our patients were successfully treated by further transoral laser microsurgery [25].

Other Treatment Options

The oncologic results of *open partial laryngectomy* (i. e., cordectomy after thyrotomy and frontolateral laryngectomy) for early glottic carcinoma are very good. The 5-year local control rate is 90–98%, and the 5-year rate for preservation of the larynx is 93–98% [10, 29–33]. These operations are associated with greater morbidity than laser microsurgery, however, due to the need for a temporary tracheotomy, the possible need for a feeding tube, and a longer hospital stay.

The 5-year local control rate that can be achieved with *primary radiotherapy* for a T1 glottic carcinoma is reportedly in the range of 81–90%, which is considerably lower than that obtained with open surgery. The 5-year rate for organ preservation is approximately 90–98% [34–40]. With T2 glottic carcinomas and a mobile vocal cord, the local control rates decline to approximately 64–87% while the rate of organ preservation falls to 75–87% [35, 41–44]. However, the most serious disadvantage of radiotherapy compared with laser microsurgery is that in the event of a local tumor recurrence, it is rarely possible to undertake a partial laryngectomy, and usually the only remaining option is total laryngectomy. Also, radiotherapy usually cannot be repeated in previously irradiated patients found to have a recurrent tumor or second primary tumor in the head and neck region.

Vocal function following laser microsurgery, conventional cordectomy, and radiotherapy is still a controversial issue. It is generally agreed that primary radiotherapy results in better voice quality than open cordectomy [32, 45]. More recent studies prove, however, that the voice is by no means "normal" in patients who have received radiotherapy for an early laryngeal carcinoma [46, 47]. As various comparative studies on voice quality indicate, the contradictory results are due mainly to differences in patient selection and methods of voice analysis. Thus, while some authors found that voice results were better after primary laser microsurgery than after conventional cordectomy [48, 49], other authors found no appreciable differences between patients who underwent laser microsurgery and radiotherapy based on perceptual voice evaluation or objective voice analysis [50–52]. Still other authors found that voice quality was significantly better after radiotherapy than after laser microsurgery [53, 54].

In our experience, the postoperative voice quality after laser microsurgery depends on a number of factors. Of particular importance are the location and extent of the tumor on the vocal cord surface and the depth of tumor invasion. These parameters determine the minimum extent of an oncologically sound resection. The voice result also depends critically on whether the tumor is resected with a narrow or wide margin of uninvolved tissue. Finally, voice quality is determined by the wound healing process, which is associated with varying degrees of granulation and scarring. Effective postoperative voice therapy is another important factor. The prospects for successful voice recovery depend ultimately on what functionally important structures the surgeon was able to preserve. These prospects are most favorable when the voice can be rehabilitated at the level of glottic phonation. Voice rehabilitation at the ventricular level results in varying degrees of dysphonia [4, 55, 56].

With the growing importance of economic considerations, various treatment modalities have been subjected to cost analysis in recent years. Myers et al. [57] found that laser surgery incurred only about one-third the costs of radiotherapy. Brandenburg [50] calculated that the costs of radiotherapy were 15 times higher compared with laser surgery. These figures confirm the importance of cost calculations and suggest that as medicine becomes more cost-conscious, laser microsurgery will become an increasingly important treatment option for early glottic carcinoma.

Glottic Carcinoma with Involvement of the Anterior Commissure

Whether laser microsurgery is appropriate for glottic carcinoma with involvement of the anterior commissure is still controversial. While carcinomas rarely arise from the anterior commissure itself, it is very common for lesions of the vocal cord to extend to the anterior commissure. The peculiar anatomy of this region, with an absence of perichondrium at the vocal cord insertion, the extension of the vocal cord fibers into the thyroid cartilage, and the connections between the intra- and extralaryngeal blood vessels and lymphatics [58–60], facilitates the infiltration of the thyroid cartilage by vocal cord lesions and their extralaryngeal spread through the cricothyroid ligament. Kirchner and Carter [61] observed in serial organ sections that T1a and T1b carcinomas rarely infiltrate the thyroid cartilage. On the other hand, carcinomas of the anterior commissure that have invaded the cartilage typically show supraglottic extension to the petiole region, subglottic extension, or both (T2 carcinomas) [61, 62].

In 1989, Krespi and Meltzer [63] reported on the laser resection of glottic carcinomas involving the anterior commissure in five patients. All the patients developed local recurrence. This prompted animal studies to investigate the possibility of microlaryngoscopic exposure of the anterior commissure. Because the resection apparently did not reach the anterior commissure in the experimental animals as well, the authors warned of the tendency for carcinomas in this region to recur after laser surgery. Other authors also reported incomplete resections of tumors involving the anterior commissure as a result of inadequate exposure and a tangential view of the operative site. Based on the numerous recurrences, the authors concluded that glottic tumors with anterior commissure extension were generally a contraindication to endoscopic laser surgery [63–66]. Other authors, however, were able to show that the adequacy of tumor resection in the anterior commissure depends on the degree of commissure exposure and that these lesions can be reliably resected by an experienced surgeon using proper instruments [16, 17, 22, 23, 67–70].

Results of Laser Microsurgery

We investigated the effect of anterior commissure extension on recurrence rates, organ preservation, and survival rates in 263 patients with previously untreated T1a, T1b, and T2a glottic carcinomas who underwent laser microsurgery at our Göttingen center between 1987 and 1996. We found that involvement of the anterior commissure by carcinoma at these T stages did affect local tumor control and

organ preservation but did not affect patient survival rates. The Kaplan–Meier 5-year local control rate for T1a lesions with anterior commissure involvement was 86%, compared with 75% for T1b lesions and 78% for T2a lesions. The larynx was preserved in 93% of the patients with T1a lesions involving the anterior commissure, 88% with T1b lesions, and 93% with T2a lesions. With carcinomas that did not involve the anterior commissure, the 5-year local control rates were 95% for T1a lesions, 93% for T1b lesions, and 83% for T2a lesions. The larynx was preserved in 99%, 94%, and 97% of the patients, respectively [71].

Some recurrences are definitely the result of inadequate primary resection. In our experience, adequate exposure of the anterior commissure is absolutely essential for prevention of tumor recurrence. Exposure can be improved by using a small, closed laryngoscope and applying external pressure to the laryngeal skeleton, providing the surgeon with a direct rather than tangential view of the subglottis. Resecting the most anterior portions of the ventricular folds can help improve exposure of the vocal cords, although uninvolved tissue in this area should be resected very sparingly as a rule, since the ventricular folds are useful for subsequent voice rehabilitation. Carcinomas of the anterior commissure should always be resected en bloc under high magnification. The vocal cord insertion on the thyroid cartilage is completely removed along with the surrounding perichondrium. If subglottic tumor growth is visible below the anterior commissure, the resection should be extended to the inferior border of the thyroid cartilage to ensure that extralaryngeal tumor spread around the inferior edge of the thyroid cartilage is not missed. The cricothyroid ligament is also completely resected if necessary (Fig. 6.5). In difficult cases, a second-look laser excisional biopsy should be performed approximately 6–8 weeks later to exclude residual tumor.

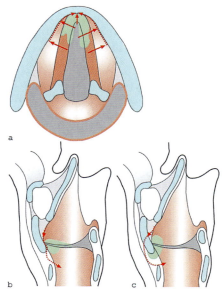

Fig. 6.5 Carcinoma of the anterior glottis. **a** Lines of resection. **b** Resection of portions of the cricothyroid ligament for subglottic tumor extension. **c** Resection of portions of the thyroid cartilage for infiltration of the cervical soft tissues (diagrams from [4]).

Other Treatment Options

Involvement of the anterior commissure is also associated with increased recurrence rates following *primary radiotherapy* and *frontolateral partial laryngectomy*. The local control rate after primary radiotherapy for a T1 carcinoma with anterior commissure extension is 57–84% [43, 72–75]. Local control rates of 80–90% have been reported after frontolateral partial laryngectomy for T1 carcinomas involving the anterior commissure [76–78]. Mallet et al. [79] achieved a 5-year local control rate of 94% in 65 patients with T1 and T2 glottic carcinomas who underwent a reconstructive anterior frontal laryngectomy with epiglottoplasty (Tucker operation).

Instead of a frontolateral partial laryngectomy, the more extensive *supracricoid partial laryngectomy* has been performed at some centers with the intention of improving the local control of anterior commissure disease. The supracricoid partial laryngectomy with cricohyoidoepiglottopexy (SCPL-CHEP) involves the resection of both vocal cords, both ventricular folds, the paraglottic space on both sides, the entire thyroid cartilage, the petiole of the epiglottis, and the lower portion of the preepiglottic fat. For reconstruction, the cricoid cartilage is first attached to the epiglottic remnant and then to the hyoid bone. This operation invariably requires a temporary tracheotomy and nasogastric tube feeding. Laccourreye et al. [80] reported on 62 cases of T1 and T2 glottic carcinomas invading the anterior commissure managed by the SCPL-CHEP operation. Eighty-one percent of the patients received neoadjuvant chemotherapy. The 5-year local control rate was excellent (98%). None of the patients had to have a laryngectomy or permanent tracheotomy for functional reasons. It should be noted, however, that the treatment is associated with considerable morbidity and therefore cannot be recommended for all patients. All the patients in the Laccourreye series were extubated, but 17 required swallowing training for aspiration, four required temporary percutaneous endoscopic gastrostomy (PEG) tube placement, and one required permanent PEG placement. SCPL-CHEP is followed by an aryepiglottic vocal compensation with correspondingly poor voice quality [81–83].

Conclusion

Comparing the results of different treatments for early carcinoma of the vocal cords, we may conclude that laser microsurgery is the method of choice for the treatment of early glottic carcinoma based on oncologic, functional, and economic considerations. We do not believe that involvement of the anterior commissure is a contraindication against laser surgery, since the local control rates are comparable to that after vertical partial laryngectomy. Excellent local control rates can be obtained with SCPL-CHEP in properly selected patients, but this is achieved at the cost of considerably higher morbidity and frequent, significant impairment of swallowing and phonation.

T2b and T3 Glottic Carcinoma

T2 carcinomas of the glottis comprise a very heterogeneous group of tumors. Some cases may show supra- and/or subglottic tumor extension with normal vocal cord mobility, while other lesions cause impaired vocal cord mobility and show considerable supra- and/or subglottic extension. The two groups differ markedly in their prognosis. T2 tumors with impaired vocal cord mobility are comparable to T3 tumors with vocal cord fixation from the standpoint of local control rates and survival. We believe, therefore, that it is important to distinguish between T2a and T2b carcinomas. In their proposal for revising the TNM classification, Kleinsasser and Glanz [84] state that glottic carcinomas with impaired vocal cord mobility should be placed in the T3 category along with tumors that cause vocal cord fixation.

Operative Technique

The resection of larger glottic carcinomas by laser microsurgery requires subdividing the tumor into several parts. Tumors that have invaded the paraglottic space are subdivided by incisions extending laterally to the thyroid cartilage and inferiorly to the cricoid cartilage. The resection can be extended to the perichondrium of the thyroid cartilage and cricoid cartilage, to the thyroid and cricoid cartilages themselves, to the arytenoid cartilage, the cricothyroid ligament and the extralaryngeal soft tissues (Figs. 6.6, 6.7).

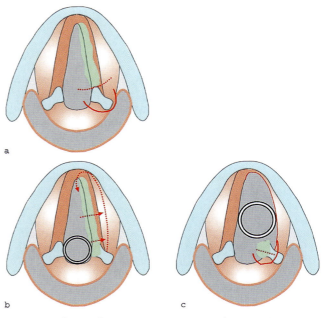

Fig. 6.**6**   Technique for resecting an extensive glottic carcinoma. **a** Incision anterior to the arytenoid cartilage. **b** Piecemeal tumor resection, proceeding from posterior to anterior. **c** (Partial) resection of the arytenoid cartilage (diagrams from [4]).

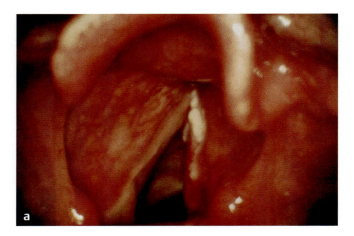

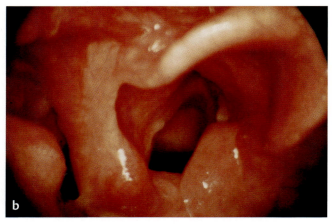

Fig. 6.7 Glottic carcinoma with fixation of the right vocal cord (T3). **a** Preoperative appearance. **b** Appearance after resection of the vocal fold, ventricular fold, and arytenoid cartilage by laser microsurgery.

Results of Laser Microsurgery

To date, we have experience with the laser microsurgery of glottic carcinomas causing impaired vocal cord mobility (T2b) or vocal cord fixation (T3) in a total of 167 patients. The postoperative TNM stage was pT2b(p)N0M0 in 97 patients and pT3(p)N0M0 in 70 patients. In patients with pT2b carcinomas, the anterior commissure was involved in 81% of cases, the contralateral vocal cord in 17%, the ipsilateral ventricular fold in 58%, and the infraglottic region in 52%. In patients with pT3 tumors, the anterior commissure was involved in 70%, the contralateral vocal cord in 28%, the ipsilateral ventricular fold in 56%, and the infraglottic region in 65%. The arytenoid cartilage was fixed in 45% of cases. Postoperatively, 10.3% of patients with stage II disease and 8.6% of patients with stage III disease underwent radiotherapy. The Kaplan–Meier 5-year local control rate was 74% for pT2b carcinomas and 68% for pT3 carcinomas. The respective secondary laryngectomy rates were 13.4% and 14.3%. The 5-year rate for definitive local tumor control was 87% in both groups, and the 5-year recurrence-free survival rate was 62% in both groups.

Postoperative voice quality in most patients was good. Speech intelligibility in the telephone test following ex-

tended laser resections was better than 90% in both groups. One patient developed glottic/subglottic cicatricial stenosis, necessitating a permanent tracheotomy. None of the patients was tracheotomized for the primary tumor surgery. Only 11% of patients with stage II disease and 44% of patients with stage III disease required nasogastric tube feeding (median of 4 days in the former group, 5 days in the latter). All patients were fully rehabilitated and had unrestricted oral intake. In summary, primary laser microsurgery can achieve a permanent cure in approximately 70% of patients, with preservation of the larynx and low morbidity [25].

Elsewhere in the literature, very little has been published on the laser microsurgery of T2 or T3 glottic carcinomas. Motta et al. [22] reported on 37 patients with T3 tumors who underwent laser microsurgery. Fifty-five percent of their patients developed locoregional recurrence, and 35% required salvage by secondary laryngectomy.

Other Treatment Options

The standard treatment for T2 glottic carcinoma with impaired vocal cord mobility is *vertical partial laryngectomy* or *radiotherapy*. Local control rates of 52–76% have been achieved with vertical partial laryngectomy for T2b neoplasms [85, 86]. Total laryngectomy is frequently done for glottic carcinomas with vocal cord fixation, and a few selected cases are managed by hemilaryngectomy. Local control rates between 73% and 83% have been reported after partial laryngectomy [87–90]. Primary total laryngectomy with a neck dissection, with or without postoperative irradiation, has a reported locoregional control rate of 69–87%, a 5-year overall survival rate of 53–56%, and a disease-specific survival rate of 71–78% [91–93].

Another organ-conserving treatment option for T2 and selected T3 glottic cancers is SCPL-CHEP, which may be performed without chemotherapy [94, 95] or with neoadjuvant chemotherapy using cisplatin and 5-fluorouracil [96–98]. Contraindications to this procedure are fixation of the arytenoid cartilage, subglottic tumor extension to the upper border of the cricoid cartilage, infiltration of the cricoid cartilage or thyroid cartilage, extensive infiltration of the preepiglottic space, and extralaryngeal tumor extension [99]. Laccourreye et al. [98] reported in 1999 on 100 patients with T2 glottic carcinoma treated by SCPL-CHEP. Preoperative vocal cord mobility was impaired in 54% of patients. The anterior commissure was involved in 42% of cases, and there was infraglottic involvement in 10%. The patients received three cycles of neoadjuvant chemotherapy with cisplatin and 5-fluorouracil at intervals of 15–21 days. Complete remission was achieved in 24% of patients and partial remission in 58%. The 5-year local control rate was 97.7% for T2a lesions and 93.8% for T2b lesions. The larynx was preserved in 95% of patients. Postoperative aspiration pneumonia developed in 9% of the patients, and one patient required a laryngectomy for functional reasons. Using the same treatment regimen for glottic carcinoma with vocal cord fixation in 20 patients, Laccourreye and his group achieved a 3-year local control rate of 89.2% and a larynx preservation rate of 90% [96]. Chevalier et al.

[94] achieved similar results in 112 patients with glottic carcinoma and impaired vocal cord mobility (n = 90) or vocal cord fixation (n = 22) without the use of neoadjuvant chemotherapy. The 5-year local control rate was 97.3 %, and the 5-year rate for larynx preservation was 95.5 %.

The local control rate after the *primary radiotherapy* of T2 glottic carcinoma with impaired vocal cord mobility is between 60 % and 76 %, and the rate of organ preservation is 70–80 % [35, 37, 41, 43, 100–102]. Fein et al. [35] achieved a 5-year local control rate of 87 % for T2 glottic carcinoma with normal vocal cord mobility. This rate declined to 76 % when vocal cord mobility was impaired. Five-year local control rates of 30–68 % are reported for the primary radiotherapy of T3 glottic carcinomas, with definitive local control rates of 80–86 %. The 5-year overall survival rate is 51–59 %. The 5-year rate for larynx preservation is 50–76 % [37, 103–106].

Another organ-preserving treatment concept, currently undergoing clinical trials, is *neoadjuvant chemotherapy followed by radiation therapy*. The first randomized study to test this regimen was conducted by the Veterans Administration Study Group on Laryngeal Cancer [107, 108]. The patients were randomized into a standard treatment group, consisting of surgery and postoperative radiation, and a study group that received two cycles of chemotherapy followed by surgery and radiotherapy in cases showing persistent or progressive tumor growth. Patients who showed partial or complete remission received a third cycle of chemotherapy followed by radiotherapy. A total of 332 patients with resectable glottic (37 %) or supraglottic (61 %) stage III or IV laryngeal carcinomas (except for T1N1) were randomly assigned to the two treatment groups. After a median follow-up of 98 months, no differences were found between the two groups with regard to local and regional recurrences, distant metastases, and survival rates. The larynx was preserved in 31 % of the patients originally assigned to the study group, representing 66 % of the survivors. On a critical note, it should be added that 9.3 % of the patients had primary tumors of the T1 or T2 category. These tumors could have been treated just as well with a partial laryngectomy using classic or laser microsurgical technique.

In a similar French study conducted by the GETTEC (Groupe d'Etude des Tumeurs de la Tete et du Cou), induction chemotherapy followed by radiotherapy was compared with surgery and postoperative radiation. A total of 68 patients with glottic or supraglottic laryngeal carcinomas with vocal cord fixation (93 % stage III, 7 % stage IV) were randomly assigned to two treatment groups. After 3 years, 20 % of the patients assigned to the chemotherapy group were still alive and still had their larynx. Significantly better disease-free survival and overall survival were documented in the group that underwent primary laryngectomy [109].

The results of the two studies were different despite similar study design. While survival in both treatment groups was the same in the Veterans Administration study, the survival rates were markedly lower in the group that received neoadjuvant chemotherapy in the French study. The cause may lie in the different patient populations. While vocal cord fixation was present in only 57 % of the patients in the Veterans Administration study, this condition was an inclusion criterion in the French study.

In another study on larynx preservation with induction chemotherapy and subsequent radiotherapy, the 5-year rate for larynx preservation was 31 % in patients who showed good response to the chemotherapy [110].

Conclusion

The role of laser microsurgery in the treatment of T2b and T3 glottic carcinomas cannot yet be definitively evaluated because data are available from only one institution and have not yet been reproduced elsewhere. Nevertheless, our results published to date indicate that approximately 70 % of patients with pT2b and pT3 carcinomas remain free of local tumor recurrence following primary treatment, with minimal morbidity and a functioning larynx. The results of laser microsurgery for T4 glottic carcinomas have not been presented because adequate data are not yet available. Comparison with the results of vertical partial laryngectomy is difficult because patients are selected for partial laryngectomy on an individual basis and total laryngectomy is already indicated in patients with T2b and T3 tumors. The local control rates achieved with supracricoid partial laryngectomy are excellent. It should be noted, however, that the patients were selected according to the criteria stated, and that this procedure is not appropriate for every patient because of its operative morbidity. In the studies that investigated the possibility of larynx preservation with radiotherapy in selected patients and on the basis of chemotherapy response, the results show that this concept cannot be established as a standard regimen at the present time.

Recurrent Glottic Carcinoma after Radiotherapy

Approximately one-half of carcinomas recurring after radiotherapy are classified as transglottic T3 or T4 tumors at the time of diagnosis [111]. Recurrences detected early can be managed with a classic partial laryngectomy, but a partial laryngectomy is rarely practiced in this subgroup for fear of postoperative complications such as cartilage necrosis, laryngeal stenosis, fistula formation, aspiration, and delayed extubation. In many cases, total laryngectomy is the only salvage option remaining for recurrent glottic carcinoma after radiotherapy.

Several authors have reported results for small numbers of patients who underwent vertical partial laryngectomy for recurrent T1 and T2 neoplasms [112–116]. Tumors in 13–24 % of the patients were not controlled by a partial resection, making it necessary to proceed with total laryngectomy. Complications occurred in up to 20 % of cases, consisting mainly of wound healing problems, and intubation had to be continued for several weeks in up to 30 % of the patients. Besides open vertical partial laryngectomy, another option for recurrence after failed radiotherapy is SCPL-

CHEP or SCPL-cricohyoidopexy (SCPL-CHP) [44, 117, 118]. In the series of 12 cases reported by Laccourreye et al. [117], five patients developed complications (perichondritis, stenosis, aspiration pneumonia). The larynx was preserved in three-fourths of the cases.

Partial laryngectomy by laser microsurgery has been described as another alternative to classic partial laryngectomy for T1 and T2 recurrent tumors [119–123]. From 13 % to 53 % of patients had subsequent total laryngectomy, usually after the first failed attempt at laser surgery. The patients who did not develop tumor recurrence were able to swallow without difficulty and were not tracheotomized. Wound healing problems resulting in cartilage loss and stenosis were much less frequent after laser microsurgery in these studies than after classic partial laryngectomy.

We have performed laser microsurgery in a total of 34 patients to treat early and advanced recurrences of glottic carcinoma after radiotherapy. Of these patients, 71 % remained disease-free after one or more laser procedures and retained a functioning larynx. Seven patients (20 %) underwent total laryngectomy, six for a tumor recurrence and one for chondronecrosis. Three patients required a temporary tracheotomy. The 5-year disease-specific survival rate was 86 % [124].

Conclusion

A comparison of the oncologic and functional results reported in the literature shows that laser microsurgery is an acceptable alternative to classic partial laryngectomy for recurrent carcinoma after radiotherapy and is even an alternative to total laryngectomy in selected cases. Laser microsurgery and classic partial laryngectomy are comparable in terms of organ preservation. The complication rates of laser microsurgery are significantly lower than those of classic partial laryngectomy, and its functional results are better.

■ Laser Microsurgery of Supraglottic Carcinoma

Supraglottic T1 and T2 Carcinoma

Early supraglottic carcinomas are defined as tumors that have not infiltrated the preepiglottic fat, have not immobilized a vocal cord, and have not yet metastasized to regional lymph nodes. Many laryngologists have shown that supraglottic laryngectomy, first described by J. M. Alonso in 1947 [125], is an effective treatment method for these lesions. Another option for early supraglottic tumors is radiotherapy. Supraglottic laryngectomy is associated with significant morbidity and postoperative functional problems, therefore it is often not an acceptable surgical treatment option, especially in elderly patients with multiple comorbidities and reduced pulmonary function. Vaughan of Boston [126] was the first surgeon to describe the CO_2 laser resection of a supraglottic carcinoma. Since 1979,

Steiner has used the CO_2 laser for the transoral endoscopic treatment of initially selected patients with supraglottic carcinoma [11, 127]. Davis et al. [128] reported in 1983 on an initial series of 20 patients who underwent laser epiglottectomy for the treatment of benign airway-obstructing lesions or small suprahyoid epiglottic carcinomas. Davis et al. [129] and Zeitels et al. [130] subsequently reported on additional transoral laser resections in selected patients with supraglottic cancers.

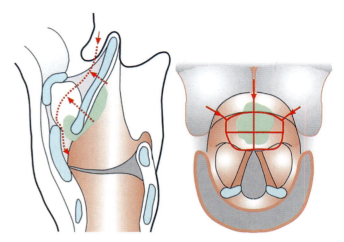

Fig. 6.**8** Lines of resection for a supraglottic carcinoma involving the preepiglottic space (diagrams from [4]).

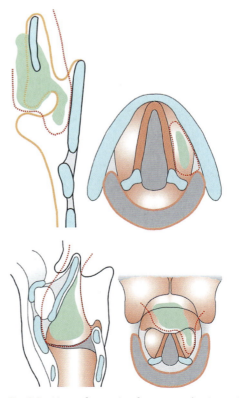

Fig. 6.**9** Lines of resection for a supraglottic carcinoma involving the pre- and paraglottic spaces (diagrams from [4]).

Operative Technique

The rare small carcinomas of the suprahyoid epiglottis or ventricular fold can usually be clearly exposed and excised en bloc. Carcinomas of the infrahyoid epiglottis are exposed with a bivalved laryngoscope and are best removed piecemeal by making an incision in the glossoepiglottic vallecula and splitting the epiglottis in the midline, including the preepiglottic fat in the resection while preserving the vocal cords and arytenoid cartilages (Fig. 6.**8**). Tumor that has spread along the inner surface of the thyroid cartilage and infiltrated the muscle tissue in the paraglottic space can be removed along with portions of the muscle (Figs. 6.**9**, 6.**10**). With advanced tumors, the resection can include portions of the base of the tongue and piriform sinus or an arytenoid cartilage. This treatment limits the possibilities for swallowing rehabilitation. Tracheotomy is generally unnecessary due to the limited tendency for postoperative edema, even after extensive supraglottic laser resections. A tracheotomy should be considered in older patients with significantly impaired pulmonary function, in patients with a bleeding diathesis (e.g., anticoagulant medication, hemodialysis), or if heavy bleeding occurred during the operation.

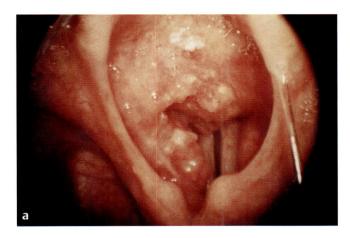

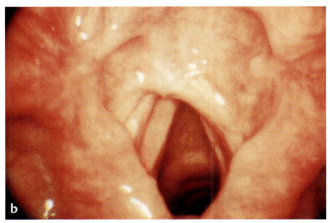

Fig. 6.**10** A supraglottic laryngeal carcinoma infiltrating the preepiglottic space (T3). **a** Preoperative appearance. **b** Appearance (inspiratory view) 2 years after tumor resection by laser microsurgery.

Results of Laser Microsurgery

While laser microsurgery is used increasingly in the treatment of glottic carcinomas, only a few reports have been published on the endoscopic resection of supraglottic cancers. Steiner [17] and Eckel and Thumfart [16] reported respectively on 30 and 15 patients with supraglottic carcinoma. Zeitels et al. [131] analyzed the results of laser microsurgery in 42 patients with supraglottic cancers in a multi-institutional study. Nineteen patients with T1 or T2 tumors treated by laser microsurgery alone developed no local recurrences. Of 23 patients, mostly with T2 tumors, who received both surgery and postoperative irradiation, four developed local recurrence and were salvaged by laryngectomy. In the latter group, the authors interpret the role of laser surgery as a "neoadjuvant therapy with a histopathologically controlled result." In 1997, Eckel [132] reported the results of supraglottic laryngectomy by laser surgery in 46 patients with T1 and T2 carcinomas. Four of the patients (8.7 %) had local or locoregional recurrence, and five (10.9 %) required secondary laryngectomy for functional reasons. Iro et al. [133] reported in 1998 on supraglottic cancer resections by laser microsurgery in 141 patients with the following Union Internationale Contre le Cancer (UICC) stage distribution: stage I, 23.4 %; stage II, 25.5 %; stage III, 16.3 %; and stage IV, 34.8 %. The authors state that the oncologic results of the laser surgery are good if clear margins (R0 resection) are obtained. Otherwise they advise transoral laser reexcision or a conventional partial or total laryngectomy. Radiotherapy is not advised because postoperative irradiation has not proved effective for R1 and R2 resections. In 1999, Rudert et al. [134] reviewed the results of transoral laser surgery in 34 patients with T1–T4 tumors, 12 of whom were treated with palliative intent. None of the patients who had the surgery for attempted cure developed local recurrence. The 3-year overall survival rate for stages I and II disease was 88 %.

We performed laser microsurgery in 48 patients with supraglottic T1 and T2 carcinomas. The 5-year local control rate was 100 % for pT1 tumors and 89 % for pT2 tumors. None of the patients required laryngectomy for tumor recurrence or functional disability. The 5-year recurrence-free survival rate in this series was 83 %, and the 5-year overall survival rate was 76 % [135].

Other Treatment Options

The reported oncologic results of *classic supraglottic laryngectomy* for early supraglottic carcinoma are very good. Local control rates of 90–100 % have been reported for T1 carcinomas and 80–97 % for T2 carcinomas [136–143]. The 5-year survival rates achieved with laser microsurgery are comparable to the rates reported for conventional supraglottic laryngectomy. Several authors have stated 3-year corrected survival rates of 67–92 % for stage I disease and 80–85 % for stage II disease [138, 140, 142–146].

Primary radiotherapy can achieve local control rates of 77–100 % in supraglottic T1 cancers and 62–83 % in T2 cancers [147–153]. While Inoue et al. [149] obtained significantly better local control rates for tumors of the epilarynx than for tumors of the infrahyoid epiglottis, other authors found no differences in local control rates for different affected areas of the supraglottis [150, 154]. However, the tumor volume determined by CT is a significant predictor of local control [155]. Published data show that patients whose tumors could have been originally treated by partial laryngectomy with preservation of the glottis will usually require a total laryngectomy if they develop a recurrence after primary radiotherapy. Johansen et al. [156] treated 117 patients with early supraglottic carcinomas by primary radiotherapy. Thirty-one percent of the patients required a laryngectomy for tumor recurrence. In the cohorts of Inoue et al. [149] and Mendenhall et al. [151], 17% and 14% of the patients, respectively, had to undergo a secondary laryngectomy.

Supraglottic T3 Carcinoma

Results of Laser Microsurgery

There are few reports on the laser treatment of supraglottic T3 carcinomas in the literature. Rudert et al. [134] reported results in nine patients with T3 carcinomas (four treated with palliative intent) and eight patients with T4 carcinomas (five treated with palliative intent). Two of the nine patients (22%) with T3 tumors and five of the eight patients (63%) with T4 tumors developed local recurrences. In the series of Iro et al. [133], a local recurrence was diagnosed in five of 15 patients (33%) with T3 carcinomas and in three of 33 patients (9%) with T4 carcinomas. While Rudert et al. [134] state that supraglottic carcinomas invading the preepiglottic space are accessible to endoscopic resection, Iro et al. [133] advise restraint in treating T3 lesions with transoral laser surgery.

We treated 50 patients with pT3 supraglottic laryngeal carcinomas (40 stage III, 10 stage IV) with transoral laser microsurgery. In 41 patients (82%), the tumor was classified as pT3 due to invasion of the preepiglottic space. Preoperative vocal cord fixation was present in nine patients (18%). Thirteen patients (26%) also had invasion of the paraglottic space, and nine cases (18%) had superficial tumor spread onto one or both vocal cords. With regard to other treatment options, it should be noted that a classic supraglottic partial laryngectomy is contraindicated in patients with findings such as vocal cord fixation, vocal cord involvement, and invasion of the paraglottic space in the glottic plane. These patients were treated by laser microsurgery as an alternative to extended supraglottic laryngectomy, SCPL-CHP, or total laryngectomy. Thirty-nine patients (78%) had a unilateral or bilateral selective neck dissection. In 17 patients (34%), the neck dissection revealed one or more positive cervical lymph nodes. Thirteen patients (26%) were selected for postoperative radiotherapy, mostly for histologically confirmed cervical lymph node metastases.

The Kaplan–Meier 5-year local control rate and definitive 5-year local control rates were 86% and 91%, respectively. Four percent of the patients underwent total laryngectomy for local tumor recurrence. Twelve percent of the patients died from tumor-related (TNM) disease. The Kaplan–Meier 5-year recurrence-free survival rate was 71%.

All patients had good vocal function. One patient developed a supraglottic web after surgery and postoperative radiation and required a permanent tracheotomy. Two patients received a prophylactic temporary tracheotomy following extended supraglottic laryngectomy. The median time for nasogastric tube feeding was 9.5 days. All patients were on an unrestricted oral diet after removal of the feeding tube. Special swallowing training was not required. None of the patients required a total laryngectomy for functional problems [25].

Other Treatment Options

Primary radiotherapy can achieve local control rates of 50–76% for supraglottic T3 carcinomas [148, 157–159]. Hinerman et al. [157] were able to preserve the larynx in 68% of their patients treated with radiotherapy for supraglottic T3 carcinomas and Nakfoor et al. [158] in 72%. The following survival rates have been reported: corrected 5-year survival rate 53% (Sykes et al. [159]), 5-year disease-free survival rate 76% (Nakfoor et al. [158]), 5-year disease-specific survival rate for stage III carcinoma 81% (Hinerman et al. [157]).

The local control rates achieved for T3 carcinomas with the *classic or extended supraglottic laryngectomy* range from 71% to 94% [137, 160, 161]. Conventional supraglottic laryngectomy is no longer possible if the cancer has invaded the floor of the Morgagni ventricle and the paraglottic space. Other contraindications are fixation of the arytenoid cartilage or vocal cord and extralaryngeal tumor extension into the base of the tongue or hypopharynx. These cases may no longer be amenable to an extended supraglottic laryngectomy, and total laryngectomy is often required. An alternative classic partial laryngectomy for tumors infiltrating the ventricle or paraglottic space is the *SCPL-CHP*. Schwaab et al. [162] reported on 146 patients who underwent SCPL and CHP for supraglottic laryngeal carcinoma (T1 in 2, T2 in 87, T3 in 53, and T4 in 4). The local control rate was very good, with only six local recurrences (4%). Nineteen percent had clinically significant postoperative aspiration and 9% (13) with intractable aspiration required total laryngectomy. The larynx was preserved in 85% of patients. The 5-year overall survival rate was 88%.

The local recurrence rate after SCPL-CHP is also very low in other series, ranging from 0% to 7% [81, 163–165]. It should be noted, however, that most of the lesions treated by SCPL-CHP consisted of T2 and T3 tumors with "minimal infiltration" of the preepiglottic space, tumors involving the paraglottic space or vocal cords, or tumors classified as T4 lesions with only circumscribed infiltration of the thyroid cartilage [162, 163, 165]. As we were able to show, laser microsurgery can be considered an effective alternative for these indications. Although the local tumor recurrence rates are higher with laser microsurgery, the survival rates are comparable. Laser microsurgery and SCPL-CHP yield similar results in terms of organ preservation considering that secondary laryngectomies were necessary after SCPL-CHP (at least in some series) due to intractable aspiration. Significantly better local control and organ preservation are achieved with laser microsurgery and with SCPL-CHP than with primary radiotherapy.

Complications

The complication rate is a major concern when evaluating a therapeutic procedure. For example, any postoperative bleeding in a non-tracheotomized patient is a serious and potentially life-threatening complication due to the risk of aspirating blood [166]. The incidence of postoperative endolaryngeal hemorrhage was 2/33 (6%) in the series of Rudert et al. [134] and 6/85 (7%) in the series of Ambrosch and Steiner [167]. The incidence of postoperative bleeding is 3.3% after SCPL-CHP [178] and 1.6–5% after classic supraglottic laryngectomy [139, 145, 168, 169]. These figures are lower than the rates after laser microsurgery, although bleeding from the base of the tongue or laryngeal remnant with a fatal outcome has been described following open supraglottic laryngectomies [168, 169]. An 18% rate of surgical complications has been reported after SCPL-CHP [162, 170].

The most frequent complications of primary radiotherapy are chondronecrosis and laryngeal edema causing airway obstruction. Complication rates of 2–7% have been reported. From 1.5% to 2% of patients receiving primary radiation for a supraglottic carcinoma require secondary laryngectomy for chondronecrosis or laryngeal edema, and another 0.6–2.5% require a permanent tracheotomy [157–159]. Postoperative adjuvant radiotherapy after supraglottic laryngectomy is indicated in cases where microscopic residual tumor is assumed to be present at the primary tumor site (R1 resection). It is also indicated in patients with more than one cervical lymph node metastasis and in cases of cervical lymph node metastasis with extracapsular spread. Whether postoperative radiotherapy after supraglottic laryngectomy has an adverse effect on laryngeal function is controversial. Steininger et al. [171] found that patients receiving postoperative irradiation were more likely to require lifelong PEG tube feeding and were also more likely to have airway obstruction due to edema. Other studies found no increase in complication rates following radiotherapy [172, 173]. It is reasonable to assume, however, that the complication rate rises when doses higher than 50 Gy are applied to the larynx [172, 174].

Functional Results

All authors who have reported on the transoral laser resection of supraglottic carcinomas are in agreement that swallowing rehabilitation proceeds more quickly and has better outcome than the Alonso operation. The rate of secondary laryngectomies for persistent aspiration after open supraglottic laryngectomy is in the range of 3.5–12.5% [136, 173, 175, 176]. The incidence of postoperative aspiration and the time needed for swallowing rehabilitation varies with the age and general health of the patient and with the degree of resection of the base of the tongue and arytenoid cartilage [177–179]. Mechanisms contributing significantly to the recovery of swallowing function after supraglottic laryngectomy are: the oropharyngeal transit time, closure of the airway at the laryngeal introitus, the position of the residual larynx in relation to the base of the tongue, and the movement of the base of the tongue toward the poste-

rior pharyngeal wall [179–181]. Patients who regain these functions postoperatively meet the requisite conditions for normal swallowing.

On the whole, the functional results of laser microsurgery for supraglottic T1–T3 tumors are considered to be very favorable based on the short duration of nasogastric tube feeding, minimal postoperative aspiration, and the reduced need for secondary permanent tracheotomies and laryngectomies due to functional problems. We attribute the early and consistently successful swallowing rehabilitation in the cases described here to the integrity of the base of the tongue and pharyngeal muscles and to the preservation of the hyoid bone with the supra- and infrahyoid muscles, enabling the larynx to move normally during swallowing. At least one mobile arytenoid cartilage was preserved in all operations, allowing for functional closure of the larynx. We also believe that preserving the extralaryngeal portions of the superior laryngeal nerves is an important factor in sensory reinnervation.

In most patients undergoing a supracricoid partial laryngectomy, the feeding tube can be removed within a month after the surgery. But the patients will require 6–12 months to return to their normal eating habits [81, 83, 164], and approximately a third of patients will have to accept permanent limitations [83]. SCPL also causes an inevitable change in voice quality, which can adversely affect the quality of life, especially in female patients [83].

Conclusion

The results of laser microsurgery in patients with early and moderately advanced supraglottic cancer are comparable to those of open supraglottic laryngectomy with regard to local control and survival rates. They are somewhat better than the results published for primary radiotherapy with regard to local control and survival, and they are superior with respect to organ preservation. A careful and precise operating technique is necessary, however, to avoid postoperative bleeding and edema. Microsurgery makes it possible to preserve functionally important structures, thereby reducing changes in the mobility of the residual larynx and pharynx and helping to facilitate earlier and better swallowing. With the low postoperative morbidity of laser microsurgery, curative surgical treatment can be offered to patients who would not have been considered as candidates for open supraglottic laryngectomy.

■ Laser Microsurgery of Hypopharyngeal Carcinoma

Hypopharyngeal carcinoma has the poorest prognosis of any carcinoma of the upper aerodigestive tract. This is due mainly to a high rate of local tumor recurrence, a high likelihood of cervical lymph node metastases at the time of diagnosis (68% in our patients), a high rate of metachronous distant metastases (13% in our patients), and a high incidence of metachronous second primary tumors (4% per year in our patients) [182].

The results of various treatment methods for hypopharyngeal carcinoma have been presented in detail [183, 184]. The literature consistently shows that recent advances in diagnostic imaging, radiotherapy, surgery, and multimodal treatment concepts are not reflected in lower mortality rates. The National Cancer Data Base Report for 1997 indicates a 5-year disease-specific survival rate of 31.4% in 3906 cases of hypopharyngeal carcinoma and a 33.6% survival rate in 822 cases of piriform sinus carcinoma [185, 186]. Regardless of treatment, the 5-year disease-specific survival rate was 63% for stage I disease, 58% for stage II, 42% for stage III, and 22% for stage IV. Further analysis of the data showed that patients with early-stage tumors treated with radiotherapy alone had lower survival rates than patients who received primary surgical treatment, with or without adjuvant radiotherapy. Advanced cancers treated with radiotherapy alone had the poorest survival rates [185].

The standard treatment for hypopharyngeal carcinoma is a combination of radical surgery—laryngectomy and (partial) pharyngectomy plus (radical) neck dissection—and postoperative radiotherapy. Because radical surgery and postoperative radiotherapy apparently cannot improve the locoregional control rate and approximately a third of patients die from distant metastases, second primaries, and intercurrent disease, it seems judicious to consider organ-conserving treatment strategies that will at least improve the quality of life for patients with a poor prognosis [183]. Innovative treatment concepts aimed at preserving the larynx, such as neoadjuvant chemotherapy followed by percutaneous radiotherapy for primarily operable tumors and concomitant radiotherapy and chemotherapy for inoperable stage IV carcinomas, have been classified as "under clinical evaluation" by the National Cancer Institute.

The results of a survey on hypopharyngeal cancer conducted by Hoffman et al. [185] showed that approximately 44% of patients were treated with a combination of surgery and radiotherapy. With regard to surgical procedures, total laryngopharyngectomy was performed in 57.5% of cases and partial laryngopharyngectomy or other partial tumor resections in 25.3% of cases. Only 4% of the patients underwent laser resection. Severe treatment-related complications arose in 6–34% of cases, and fatal complications occurred in 2.4–14%.

Besides the therapeutic procedures listed above, laser use represents another approach to organ- and function-conserving treatment. Before lasers were introduced in laryngology, hypopharyngeal carcinomas were rarely resected by the transoral route [187]. To our knowledge, the CO_2 laser has been used at various centers in the U.S., India, and Europe (especially Germany) for the resection of hypopharyngeal cancers, however, few reports have been published on the treatment results.

The first results in 36 patients treated by laser microsurgery were presented in 1985 and published by Steiner and Herbst in 1987 [188]. These were followed by a report on 42 patients treated at the Department of Otorhinolaryngology of Erlangen-Nuremberg University Hospital between 1981 and 1986 [184]. Several more studies were published

between 1988 and 2001 on the results of transoral laser microsurgery for hypopharyngeal carcinoma [115, 182, 189, 190]. Besides the figures reported by Steiner and his group, additional results of laser microsurgery for hypopharyngeal carcinoma were published by Rudert [191, 192].

Operative Technique

Optimum exposure of the larynx and piriform sinus is essential for an adequate endoscopic tumor resection. The

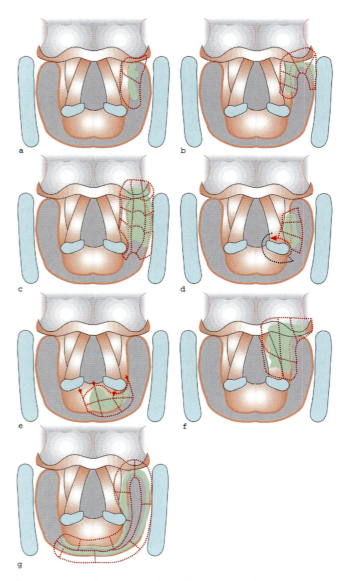

Fig. 6.**11** Lines of resection for hypopharyngeal carcinoma. **a** Carcinoma of the aryepiglottic fold. **b** Carcinoma of the medial, anterior, and lateral walls of the piriform sinus. **c** Piriform sinus completely filled by carcinoma. **d** Carcinoma of the aryepiglottic fold with possible infiltration of the arytenoid cartilage. **e** Carcinoma of the postcricoid region. **f** Carcinoma of the piriform sinus with involvement of the oropharynx. **g** Carcinoma of the piriform sinus with involvement of the postcricoid region and posterior wall of the hypopharynx (diagrams from [4]).

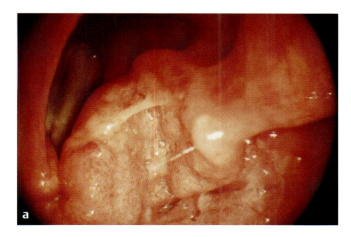

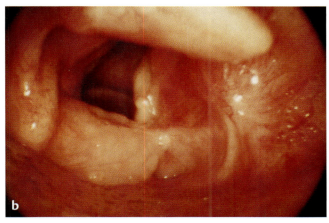

Fig. 6.**12** Carcinoma of the right piriform sinus (T2). **a** Preoperative appearance. **b** Appearance 8 months after tumor resection by laser microsurgery.

tumor is exposed with a bivalved laryngoscope and progressively resected in the cranial-to-caudal direction. The position of the laryngoscope is adjusted several times as the resection proceeds in order to keep both the tumor and the surrounding healthy tissue within the visual field of the microscope. Carcinomas of the piriform sinus are resected en bloc to assess the extent of local tumor infiltration and, aided by frozen section margins, preserve a maximum amount of normal, healthy tissue. Piriform sinus tumors are encompassed with a safety margin of approximately 5–10 mm (Figs. 6.**11**, 6.**12**).

Results of Laser Microsurgery

Between 1981 and 1996, we performed primary laser microsurgery in curative intent in 129 previously untreated patients with squamous cell carcinoma of the piriform sinus [182]. The goal of the operation was complete tumor removal with preservation of functionally important laryngeal structures. The primary tumors were categorized as pT1 in 24 patients, pT2 in 74, pT3 in 17, and pT4 in 14 (UICC 1992). Cervical lymph node metastases were present in 88 patients (68.2%) at the time of diagnosis. The tumors were distributed by stages as follows: stage I in 10 patients (7.7%), stage II in 23 (17.8%), stage III in 26 (20.2%), and stage IV in 70 (54.3%).

Unilateral or bilateral predominantly selective neck dissection was performed in 110 patients a median period of 10 days after the primary tumor surgery. Twenty-seven patients (81.8%) with stage I or II disease were treated by surgery alone, and only six patients (18.2%) received a combination of surgery and postoperative radiation. In contrast, 44 patients (28.2%) with stage III or IV disease received only surgical treatment while 69 (71.8%) received a combined regimen. Radiation was always delivered to the primary tumor area and both sides of the neck. The median follow-up period was 44 months.

Local and locoregional recurrences developed in a total of 17 patients (13.2%) (stage I and II: 3/33, 9.1%; stage III and IV: 14/96, 14.6%). The Kaplan–Meier 5-year local control rate was 82% (95% confidence interval [CI] 66% to 98%) for stage I and II and 69% (95% CI 48% to 72%) for stage III and IV. Eighteen patients (14.0%) had late or recurrent metastases in the neck and eight patients (6.2%) developed metachronous distant metastases with locoregional tumor control. A metachronous second primary was diagnosed in 24 patients (18.6%).

Fifty-seven (44.2%) patients (one with tumor) were alive at the end of follow-up while 72 (55.8%) died during the follow-up period: 26 (20.1%) died from their cancer (stage I and II: 1/33, 3.0%; stage III and IV: 25/96, 26.0%), 26 (20.1%) died of incurrent disease, 18 (14.0%) from a second primary tumor, and 2 (1.6%) due to unknown causes. The Kaplan–Meier 5-year overall survival rate was 71% for stages I and II and 47% for stages III and IV. The 5-year recurrence-free survival rate was 95% for stages I and II and 69% for stages III and IV.

Five patients (3.9%) had postoperative endolaryngeal bleeding, which was controlled endoscopically in all cases. Three patients required PEG tube feeding, one for a hypopharyngeal stenosis and two for aspiration. Except for these cases, all patients regained normal swallowing function.

Rudert [192] reported the results of 29 patients with hypopharyngeal carcinoma whom he treated with laser microsurgery at the University of Kiel between 1991 and 1995. Twenty-seven patients had T1 or T2 tumors. Eight patients (28%) developed local recurrence. The overall 5-year survival rate was 58%, and the disease-specific survival rate was also 58%. In this study as in others, analysis showed that the survival rates depended strongly on cervical lymph node involvement. The 5-year survival rate was 74% for patients with a N0 neck but only 34% for patients with cervical lymph node metastases. Accordingly, the survival rate was 78% for patients with stage I or II disease vs. 35% for patients with stage III or IV disease. None of the patients required a tracheotomy together with the primary tumor surgery, and all patients had normal postoperative swallowing.

Other Treatment Options

Although radical surgery is still advocated today, even for T1 and T2 carcinomas [193], there has been a definite trend in recent years toward less radical treatment options. With their high complication and death rates, however, *partial laryngopharyngectomies* did not gain much acceptance initially. Ogura et al. first reported on the successful treatment of hypopharyngeal carcinomas by partial laryngopharyngectomy in 1960 [194].

Successful organ-preserving partial laryngopharyngectomy for carcinoma of the piriform sinus requires precise knowledge of tumor extent and growth patterns of carcinomas in this region. In recent years, various authors have performed histomorphologic studies of laryngectomy specimens showing that, based on actual tumor extent, a partial laryngopharyngectomy with preservation of the contralateral, uninvolved hemilarynx would have been possible in at least some cases [195–197]. Ogura et al. [194] were the first to report on piriform sinus carcinomas treated with organ-preserving partial laryngopharyngectomies. They achieved a 3-year survival rate of 53% in highly selected patients with early piriform sinus carcinoma (mobile vocal cords, no tumor involvement of the piriform sinus apex, postcricoid region, or thyroid cartilage). However, 34% of patients required a secondary total laryngectomy for local tumor recurrence [198]. Ogura's indications were subsequently adopted by several other laryngologists.

Henri Laccourreye et al. [199] reported in 1987 on 240 patients who underwent *supracricoid hemilaryngopharyngectomy* for early piriform sinus carcinoma. Local recurrences developed in 5.2% of cases. Eight percent of the patients required a tracheostomy and 15% had dysphagia. Spector et al. [200] reported the results of 408 patients treated by various modalities from 1964 to 1991. A partial laryngopharyngectomy, with or without postoperative radiation, was performed in 207 patients. Outstanding results were achieved in terms of local tumor control and survival. The 5-year disease-specific survival rates ranged from 46% to 77%, depending on the location and extent of the tumor. The authors state that the good results were the effect of selection since only patients with early tumors were selected for partial laryngopharyngectomy. It should be noted, however, that the rates of surgical complications and treatment-related deaths were high. The authors noted that by reconstructing the pharynx with a myocutaneous pectoralis major island flap and omitting preoperative radiotherapy, the incidence of complications was reduced to 19% and the incidence of fatal complications to 4.6%.

Chevalier et al. [201] reported further treatment results in 31 patients with T1 and T2 piriform sinus carcinomas treated over a period of 15 years. Treatment consisted of a supraglottic hemilaryngopharyngectomy and postoperative radiotherapy. While very good local tumor control was achieved with this combination (only a 2% incidence of local recurrences), the survival rates were low, especially in patients with T2 tumors, due to a high incidence of recurrent metastases in the neck and distant metastases. All patients required a temporary tracheotomy and nasogastric tube feeding. It is noteworthy that, in contrast with the various treatment methods cited above, none of the patients we treated by laser microsurgery required a tracheotomy. We also documented a markedly lower complication rate, better postoperative swallowing function, and better survival rates. Kraus et al. [202] reported on 39 patients, mostly with piriform sinus carcinomas treated by partial laryngopharyngectomy and postoperative radiotherapy. The local control rate was 79% and the 5-year disease-specific survival rate was 54%.

Another organ-conserving treatment option is *neoadjuvant chemotherapy* followed by a *partial hemilaryngopharyngectomy* and *postoperative radiotherapy*. Laccourreye et al. [203] used this regimen to treat 34 patients with selected T2 carcinomas of the piriform sinus between 1964 and 1985. Only one patient had a local tumor recurrence. Two patients developed recurrent metastases in the neck, and three patients developed distant metastases. The 5-year disease-specific survival rate was 56%. On a critical note it should be added that the authors did not report either the clinical response to chemotherapy or the histopathologic results for the surgical specimens. Complications arose in 85% of patients, and 20% had severe aspiration resulting in pulmonary complications. Secondary laryngectomy was unavoidable in three patients due to severe aspiration.

For carcinomas of the upper piriform sinus with mobile vocal cords, organ-preserving hemilaryngopharyngectomy with neck dissection and postoperative irradiation yields oncologic results comparable with those produced by total laryngectomy with partial pharyngectomy [198, 200, 201, 203]. On comparing transoral laser microsurgery plus selective neck dissection and postoperative radiotherapy with classic partial laryngopharyngectomy, we found that the former was associated with markedly fewer complications, particularly an absence of fatal complications. The postoperative morbidity was far lower, and the 5-year disease-specific and overall survival rates were significantly better.

Primary radiotherapy delivered to the primary tumor and both sides of the neck is viewed as an alternative to surgery, especially for early carcinomas of the upper piriform sinus [204–207]. Pameijer et al. [208] reported a local control rate of 78% for 23 T1 and T2 carcinomas which they treated between 1984 and 1993. The local control rate declined when the apex of the piriform sinus was involved by carcinoma and the tumor volume exceeded 6.5 mL. In a subsequent publication from the same institution, the 5-year local control rate was 90% for T1 tumors and 80% for T2 tumors. Local control with organ preservation was 86% for patients with T1 carcinomas and 82% for patients with T2 carcinomas [209]. Garden et al. [210] achieved a local control rate of 75.5% in 57 T1 and T2 carcinomas. Wang [211] reported a 5-year local control rate of 74% for T1 carcinomas and 76% for T2 carcinomas. The 5-year disease-free survival rates were 73% for T1 tumors and 68% for T2 tumors. Jones [205] found a 5-year disease-specific survival rate of only 40% for T1 carcinomas and 28% for T2 carcinomas.

It is known that operations for tumors recurring after primary, conventional radiotherapy are associated with serious complications in a high percentage of cases [210, 212, 213]. For example, Davidson et al. [214] reported that complications arose in 27% of 108 patients who underwent total laryngectomy for tumor recurrence after primary radiation. The 3-year overall survival rate was 22%.

Primary radiotherapy of advanced hypopharyngeal cancers yields considerably poorer results. The 5-year survival rates range from 5% to 30% [185, 205, 211, 215]. Combining radiotherapy with chemotherapy in patients with locally advanced head and neck cancers has only slightly improved survival rates, though it has been found that concomitant chemoradiotherapy offers advantages over other treatment regimens [216–219]. Another approach consisting of intraarterial chemotherapy with cisplatin and percutaneous radiotherapy is currently undergoing clinical trials. Initial results in 25 patients with advanced hypopharyngeal carcinomas show that while complete remissions were achieved, the 5-year overall survival rate was only 23% [220].

It should be added that severe functional disabilities, especially swallowing difficulties, can occur as a side effect of chemoradiotherapy [221–223]. While results of the treatment of recurrent tumors after conventional fractionated radiotherapy have been reported [210, 212–214], there have been no reports on the results of recurrent tumor treatment after irradiation with a modified fractionation schedule or after chemoradiotherapy.

Another, nonsurgical organ-conserving approach for the treatment of head and neck cancer is *neoadjuvant chemotherapy with 5-fluorouracil and cisplatin combined with radiation therapy*. A review of clinical trials conducted between 1970 and 1995 and a meta-analysis of previously published data show no clear evidence for an improvement in locoregional tumor control or survival rates or a decrease in incidence of metachronous distant metastases [224, 225]. Nevertheless, induction chemotherapy has become a widely accepted modality for the treatment of advanced head and neck cancers, particularly in the USA [224].

A randomized phase III study was conducted by the European Organization for Research and Treatment of Cancer (EORTC) to compare a combination of larynx-preserving chemotherapy and radiotherapy with a combination of radical surgery and radiotherapy in the treatment of hypopharyngeal cancer [226]. Approximately 200 patients were randomly assigned to the chemotherapy and surgery arms of the study. In the chemotherapy arm (n = 100), 54% of patients had complete remission of the primary tumor and 51% had complete remission of regional lymphatic involvement. Every other patient with a complete response had a functionally competent larynx at the end of 5 years. Patients who did not respond to chemotherapy underwent surgery (total laryngectomy with partial pharyngectomy) and postoperative irradiation. Patients who had tumor recurrence following chemotherapy and radiation also underwent surgery. No differences were found between the two treatment arms with respect to local and regional tumor control. The 5-year disease-specific survival rates were 29% in the chemotherapy arm and 36% in the surgery arm. When only local recurrence was considered a treat-

ment failure, the likelihood of a patient in the chemotherapy arm surviving 5 years with a functional larynx was 35%. When deaths were considered without regard for cause, this likelihood declined to 17%. The authors concluded from their results that chemotherapy could be used for organ preservation in patients with hypopharyngeal carcinoma without compromising survival rates. A critical analysis of the study, however, shows that for various reasons only 52 of 100 patients completed their chemotherapy cycles according to protocol. This resulted in a relatively small base for making a definitive evaluation. The complication rate, including two treatment-related deaths, was remarkably high. While 94% of the patients had stage III or IV disease, 38 patients had T2 primary tumors. Conservation surgery would have been an option for these patients according to our criteria, and "needing radical surgery" thus appears to have been a very subjective criterion for inclusion in the trial.

A study was done at the University of Michigan on the efficacy of neoadjuvant chemotherapy with carboplatin and 5-fluorouracil followed by radiotherapy in 55 patients with oropharyngeal cancer and 34 patients with hypopharyngeal cancer stages II—IV [227]. In 59% of the patients with hypopharyngeal cancer, larynx preservation was achieved at the end of treatment. At the time the study was evaluated, 29% of the patients with hypopharyngeal cancer were still alive with a functioning larynx. The 5-year survival rate was 24%. It should also be noted that 26% of the patients overall had T1 or T2 primary tumors and presumably would have been candidates for organ-preserving surgery.

Conclusion

In summary, these data show that the results of laser microsurgery for early piriform sinus carcinomas are better than the results of primary radiotherapy from an oncologic standpoint (local control and survival rates). The morbidity and complication rates are lower, organ function is comparable, but the rate of organ preservation is higher. The same pattern emerges when laser microsurgery is compared with the results of partial laryngopharyngectomy, with or without neoadjuvant chemotherapy or adjuvant radiotherapy. Compared with standard surgical treatment and newer organ preservation protocols (neoadjuvant chemotherapy combined with radiation), the results of laser microsurgery in the treatment of advanced piriform sinus cancers are again better from an oncologic standpoint. Morbidity is less, complication rates are lower, and the rate of organ preservation is higher. The functional results of laser microsurgery were comparable to those of neoadjuvant chemotherapy and radiotherapy and better than those of standard surgery.

■ Laser Microsurgery of Oral and Oropharyngeal Carcinoma

Soon after the CO_2 laser was introduced into microsurgery of the larynx, the new treatment modality was applied to the soft tissues of the oral cavity [228]. Initially, laser use was limited to the excision of leukoplakia [229–231] and small, superficial carcinomas [232–235]. One of the earliest discoveries was that laser use in the oral cavity did not result in wound healing problems [228, 233].

Operative Technique

Every lesion in the oral cavity and oropharynx that is resectable by the intraoral or transoral route should be removed with a laser under the operating microscope and not grossly with a scalpel or cautery needle, since operating under the microscope improves the precision of the tumor resection. For excising carcinomas of the oral cavity, soft palate, or tonsils, instruments such as mouth gags, spatulas, and retractors are used to expose the tumor site. Surgery of the base of the tongue is a particular challenge due to the difficulties of topographic orientation. Bivalved laryngoscopes are used in resecting carcinomas of the base of the tongue and posterior oropharyngeal wall. The only useful landmarks are the glossoepiglottic fold, vallecula, foramen cecum, and the hyoid bone, which can be visualized as the operation proceeds. The differentiation between involved and uninvolved tissue is particularly challenging at the base of the tongue due to the difficulty in defining the lingual tonsils.

With its coagulating properties, the CO_2 laser can seal blood vessels and lymphatics up to 0.5 mm in diameter. This creates an almost bloodless incision, minimizes postoperative edema, and eliminates the need for a tracheotomy. The reepithelialization of a laser-produced wound proceeds more slowly than of a lesion made with a scalpel. Superficial excisions in the oral cavity and oropharynx heal with smooth scar formation and without contractures. Local wound infections are very rare, and even large defects can be left to heal spontaneously, without the need for flap or graft coverage. The CO_2 laser can transect the Wharton or Stenon duct without causing stenosis.

When intraoral carcinomas reach the gingiva, the gingiva should be resected along with the periosteum. We dissect the periosteum with a periosteal elevator to preserve it for histologic study and facilitate the detection of cortical erosions. The cortex is treated with the laser after tumor excision. If cortical infiltration is noted, a partial mandibulectomy must be carried out. It is not necessary to cover exposed bone. Even larger wound defects with exposed bone will heal by secondary intention within 6–8 weeks.

Laser Microsurgery of Oral Carcinoma and Other Treatment Options

Cancers of the oral cavity are most commonly located at the tongue and floor of the mouth. Ben-Bassat et al. [236] and Strong et al. [228] were the first authors, in the late 1970s, to describe laser resection of tongue cancer. The first long-term results were published by Carruth [237], Hirano et al. [238], and Williams and Carruth [239]. Eckel et al. [240] reported additional long-term results. They carried out laser resections of T1–T4 oral cavity carcinomas in

64 patients. The local recurrence rate was 36%. The tumor-related survival rate at 5 years was 81% for stage I and II lesions, 73% for stage III disease, and 21% for stage IV disease. The functional results (without plastic coverage of the defect) were very satisfactory. Bier-Laning and Adams [241] reported on the microsurgical laser excision of intraoral carcinomas in 51 patients. The incidence of local recurrences was 34%.

Between 1986 and 1997, we carried out primary laser microsurgery for cure in 81 patients with *tongue cancer*. The tumors were distributed by stage as follows: stage I in 27 patients (33%), stage II in 21 (27%), stage III in 19 (23%), and stage IV in 14 (17%) (UICC 1992). Local or locoregional tumor recurrence was observed in a total of 15 patients (18.5%). The 5-year local control rate was 78%. The 5-year overall survival rates were 64% for stage I and II tumor and 40% for stage III and IV tumors (unpublished data).

Similar oncologic results have been reported in the literature for conventional surgical treatment. Five-year local control rates of 60–80% are reported for stage I and II tongue cancers [242–245]. The local control rate for stage III and IV cancers treated by surgery and postoperative radiation is approximately 50% [242, 244]. The 5-year survival rate for patients with stage I and II tongue cancers is approximately 80%, decreasing to about 50% in patients with stage III and IV tumors [244, 246].

Even relatively large defects in the oral cavity can be left to heal spontaneously and do not require coverage with local, regional or free flaps, which is beneficial in terms of functional outcome. As early as 1987, McConnel et al. [247] compared different reconstructive techniques in patients with T2 and T3 tongue cancers. Postoperative function was best following repair of the defect with split-thickness skin grafts and after primary wound closure. The functional results were poorest when local or regional flaps had been used for reconstruction. In a multicenter prospective study, three different methods of reconstructing defects in the tongue and the base of the tongue (of comparable location and extent) were compared with respect to speech and swallowing function: primary wound closure, myocutaneous flap, and microvascular free flap. Contrary to popular beliefs, the authors found that primary wound closure resulted in equal or better function than the use of myocutaneous or free flaps [248]. Other authors have published similar observations [249–251].

Surgical treatment is preferred for T1 and T2 *floor of the munth cancers* due to the complications that can result from irradiating a tumor in such close proximity to the lower jaw. Stage III and IV oral floor cancers are generally managed by surgical excision and postoperative radiotherapy. Between 1986 and 1997, we carried out primary laser microsurgery for cure in 53 patients with squamous cell carcinoma of the floor of the month. The distribution of the lesions by stage was as follows: stages I and II in 11 patients (21%) each, stage III in 15 (28%), and stage IV in 16 (30%) (UICC 1992). Local or locoregional tumor recurrence was observed in a total of 13 patients (23%) (stages I and II 18%, stages III and IV 29%). The 5-year overall survival rate was 61% (unpublished data).

Comparable rates of local recurrence in floor of the mouth carcinoma were observed after conventional tumor resection with or without partial mandibulectomy and with or without defect repair [245, 252, 253]. Hicks et al. [252] treated 96 patients with oral floor cancers (43% stage I and II) with primary conventional surgery. A marginal or segmental mandibulectomy was done in half of the patients. Despite this aggressive approach, 16% of the patients with a T2 or T1 tumor and 27% of the patients with a T3 or T4 tumor developed local recurrence. Sessions et al. [254] observed a local recurrence rate of 17.5% in 280 patients with oral floor cancers (50% with a stage I or II lesion) who had been treated with various modalities.

Local control rates of 80%, 56%, and 17% have been reported for T1, T2, and T3 floor of the mouth cancers, respectively, treated by percutaneous radiotherapy alone [255]. The use of interstitial brachytherapy alone in 160 patients with T1 and T2 oral floor cancers resulted in a local control rate of 89% and a 5-year survival rate of 76%. Soft-tissue necrosis occurred in 10% of the patients, however, and bone necrosis developed in 18% [256].

Laser Microsurgery of Oropharyngeal Carcinoma and Other Treatment Options

The poor prognosis in patients with oropharyngeal cancer, which usually involves the tonsil or base of the tongue, is attributed to the fact that most cases are diagnosed at an advanced stage due to the absence of early symptoms. While it is true that therapeutic advances in recent years have resulted in improved locoregional tumor control, survival rates have not improved due to the frequency of distant metastasis.

Eckel et al. [240] reported on 53 patients who underwent laser microsurgery for the resection of stage I–IV oropharyngeal cancers. The local recurrence rate was 38%. The 5-year tumor-related survival rates were 86% for stage I and II tumors, 65% for stage III tumors, and 21% for stage IV tumors. Between 1986 and 1996 we performed primary microsurgical laser resections for cure in 90 patients with *tonsillar carcinoma*. The stage distribution was as follows: stage I in 5 patients (6%), stage II in 8 (9%), stage III in 22 (24%), and stage IV in 55 (61%) (UICC 1992). Local or locoregional tumor recurrence was observed in a total of 27 patients (30%) (stages I and II 8%, stages III and IV 34%). The 5-year overall survival rate was 63% for stage I and II lesions and 35% for stage III and IV lesions (unpublished data).

Similar oncologic results have been reported in the literature for conventional operations, in which the resulting defects were reconstructed with local flaps or microvascular free flaps. Five-year local control rates of 75–80% are reported for stage I and II tonsillar carcinoma [257, 258]. The local tumor control rate for stage III and IV cancers treated by surgery and postoperative radiation is approximately 60–65% [258–260]. The 5-year overall survival rate after a combined treatment regimen (30–65% of patients had stage IV disease) is 38–54% [260–262].

Radiotherapy alone, with or without a planned neck dissection (the percentage of patients with T4 tumors was 5–23%), is associated with a 5-year local control rate of 44–76% [260, 261, 263, 264] and a 5-year overall survival rate of 48–60% after radiotherapy alone [263–265]. A review of the literature by Parsons et al. [266] indicates that the oncologic results of primary radiotherapy, with or without a planned neck dissection, for all stages of tonsillar carcinoma are comparable with the results achieved with surgery and postoperative radiotherapy.

Only a few studies have been done on postoperative swallowing and speech function after radical surgery and postoperative radiation [248, 267]. Contrary to expectations, the functional results are not always satisfactory despite improved modern reconstructive techniques using microvascular free flaps. The majority of patients can eat only soft foods after the radical excision of oropharyngeal cancer and avoid eating in public. The stage of the primary tumor has no effect on the degree of postoperative functional disability [267].

Many articles on the surgery of *cancer of the base of the tongue* note the morbidity of the surgery and the frequently poor functional results in patients who already have a poor prognosis. We analyzed the data from 48 patients with tongue base cancers who underwent primary laser microsurgery with curative intent between 1986 and 1997. One patient had a pT1 primary tumor, 12 had a pT2 tumor, 7 had a pT3 tumor, and 28 had a pT4 tumor (UICC 1997). Cervical lymph node metastases were detectable in 33 patients (69%) at the time of diagnosis. Ninety-four percent of the patients were classified as having stage III or IVa disease. Forty-three patients underwent selective neck dissection, and 23 patients received postoperative radiotherapy. The 5-year local control rate was 85%, the 5-year overall survival rate was 52%, and recurrence-free survival was 73%. None of the patients required a peri- or postoperative tracheotomy, and none required total laryngectomy for functional problems. Oral intake was possible in all but three patients, who required a PEG feeding tube [268].

To date there have been no other published reports on the results of laser microsurgery for carcinoma of the base of the tongue, and so we are unable to compare our results with those of other authors. There are also very few comparable data on cancers of the base of the tongue treated entirely with conventional surgery. Most of the patients treated to date had a T1 or T2 primary tumor and underwent tongue base resection with a temporary mandibulotomy or partial mandibulectomy. The 5-year local control rates range from 74% to 100%, and the 5-year overall survival rate is approximately 50% [269–271].

Although the combination of surgery and postoperative radiotherapy (30–61% of the patients had T3 and T4 tumors) yielded better local control rates of 77–94%, the 5-year overall survival rates were still only 41–55% [262, 270, 272, 273]. Fifteen to 20% of the patients required a total laryngectomy [269, 271–273], 11–35% required a partial mandibulectomy [262, 269, 271–273], and 10–25% required a permanent tracheotomy and/or a PEG tube [269, 274]. Serious complications such as bleeding, pharyngocutaneous fistulas, osteomyelitis, flap necrosis, and pulmonary complications from chronic aspiration occurred in 17–49% of the patients treated [269, 271, 272, 273].

In patients treated by primary radiotherapy, local control is dependent on the tumor volume. Local control rates of 80–100% have been reported for T1 tumors, 57–96% for T2 tumors, 45–82% for T3 tumors, and 18–50% for T4 tumors [271, 275–278]. More than half the patients treated had T3 or T4 tumor, and the 5-year local control rate was 44–79%, regardless of the tumor stage [275, 276, 278]. The 5-year overall survival rates in these studies ranged from 27% to 50%. Results on swallowing function show that a higher percentage of patients were eating normally after primary radiotherapy (74–94%) than after surgery and postoperative radiation [279–281].

In two studies the prevalence of T3 and T4 tumors was less than 50% and treatment consisted of primary external-beam irradiation followed by a brachytherapy boost with I-125 [282] or Ir-92 [283]. The 5-year local control rates in these studies were 88% and 89%, and the 5-year overall survival rates were 72% and 86%, respectively. Almost all the patients had a temporary tracheotomy, and complications such as osteoradionecrosis of the mandible, soft-tissue necrosis, bleeding after removal of the brachytherapy applicators, and hypoglossal nerve palsy occurred in 20% and 19% of the cases, respectively. Vokes et al. [284] conducted a phase II trial to evaluate the concomitant chemoradiotherapy of stage IV head and neck cancers (53% oropharyngeal cancers). Local control was excellent, at 92%, but overall survival was only 55%, and more than 60% of the patients had moderate to severe swallowing difficulties.

Conclusion

The intra- or transoral approach for cancers of the oral cavity and oropharynx eliminates the need for pharyngotomy, mandibulotomy or partial mandibulectomy, and tracheotomy, resulting in far less morbidity for the patient. The limitations of this approach are inadequate tumor exposure and contiguous tumor spread into the soft tissues of the neck, since exposing the major vessels in the neck through a transoral route poses a serious risk of hemorrhage. At least one hypoglossal nerve should be preserved in the operative treatment of cancers of the base of the tongue. In our experience, even large surgical defects in the oral cavity and oropharynx do not require plastic repair. Eliminating flap surgery avoids additional morbidity. Our own experience and the studies on postoperative function cited in this article have shown that primary wound closure has no adverse effects on postoperative swallowing and speech function.

■ Palliative Laser Microsurgery of Head and Neck Cancers

One of the first applications of the CO_2 laser in laryngology was for debulking obstructing laryngeal cancers [126, 285]

and larynx-obstructing tumors of the oropharynx and hypopharynx as an alternative to tracheotomy. The laser can still be used for this purpose today to reestablish a safe airway and avoid emergency tracheotomy. A prerequisite for laser surgery in these cases is endotracheal intubation, which can generally be accomplished fiberoptically in the sedated patient even when is present. Other options are orotracheal intubation or the intubation of a rigid bronchoscope using a guidewire to facilitate the intubation. Definitive diagnosis and treatment can then be planned in an unhurried fashion.

Laccourreye et al. [286] used the CO_2 laser to debulk obstructing endolaryngeal carcinomas in 42 patients as a prelude to definitive curative treatment. Tracheotomy was avoided in 39 of the 42 patients (93%) with one or two laser procedures. Perioperative complications are rare [126, 285, 287–289]. Especially in cases where laser tumor debulking is done with palliative intent as an alternative to tracheotomy, the patient's quality of life can be significantly improved. The difficulty with this surgery lies in determining the extent of the resection. If too little tissue is resected, the obstruction will persist and a tracheotomy will be required. On the other hand, resecting too much tissue can lead to massive aspiration necessitating a secondary tracheotomy. In both cases the procedure fails to meet the goal of improving the quality of life [4].

When dysphagia is present, one should hesitate to recanalize the upper digestive tract by CO_2 laser ablation of tumor tissue from the hypopharynx and esophageal inlet. In our experience, this type of procedure improves swallowing function only temporarily and is associated with a serious bleeding risk. The placement of a PEG tube is a better option for these patients.

Ideally, a palliative measure should relieve obstructive symptoms for an extended period of time. But the actual value of a palliative CO_2 laser procedure is difficult to evaluate in terms of the length of the remission and possible side effects, because the assessment is based on the individual experience of the surgeon without benefit of systematic retrospective or prospective studies. Although Laccourreye et al. [259], in a retrospective study of eight patients, were able to avoid tracheotomy for the remainder of the patients' lives (up to 8 months) by palliative laser debulking of their tumors, other authors state that, in their experience, tracheotomy can only be postponed for a few months [290].

■ References

1 Braun U. Anestheiological aspects of laser surgery in otorhinolaryngology. In: Steiner W, Ambrosch P. Endoscopic laser surgery of the upper aerodegistive tract. With special emphasis on cancer surgery. Stuttgart, New York: Georg Thieme Verlag, 2000: 116–123

2 Shikowitz MJ, Abramson AL, Liberatore L. Endolaryngeal jet ventilation: a 10-year review. Laryngoscope 1991; 101: 455–461

3 Claes J, Vermeyen K, van der Heyning PH, Boeckx E. Preglottic low-frequency Venturi jet ventilation in laryngoscopic microsurgery in adults. The influence of inspiratory time and frequency of ventilation. Clin Otolaryngol 1989; 14: 433–440

4 Steiner W, Ambrosch P. Endoscopic Laser surgery of the upper aerodigestive tract. Stuttgart, New York: Georg Thieme, 2000

5 Ambrosch P, Brick U, fischer G, Steiner W. Spezielle Aspekte der histopathologischen Diagnostik bei der Lasermikrochirurgie von Karzinomen des oberen Aerodegistivtraktes. Laryngorhinootologie 1994; 73: 78–83

6 Davidson TM, Nahum AM, Haghighi P, Astarita SL, Saltzstein S, Seagren S. The biology of head and neck cancer. Detection and control by parallel histologic sections. Arch Otolaryngol 1984; 110: 193–196

7 Davidson TM, Haghighi P. Parallel histologic section for head and neck mucosal cancer. Facial Plast Surg 1987 1987; 5: 67–90

8 Kleinsasser O, Glanz H. Histologisch kontrollierte Tumorchirurgie. HNO 1984; 32: 234–236

9 Strong MS, Jako J. Laser surgery in the larynx. Early clinical experience with continuous CO_2 laser. Ann Otol Rhinol Laryngol 1972; 81: 791–798

10 Kleinsasser O, Glanz H, Kimmich T. Endoskopische Chirurgie des Stimmlippenkarzinoms. HNO 1988; 36: 412–416

11 Steiner W. Experience in endoscopic laser surgery of malignant tumours of the upper aerodigestive tract. Adv Otorhinolaryngol 1988; 39: 134–144

12 Remacle M, Lawson G, Jamart J, Minet M, Watelet JB, Delos M. CO_2 laser in the diagnosis and treatment of early cancer of the vocal fold. Eur Arch Otorhinolaryngol 1997; 254: 169–176

13 Thumfart WF, Eckel HE. Endolaryngeale Laserchirurgie zur Behandlung von Kehlkopfkarzinomen. HNO 1990; 38: 174–178

14 Remacle M, Eckel HE, Antonelli A, Brasnu D, Chevalier D, Friedrich G, Olofsson J, Rudert HH, Thumfart WF, de Vincentiies M, Wustrow TPU. Endoscopic cordectomy. A proposal for a classification by the working committee. European Laryngological Society. Eur Arch Otorhinolaryngol 2000; 257: 227–231

15 Shapshay SM, Hybels RL, Bohigian RK. Laser excision of early vocal cord carcinoma: indications, limitations, and precautions. Ann Otol Rhinol Laryngol 1990; 99: 46–50

16 Eckel HE, Thumfart WF. Laser surgery for the treatment of larynx carcinomas: indications, techniques, and preliminary results. Ann Otol Rhinol Laryngol 1992; 101: 113–118

17 Steiner W. Results of curative laser microsurgery of laryngeal carcinomas. Am J Otolaryngol 1993; 14: 116–121

18 Czigner J, Sávay L. Primäre CO_2-Laser-Chordektomie beim Stimmlippenkarzinom. Laryngo-Rhino-Otol 1994; 73: 432–436

19 Rudert HH, Werner JA. Endoscopic resections of glottic and supraglottic carcinomas with the CO_2 laser. Eur Arch Otorhinolaryngol 1995; 252: 146–148

20 Lindholm CE, Elner A. Transoral laser surgery of laryngeal carcinomas: In: Rudert H, Werner JA (Eds). Lasers in otorhinolaryngology and in head and neck surgery. Adv Otorhinolaryngol 49. Basel: Karger, 1995: 250–253

21 Thumfart WF, Scholtz AW, Eckel HE, Gunkel AR, Pototschnig C. Early cancer of the larynx. Proceedings of the Fourth International Conference on Head and Neck Cancer, Toronto, July 28–August 1. 1996: 289–297

22 Motta G, Esposito E, Cassiano B, Motta S. T1-T2-T3 glottic tumors: fifteen years experience with CO_2 laser. Acta Otolaryngol (Stockh) 1997; 527: 155–159

23 Peretti G, Cappiello J, Berlucchi M, Ansarin M, Antonelli AR. Transoral CO_2 laser surgery for Tis, T1 and T2 glottic cancer. In: Kleinsasser O, Glanz H, Olofsson J (Eds). Advances in Laryngology in Europe. Amsterdam, the Netherlands: Elsevier, 1997: 270–275

24 Mahieu H, Peeters J, Snel F, Leemans R. Transoral endoscopic surgery for early glottic cancer. Proceedings of the Fifth International Conference on Head and Neck Cancer, San Francisco, July 29–August 2. 2000: 165–172

25 Ambrosch P, Rödel R, Kron M, Steiner W. Die transorale Lasermikrochirurgie des Larynxkarzinoms. Eine retrospektive Analyse von 657 Patientenverläufen. Onkologe 2001; 7: 505–512

26 Peretti G, Nicolai P, Piazza C, Redaelli de Zinis LO, Valentini S, Antonelli AR. Oncological results of endoscopic resections of Tis and T1 glottic carcinomas by carbon dioxide laser. Ann Otol Rhinol Laryngol 2001; 110: 820–826

27 Gallo A, de Vincentiis M, Manciocco V, Simonelli M, Fiorella ML, Shah JP. CO_2 laser cordectomy for early-stage glottic carcino-

ma: a long-term follow-up of 156 cases. Laryngoscope 2002; 112: 370–374

28 Eckel HE. Local recurrences following transoral laser surgery for early glottic carcinoma: frequency, management, and outcome. Ann Otol Rhinol Laryngol 2001; 110: 7–15

29 Glanz H, Kimmich T, Eichhorn T, Kleinsasser O. Erebnisse der Behandlung von 584 Kehlkopfkarzinomen an der HNO-Klinik Marburg. HNO 1989; 37: 1–10

30 Johnson JT, Myers EN, Hao SP, Wagner RL. Outcome of open surgical therapy for glottic carcinoma. Ann Otol Rhinol Laryngol 1993; 102: 752–755

31 Neel HB III, Devine KD, DeSanto LW. Laryngofissure and cordectomy for early cordal carcinoma: Outcome in 182 patients. Otolaryngol Head Neck Surg 1980; 88: 79–84

32 Thomas JC, Olsen KD, Neel HB 3rd, De Santo LW, Suman VJ. Recurrences after endoscopic management of early (T1) glottic carcinoma. Laryngoscope 1994; 104: 1099–1104

33 Ton-Van J, Lefebvre JL, Stern JC, Buisset E, Coche-Dequeant B, Vankemmel B. Comparison of surgery and radiotherapy in T1 and T2 glottic carcinomass Am J Surg 1991; 162: 337–340

34 Epstein BE, Lee DJ, Kashima H, Johns ME. Stage T1 glottic carcinoma: results of radiation therapy or laser excision. Radiology 1990; 175: 567–570

35 Fein DA, Mendenhall WM, Parsons JT, Million RR. T1–T2 squamous cell carcinoma of the glottic larynx treated with radiotherapy: a multivariate analysis of variables potentially influencing local control. Int J Radiat Oncol Biol Phys 1993; 25: 605–611

36 Grant DG, Hussain A, Hurman D. Pre-treatment anaemia alters outcome in early squamous cell carcinoma of the larynx treated by radical radiotherapy. J Laringol Otol 1999; 113: 829–833

37 Jorgensen K, Godballe C, Hansen O, Bastholt L. Cancer of the larynx. Treatment results after primary radiotherapy with salvage surgery in a series of 1005 patients. Acta Oncol 2002; 41: 69–76

38 Mendenhall WM, Parsons JT, Stringer SP, Cassissi NJ. Management of Tis, T1 and T2 squamous cell carcinoma of the glottic larynx. Am J Otolaryngol 1994; 15: 250–257

39 Rosier JF, Grégoire V, Counoy H, Octave Prignot M, Rombaut P, Scalliet P, Vanderlinden F, Hamoir M. Comparison of external radiotherapy, laser microsurgery and partial laryngectomy for the treatment of T1N0M0 glottic carcinomas; a retrospective evaluation. Radiother Oncol 1998; 48: 175–183

40 van der Voet JC, Keus RB, Hart AA, Hilgers FJ, Bartelink H. The impact of treatment time and smoking on local control and complications in T1 glottic cancer. Int J Radiat Oncol Biol Phys 1998; 42: 247–255

41 Barthel SW, Esclamado RM. Primary radiation therapy for early glottic cancer. Otolaryngol Head Neck Surg 2001; 124: 35–39

42 Dinshaw KA, Sharma V, Agarwal JP, Ghosh S, Havaldar R. Radiation therapy in T1–T2 glottic carcinoma: influence of various treatment parameters on local control/complications. Int J Radiat Oncol Biol Phys 2000; 48: 723–735

43 Marshak G, Brenner B, Shvero J, Shapira J, Ophira D, Hochman I, Marshak G, Sulkes A, Rakowsky E. Prognostic factors for local control of early glottic cancer: the Rabin medical center retrospective study on 207 patients. Int J Radiat Oncol Biol Phys 1999; 43: 1009–1013

44 Schwaab G, Mamelle G, Lartigau E, Parise O, Wibault P, Luboinski B. Surgical salvage treatment of T1/T2 glottic carcinoma after failure of radiotherapy. Am J Surg 1994; 168: 474–475

45 Reker U. Phoniatory ability after surgery of vocal cord carcinoma of limited extension. A comparison between transoral laser microsurgery and frontolateral partial laryngeal resection Adv Otorhinolaryngol 1995; 49: 215–218

46 Dagli AS, Mahieu HF, Festen JM. Quantitative analysis of voice quality in early glottic laryngeal carcinomas treated with radiotherapy. Eur Arch Otolaryngol 1997; 254: 78–80

47 Verdonck-De Leeuw IM, Keus RB, Hilgers FJM, Koopmans-van Beinum FJ, Greven AJ, Jongde JMA, Vreeburg G, Bartelink H. Consequences of voice impairment in daily life for patients following radiotherapy for glottic cancer: voice quality, vocal function, and vocal performance. Int J Rad Oncol Biol Phys 1999; 44: 1071–1978

48 Keilmann A, Bergler W, Artzt M, Hörmann K. Vocal function following laser and conventional surgery of small malignant vocal

fold tumours. J Laryngol Otol 1996; 110: 1138–1141

49 Pia F, Gonella ML, Boggero R, Ponzo S, Giordano C. Valutazione obiettivo-instrumentale della funzionalità glottica residua dopo cordectomia tradizionale e coredectomia CO_2 laser. Acta Otorhinolaryngol Ital 1994; 14: 329–338

50 Brandenburg JH. Laser cordotomy versus radiotherapy: an abjective cost analysis. Ann Otol Rhinol Laryngol 2001; 110: 312–317

51 Delsupehe KG, Zink I, Lejaegere M, Bastian RW. Voice quality after narrow-margin laser cordectomy compared with laryngeal irradiation. Otolaryngol Head Neck Surg 1999; 121: 528–533

52 McGuirt WF, Blalock D, Koufman JA, Feehs RS, Hilliard AJ, Greven K, Randall M. Comparative voice results after laser resection or irradiation of T1 vocal cord carcinoma. Arch Otolaryngol Head Neck Surg 1994; 120: 951–955

53 Haraf DJ, Weichselbaum RR. Treatment selection in T1 and T2 vocal cord carcinoma. Acta Oncol 1991; 30: 357–362

54 Rydell R, Schalén L, Fex S, Elner A. Voice evaluation before and after laser excision vs. radiotherapy of T1A glottic carcinoma. Acta Otolaryngol (Stockh) 1995; 115: 560–565

55 Kruse E. The role of the poniatrician in laser surgery of the larynx. In: Steiner W, Ambrosch P (Eds). Endoscopic laser surgery of the upper aerodigestive tract. With special emphasis on cancer surgery. Stuttgart, New York: Georg Thieme Verlag, 2000: 124–129

56 Steiner W, Aurbach G, Ambrosch P. Minimally invasive therapy in otorhinolaryngology and head and neck surgery. MITAT 1991; 108: 57–70

57 Myers EN, Wagner RL, Johnson JT. Microlaryngoscopic surgery for T1 glottic lesions: a cost-effective option. Ann Otol Rhinol laryngol 1994; 103: 28–30

58 Paulsen F, Tillmann B. Struktur und Funktion des ventralen Stimmlippenansatzes. Unter klinischen Gesichtspunkten. Laryngo-Rhino-Otol 1996; 75: 590–596

59 Rucci L, Gammarota L, Borghi Cirri MB. Carcinoma of the anterior commissure of the larynx: I. Embryological and anatomic considerations. Ann Otol Rhinol Laryngol 1996; 105: 303–308

60 Rucci L, Gammarota L, Gallo O. Carcinoma of the anterior commissure of the larynx: II. Proposal of a new staging system. Ann Otol Rhinol Laryngol 1996; 105: 391–396

61 Kirchner JA, Carter D. Intralaryngeal barriers to the spread of cancer. Acta Otolaryngol (Stockh) 1987; 103: 503–513

62 Kirchner JA. What have wohe organ sections contributed to the treatment of laryngeal cancer? Ann Otol Rhinol Laryngol 1989; 98: 661–667

63 Krespi YP, Meltzer CJ. Laser surgery for vocal cord carcinoma involving the anterior commissure. Ann Otol Rhinol Laryngol 1989; 98: 105–109

64 Casiano R, Cooper JD, Lundy DS, Chandler JR. Laser cordectomy for T1 glottic carcinoma: a 10-year experience and videostroboscopic findings. Otolaryngol Head Neck Surg 1991; 104: 831–837

65 Wetmore SJ, Key M, Suen JY. Laser therapy for T1 glottic carcinoma of the larynx. Arch Otolaryngol Head Neck Surg 1986; 112: 853–855

66 Wolfensberger M, Dort JC. Endoscopic laser surgery for early glottic carcinoma: a clinical and experimental study. Laryngoscope 1990; 100: 1100–1105

67 Davis RK, Jako GJ, Hyams VJ, Shapshay SM. The anatomic limitations of CO_2 laser cordectomy. Laryngoscope 1982; 92: 980–984

68 Desloge RB, Zeitels SM. Endolaryngeal microsurgery at the anterior glottal commissure: controversies and observations. Ann Otol Rhinol Laryngol 2000; 109: 385–392

69 Kashima HK, Lee D-J, Zinreich SJ. Vestibulectomy in early vocal fold carcinoma. Trans Am Broncho-Esophagol Assoc 1991; 71: 28–32

70 Rudert HH. Transoral CO_2-laser surgery of early glottic cancer (CIS-T2). In: Smee R, Bridger P (Eds). Laryngeal Cancer: Proceedings of the 2nd World Congress on Laryngeal Cancer. Amsterdam, the Netherlands: Elsevier, 1994: 389–392

71 Steiner W, Ambrosch P, Rödel RMW, Kron M. Impact of anterior commissure involvement on local control of early glottic carcinoma treated by laser microresection. Laryngoscope 2004; 114: 1485–91

72 Hirota S, Soejima T, Obayashi K, Hishikawa Y, Honda K, Okamoto Y, Maed H, Takada Y, Innoue K, Kinishi M, Amatsu M, Kimura S. Radiotherapy of T1 and T2 glottic cancer: analysis of anterior commissure involvement. Radiat Med 1996; 14: 297–302

73 Maheshwar AA, Gaffney CC. Radiotherapy for T1 glottic carcinoma: impact of anterior commissure involvement. J Laryngol Otol 2001; 115: 298–301

74 Reddy SP, Mohideen N, Marra S, Marks JE. Effect of tumour bulk on local control and survival of patients with T1. Radiother Oncol 1998; 47: 161–166

75 Rudoltz MS, Benammar A, Mohiuddin M. Prognostic factors for local control and survival in T1 squamous cell carcinoma of the glottis. Int J Radiat Oncol Biol Phys 1993; 26: 767–772

76 Rucci L, Gallo O, Fini-Storchi O. Glottic cancer involving anterior commissure: surgery vs. radiotherapy. Head Neck 1991; 13: 403–410

77 Woodhause RJ, Quivey JM, Fu KK, Sein PS, Dedo HH, Phillips TL. Treatment of carcinoma of the vocal cord. A review of 20 years experience. Laryngoscope 1981; 91: 1155–1162

78 Zohar Y, Rahima M, shvili Y, Talmi YP, Lurie H. The controversial treatment of anterior commissure carcinoma of the larynx. Laryngoscope 1992; 102: 69–72

79 Mllet Y, Chevalier D, Darras JA, Wiel E, Desaulty A. Near total laryngectomy with epiglottic reconstruction. Our experience of 65 cases. Eur Arch Otorhinolaryngol 2001; 258: 488–491

80 Laccourreye O, Muscatello L, Laccourreye L, Naudo P, Brasnu D, Weinstein G. Supracicroid partial laryngectomy with cricohyoidoepiglottopexy for „early" glottic carcinoma classified as T1–T2N0 invading the anterior commissure. Am J Otolaryngol 1997; 18: 385–390

81 Bron L, Brossard E, Monnier P, Pasche P. Supraglottic partial laryngectomy with cricohyoidoepiglottopexy and cricohyoidopexy for glottic and supraglottic carcinomas. Laryngoscope 2000; 110: 27–634

82 Bron LP, Soldati D, Zouhair A, Ozsahin M, Brossard E, Monnier P, Pasche P. Treatment of early stage squamous-cell carcinoma of the glottic larynx: endoscopic surgery or cricohyoidoepiglottopexy versus radiotherapy. Head Neck 2001; 23: 823–829

83 Bron L, Pasche P, Brossard E, Monnier P, Schweizer V. Functional analysis after supracricoid partial laryngectomy with cricohyoidoepiglottopexy. Laryngoscope 2002; 112: 1289–1293

84 Kleinsasser O, Glanz H. Optional proposals for test new telescopic ramifications of TNM. In: Hermanek P, Henson DE, Hutter RVP, Sobin LH (Eds). TNM Supplement 1993. Berlin, Heidelberg, New York: Springer, 1993: 112–117

85 Laccourreye O, Weinstein G, Brasnu D, Trotoux J, Laccourreye H. Vertical partial laryngectomy: a critical analysis of local recurrence. Ann Otol Rhinol Laryngol 1991; 100: 68–71

86 Som ML. Cordal cancer with extension to vocal process. Laryngoscope 1975; 85: 1298–1307

87 Biller HF, Lawson W. Partial laryngectomy for vocal cord cancer with marked limitation or fixation of the vocal cord. Laryngoscope 1986; 96: 61–64

88 Lesinski Sg, Bauer WC, Ogura FH. Hemilaryngectomy for T3 (fixed cord) epidermoid carcinoma of the larynx. Laryngoscope 1976; 86: 1563–1571

89 Piquet JJ, Desaulty A, Pilliaert JM, Decroix G. Results of surgical treatment of cancers of the endolarynx. Acta Otorhinolaryngol Belg 1973; 27: 916–923

90 Vega SF, Scola B, Vega MF, Martinez T, Scola E. Laryngeal vertical partial surgery. Surgical techniques. Oncological and functional results. Acta Otorhinolaryngol Ital 1996; 16: 272–280

91 Bryant GP, Poulsen MG, Tripcony L, Dickie GJ. Treatment decisions in T3N0M0 glottic carcinoma. Int J Radiat Oncol Biol Phys 1995; 31: 285–293

92 Foote RL, Olsen KD, Buskirk SJ, Stanley RJ, Suman VJ. Laryngectomy alone for T3 glottic cancer. Head Neck 1994; 16: 406–412

93 Razack MS, Maipang T, Sako K, Bakamjian V, Shedd DP. Management of advanced glottic cancer. Am J Surg 1989; 159: 318–320

94 Chevalier D, Laccourreye O, Brasnu D, Laccourreye H, Piquet JJ. Cricohyoidoepiglottopexy for glottic carcinoma with fixation or impaired motion of the true vocal cord: 5-year oncologic results with 112 patients. Ann Otol Rhinol Laryngol 1997; 106: 364–369

95 Piquet JJ, Chevalier D. Subtotal laryngectomy with crico-hyo-do-epiglotto-pexy for the treatment of extended glottic carcinoma. Am J Surg 1991; 162: 357–361

96 Laccourreye O, Salzer SJ, Brasnu D, Shen W. Laccourreye H, Weinstein GS. Glottic carcinoma with a fixed true vocal cord: Outcomes after neoadjuvant chemotherapy and supracricoid partial laryngectomy with cricohyoidoepiglottopexy. Otolaryngol Head Neck Surg 1996; 114: 400–406

97 Laccourreye O, Brasnu D, Biacabe B, Hans S, Seckin S, Weinstein G. Neo-adjuvant chemotherapy and supracricoid partial laryngectomy with cricohyoidopexy for advanced endolaryngeal carcinoma classiefied as T3–T4: 5-year oncologic results. Head Neck 1998; 20: 595–599

98 Laccourreye O, Diaz EM, Muscatello L, Garcia D, Brasnu D. A multimodal strategy for the treatment of patients with T2 invasive squamous cell carcinoma of the glottis. Cancer 1999; 85: 40–46

99 Laccourreye O, Laccourreye L, Muscatello L, Périé S, Weinstein G, Brasnu D. Local failure after supracricoid partial laryngectomy: symptoms, management, and outcome. Laryngoscope 1998; 108: 339–344

100 Burke LS, Greven KM, McGuirt WT, Case D, Hoen HM, Raben M. Definitive radiotherapy for early glottic carcinoma: prognostic factors and implications for treatment. Int J Radiat Oncol Biol Phys 1997; 38: 1001–1006

101 Mendenhall WM, Parsons JT, Stringer SP, Cassisi NJ, Million RR. T1–T2 vocal cord carcinoma: a basis for comparing the results of radiotherapy and surgery. Head Neck Surg 1988; 10: 373–377

102 Turesson I, Sandberg N, Mercke C, Johansson KA, Sandin I, Wallgren A. Primary radiotherapy for glottic laryngeal carcinoma stage I and II. A retrospective study with special regard to failure patterns. Acta Oncol 1991; 30: 357–362

103 Harwood AR, Bryce DP, Rider WD. Management of T3 glottic cancer. Arch Otolaryngol 1980; 106: 697–699

104 Mendenhall WM, Parsons JT, Mancuso AA, Pameijer FJ, Stringer SP, Cassissi NJ. Definitive radiotherapy for T3 squamous cell carcinoma of the glottic larynx. J Clin Oncol 1997; 15: 2394–2402

105 Parsons JT, Mendenhall WM, Mancuso AA, Cassisi NJ, Stringer SP, Million RR. Twice-a-day radiotherapy for T3 squamous cell carcinoma of the glottic larynx. Head Neck 1989; 11: 123–128

106 Wylie JP, Sen M, Swindell R, Sykes AJ, Farrington WT, Slevin NJ, Definitive radiotherapy for 114 cases of T3N0 glottic carcinoma: influence of dose-volume parameters on outcome. Radiotherapy and Oncology 1999; 53: 15–21

107 Department of Veterans Affairs Laryngeal Cancer Study Group. Induction chemotherapy plus radiation compared with surgery plus radiation in patients with advanced laryngeal cancer. N Enl J Med 1991; 324: 1685–1690

108 Wolf GT, Hong WK, Fisher SG. Neoadjuvant chemotherapy for organ preservation: current status. Proceedings 4th International Conference on Head and Neck Cancer 1996; 4: 89–97

109 Richard JM, Sancho-Garnier H, Pessey JJ, Luboinski B, Lefebvre JL, Dehesdin D, Stromboni-Luboinski M, Hill C. Randomized trial of induction chemotherapy in larynx carcinoma. Oral Oncol 1998; 34: 224–228

110 Janot F, Rhein B, Koka VN, Wibault P, Domenge C, Bessede JP, Marandas P, Schwaab G, Luboinski B. Laryngeal preservation with induction chemotherapy. Experience of two GETTEC Centers, between 1985 and 1995. Ann Otolaryngol Chir Cervicofac 2002; 119: 12–20

111 Viani L, Stell PM, Dalby JE. Recurrence after radiotherapy for glottic carcinoma. Cancer 1991; 67: 577–584

112 Kooper DP, van den Broek P, Manni JJ, Tiwari RM, Snow GB. Partial vertical laryngectomy for recurrent glottic carcinoma. Clin Otolaryngol 1995; 20: 167–170

113 Nibu K, Kamata S, Kawabata K, Nakamizo M, Nigauri T, Hoki K. Partial laryngectomy in the treatment of radiation-failure of early glottic carcinoma. Head Neck 1997; 19: 116–120

114 Rodriguez-Cuevas S, Labstida S, Gonzalez D, Briseno N, Cortes H. Partial laryngectomy as salvage surgery for radiation failure in T1–T2 laryngeal cancer. Head Neck 1998; 20: 630–633

115 Steiner W, Ambrosch P, Uhlig P, Kron M. CO_2 laser microsurgery for hypopharyngeal carcinoma. Proceedings of the 3red

European Congress of the European Federation of Oto-Rhino-Laryngological Societies „EUFOS", Budapest, 9–14 June 1996. Bologna: Monduzzi Editore S. p. a., 1996: 669–672

116 Watters GWR, Patel SG, Rhys-Evans PH. Partial laryngectomy for recurrent laryngeal carcinoma. Clin Otolaryngol 2000; 25: 146–152

117 Laccourreye O, Weinstein G, Naudo P, Brasnu D, Cauchois R, Laccourreye H. Supracricoid partial laryngectomy after failed laryngeal radiation therapy. Laryngoscope 1996; 106: 495–498

118 Spriano G, Pellini R, Romano G, Muscatello L, Roselli R. Supracricoid partial laryngectomy as salvage surgery after radiation failure. Head Neck 2002; 24: 759–765

119 Annyas AA, Overbeek JJM, Escajadillo JR, Hoeksema PE. CO_2 laser in malignant lesions of the larynx. Laryngoscope 1984; 94: 836–838

120 Blakeslee D, Vaughan CW, Shapshay SM, Simpson GT, Strong MS. Excisional biopsy in the selective management of T1 glottic cancer: A three-year follow-up study. Laryngoscope 1984; 94: 488–494

121 De Gier HHW, Knegt PPM, de Boer MF, Meeuwis CA, van der Velden L, Kerrebijn JDF. CO_2 laser treatment of recurrent glottic carcinoma. Head Neck 2001; 23: 177–180

122 Outzen KE, Illum P. CO_2 laser therapy for carcinoma of the larynx. J Laryngol Otol 1995; 109: 111–113

123 Quer M, Leon X, Orus C, Venegas P, Lopez M, Burgues J. Endoscopic laser surgery in the treatment of radiation failure of early laryngeal carcinoma. Head Neck 2000; 8: 520–523

124 Steiner W, Ambrosch P, Vogt P. Transoral carbon dioxide laser microsurgery for recurrent glottic carcinoma after radiotherapy, Head Neck 2004; 26:477–84

125 Alonso JM. Conservative surgery of cancer of the larynx. Trans Am Acad Ophthalmol Otolaryngol 1947; 51: 633–645

126 Vaughan CW. Transoral laryngeal surgery using the CO_2 laser. Laboratory experiments and clinical experience. Laryngoscope 1978; 88: 1399–1420

127 Steiner W, Jaumann MP, Pesch HJ. Endoskopische Therapie von Krebsfrühstadien im Larynx – vorläufige Ergebnisse. Arch Otorhinolaryngol 1981; 231: 637–643

128 Davis RK, Shapshay SM, Strong MS, Hyams VJ. Transoral partial supraglottic resection using the CO_2 laser. Laryngoscope 1983; 93: 429–432

129 Davis RK, Kelly SM, Hayes J. Endoscopic CO_2 laser excisional biopsy of early supraglottic cancer. Laryngoscope 1991; 101: 680–683

130 Zeitels SM, Vaughan CW, Domanowski GF. Endoscopic management of early supraglottic cancer. Ann Otol Rhinol Laryngol 1990; 99: 951–956

131 Zeitels SM, Koufman JA, Davis RK, Vaughan CW. Endoscopic treatment of supraglottic and hypopharynx cancer. Laryngoscope 1994; 104: 71–78

132 Eckel HE. Endoscopic laser resection of supraglottic carcinoma. Otolaryngol Head Neck Surg 1997; 117: 681–687

133 Iro H, Waldfahrer F, Altendorf-Hofmann A, Weidenbecher M, Sauer R, Steiner W. Transoral laser surgery of supraglottic cancer. Arch Otolaryngol Head Neck Surg 1998; 124: 1245–1250

134 Rudert HH, Werner JA, Höft S. Transoral carbon dioxide laser resection of supraglottic carcinoma. Ann Otol Rhinol Laryngol 1999; 108: 819–827

135 Ambrosch P, Kron M, Steiner W. Carbon dioxide laser microsurgery for early supraglottic carcinoma. Ann Otol Rhinol Laryngol 1998; 107: 680–688

136 Bocca E, Pignataro O, Oldini C. Supraglottic laryngectomy: 30 years of experience. Ann Otol Rhinol Laryngol 1983; 92: 14–18

137 Bocca E. Surgical management of supraglottic cancer and its lymph mode metastases in a conservative perspective. Ann Otol Rhinol Laryngol 1991; 100: 261–267

138 DeSanto LW. Early supraglottic cancer. Ann Otol Rhinol Laryngol 1990; 99: 593–597

139 Herranz-Gonzales J, Gavilan J, Martinez-Vidal J, Gavilan C. Supraglottic laryngectomy: functional and oncologic results. Ann Otol Rhinol Laryngol 1996; 105: 18–22

140 Lutz CK, Johnson JT, Wagner RL, Myers EN. Supraglottic carcinoma: patterns of recurrence. Ann Otol Rhinol Laryngol 1990; 99: 12–17

141 Robbins KT, Davidson W, Peters LJ, Goepfert H. Conservation surgery for T2 and T3 carcinomas of the supraglottic larynx. Arch Otolaryngol Head Neck Surg 1988; 114: 421–426

142 Soo KC, Shah JP, Gopinath KS, Gerold FP, Jacques DP, Strong EW. Analysis of prognostic variables and results after supraglottic partial laryngectomy. Am J Surg 1988; 156: 301–305

143 Suarez C, Rodrigo JP, Herranz J, Llorente JL, Martinez JA. Supraglottic laryngectomy with or without postoperative radiotherapy in supraglottic carcinomas. ann Otol Rhinol Laryngol 1995; 104: 358–363

144 Martinez T, Escamilla Y, Gutierrez M, Bodoque M, Scola B, Vega MF. La cirugia parcial en el carcinoma supraglotico. Resultados oncologicos y functionales. Acta Otorinolaring Esp 1996; 48: 125–128

145 Maurizi M, Paludetti G, Galli J, Attaviani F, D'Abramo G, Almadori G. Oncological and functional outcome of conservative surgery for primary supraglottic cancer. Eur Arch Otorhinolaryngol 1999; 256: 283–290

146 Myers EN, Alvi A. Management of carcinoma of the supraglottic larynx: evolution, current concepts, and future trends. Laryngoscope 1996; 106: 559–567

147 Fletcher GH, Jesse RH, Lindberg RD, Koons CR. The place of radiotherapy in the management of the squamous cell carcinoma of the supraglottic larynx. Am J Roentgenol 1970; 108: 19–26

148 Harwood AR, Beale FA, Cummings BJ, Keane TJ, Payne DG, Rider WD. Management of early supraglottic laryngeal carcinoma by irradiation with surgery in reserve. Arch Otolaryngol 1983; 109: 583–585

149 Inoue Ta, Matayoshi Y, Inoue TO, Ikeda H, Teshima T, Murayama S. Prognostic factors in telecobalt therapy for early supraglottic carcinoma. Cancer 1993; 72: 57–61

150 Mendenhall WM, Parsons JT, Stringer SP, Cassisi NJ, Million RR. Carcinoma of the supraglottic larynx: a basis for comparing the results of radiotherapy and surger<. Head Neck 1990; 12: 204–209

151 Mendenhall WM, Parsons JT, Mancuso AA, Stringer SP, Cassisi NJ. Radiotherapy for squamous cell carcinoma of the supraglottic larynx: an alternative to surgery. Head Neck 1996; 18: 24–35

152 Shimm DS, Coulthard SW. Radiation therapy for squamous cell carcinoma of the supraglottic larynx. Am J Clin Oncol 1989; 12: 17–23

153 Spaulding CS, Krochak RJ, Hahn SS, Constable WC. Radiotherapeutic management of cancer of the supraglottis. Cancer 1986; 57: 1292–1298

154 Borgaert WVD, Ostyn F, Schueren EVD. The diffeent clinical presentation, behavior and prognosis of carcinomas originating in the epilarynx and the lower supraglottis. Radiother Oncol 1983; 1: 117–131

155 Mancuso AA, Mukherji SK, Schmalfuss I, Mendenhall W, Parsons J, Pameijer F, Hermans R, Kubilis P. Preradiotherapy computed tomography as a predictor of local control in supraglottic carcinoma. J clin Oncol 1999; 17: 631–637

156 Johansen LV, Overgard J, Hjelm-Hansen M, Gadeberg C. Primary radiotherapy of T1 squamous cell carcinoma of the larynx: analysis of 478 patients treated from 1963 to 1985. Int J Radiat Oncol Biol Phys 1990; 18: 1307–1313

157 Hinerman RW, Mendenhall WM, Amdur RJ, Stringer SP, Villaret DB, Robbins KT. Carcinoma of the supraglottic larynx: treatment results with radiotherapy alone or with planned neck dissection. Head Neck 2002; 24: 456–467

158 Nakfoor BM, Spiro IJ, Wang CC, Martins P, Montgomery W, Fabian R. Results of accelerated radiotherapy for supraglottic carcinoma: a Massachusetts General Hospital and Massachusetts Eye and Ear Infirmary experience. Head Neck 1998; 20: 379–384

159 Sykes AJ, Slevin NJ, Gupta NK, Brewster AE. 331 cases of clinically node-negative supraglottic carcinoma of the larynx: a study of a modest size fixed field radiotherapy approach. Int J Radiat Oncol Biol Phys 200; 46: 1109–1115

160 Isaacs JH, Slattery III WH, Mendenhall WM, Cassisi NJ. Supraglottic laryngectomy. Am J Otolaryngol 1998; 19: 118–123

161 Burstein FD, Calcaterra TC. Supraglottic laryngectomy: Series report and analysis of results. Laryngoscope 1985; 95: 833–836

162 Schwaab G, Kolb F, Julieron M, Janot F, Le Ridant AM, Mamelle G, Marandas P, Koka VN, Luboinski B. Subtotal laryngectomy with cricohyoidopexy as first treatment precedure for supraglottic carcinoma: Institute Gustave-Roussy experience (146 cases, 1974–1997). Eur Arch Otorhinolaryngol 2001; 258: 246–249

163 Chevalier D, Piquet JJ. Subtotal laryngectomy with cricohyoidopexy for supraglottic carcinoma: review of 61 cases. Am J Surg 1994; 168: 472–473

164 De Vincentiis M, Minni A, Gallo A, Di Nardo A. Supracricoid partial laryngectomies: oncologic and functional results. Head Neck 1998; 20: 504–509

165 Lacourreye O, Brasnu D, Merite-Drancy A, Cauchois R, Chabardes E, Menard M, Laccourreye H. Cricohyoidopexy in selected infrahyoid epiglottic carcinomas presenting with pathological preepiglottic space invasion. Arch Otolaryngol Head Neck Surg 1993; 119: 881–886

166 Kremer B, Schlöndorff G. Late lethal secondary hemorrhage after laser supraglottic laryngectomy. Arch Otolaryngol Head Neck Surg 2001; 127: 203–205

167 Ambrosch P, Steiner W. Komplikationen nach transoraler Lasermikrochirurgie von Mundhöhlen-, Rachen- und Kehlkopfkarzinomen. Otorhinolaryngologia Nova 1995; 5: 268–274

168 Serafini I. Results of supraglottic horizontal laryngectomy. In: Wigand ME, Steiner W, Stell PM (Eds). Functional Partial Laryngectomy. Berlin, Heidelberg, New York: Springer, 1984: 223–225

169 Vega MF. Early and late complications after partial resections of the larynx. In: Wigand ME, Steiner W, Stell PM (Eds). Functional Partial Laryngectomy. Berlin, Heidelberg, New York: Springer, 1984: 295–298

170 Naudo P, Laccourreye O, Weinstein G, Hans S, Lyccourreye H, Brasnu D. Functional outcome and prognostic factors after supracricoid partial laryngectomy with cricohyoidopexie. Ann Otol Rhinol Laryngol 1997; 106: 291–296

171 Steininger JR, Parnes SM, Gardner GM. Morbidity of combined therapy for the treatment of supraglottic carcinoma: supragottic laryngectomy and radiotherapy. Ann Otol Rhinol Laryngol 1997; 106: 151–158

172 Spriano G, Antognoni P, Sanguineti G, Sormani M, Richetti A, Ameli F, Piantanida R, Luraghi R, Magli A, Corvo R, Tordiglione M, Vitale V. Laryngeal long-term morbidity after supraglottic laryngectomy and postoperative radiation therapy. Am J Otolaryngol 2000; 21: 14–21

173 Suarez C, Rodrigo JP, Herranz J, Diaz C, Fernandez JA. Complications of supraglottic laryngectomy for carcinomas of the supraglottis and the base of the tongue. Clin Otolaryngol 1996; 21: 87–90

174 Laccourreye O, Hans S, Borzog-Grayeli A, Maulard-Durdux C, Brasnu D, Housset M. Complications of postoperative radiation therapy after partial laryngectomy in supraglottic cancer: a long-term evaluation. Otolaryngol Head Neck Surg 2000; 122: 752–757

175 Flores TC, Wood BG, Koegel L, Levine HL, Tucker HM. Factors in successful deglutition following supraglottic laryngeal surgery. Ann Otol Rhinol Laryngol 1982; 91: 579–583

176 Lee NK, Goepfert H, Wendt CD. Supraglottic laryngectomy for intermediate stage cancer: UT.M.D. Anderson Cancer Center experience with combined therapy. Laryngoscope 1990; 100: 831–836

177 Beckhardt RN, Murray JG, Ford CN, Grossman JE, Brandenburg JH. Factors influencing outcome in supraglottic laryngectomy. Head Neck 1994; 16: 232–239

178 Hirano M, Tateishi M, Kurita S, Matsuoka H. Deglutition following supraglottic horizontal laryngectomy. Ann Otol Rhinol Larygol 1987; 96: 7–11

179 Logemann JA, Gibbons P, Rademaker AW, Poulski BR, Kahrilas PJ, Bacon M, Bowman J, McCracken E. Mechanisms of recovery of swallow after supraglottic laryngectomy. J Speech Hear Res 1994; 37: 965–974

180 Rademaker AW, Logemann JA, Pauloski BR, Bowman JB, Lazarus CL, Sisson GA, Milianti FJ, Graner D, Cook BS, Collin SL. Recovery of postoperative swallowing in patients undergoing partial laryngectomy. Head Neck 1993; 15: 325–334

181 Schweinfurth JM, Silver SM. Patterns of swallowing after supraglottic laryngectomy. Laryngoscope 2000; 110: 1266–1270

182 Steiner W, Ambrosch P, Hess CF, Kron M. Organ preservation by transoral laser microsurgery in piriform sinus carcinoma. Otolaryngol Head Neck Surg 2001; 124: 58–67

183 Allal AS. Cancer of the pyriform sinus: the trend towards conservative treatment. Bull Cancer 1997; 84: 757–762

184 Steiner W. Therapie des Hypopharynxkarzinoms. HNO 1994; 42: 4–13

185 Hoffman HT, Karnell LH, Shah J, Ariyan S, Brown S, Fee WE, Glass AG, Goepfert H, Ossoff RH, Fremgen AM. Hypopharyngeal cancer patient care evaluation. Laryngoscope 1997; 107: 1005–1017

186 Hoffman HT, Karnell LH, Funk GF, Robinson RA, Menck HR. The national cancer data base report on cancer of the head and neck. Arch Otolaryngol Head Neck Surg 1998; 124: 951–962

187 Carpenter RJ, DeSanto LW, Devine KD, Taylor WF. Cancer of the hypopharynx: analysis of treatment and results in 162 patients. Arch Otolaryngol 1976; 102: 716–721

188 Steiner W, Herbst M. Combined therapy of hypopharyngeal carcinoma consisting of endoscopic laser surgery and postoperative radiotherapy. In: Sauer R, Schwab W (Eds). Combined therapy of oropharyngeal and hypopharyngeal carcinoma. München, Wien, Baltimore: Urban & Schwarzenberg, 1987: 108–113

189 Steiner W. Therapy of hypopharyngeal carcinoma. In: Johnson JT Didolkar MS (Eds). Head and Neck Cancer, Vol III. Proceedings of the Third International Conference on Head and Neck Cancer, San Francisco, 26–30 July 1992. Amsterdam, London, New York, Tokyo: Excerpta Medica, 1993: 101–109

190 Steiner W, Ambrosch P. CO_2 laser microsurgery for hyperpharyngeal carcinoma. In: Smee R, Bridger GP (Eds). Laryngeal Cancer. Proceedings of the 2nd World Congress on Laryngeal Cancer, Sydney, 20–24 February 1994. Amsterdam, Lausanne, New York, Oxford, Shannon, Tokyo: Elsevier, 1994: 606–609

191 Rudert HH. Laser surgery in the management of carcinoma of the supraglottic larynx and hypopharynx. In: Myers EN, Bluestone CD, Brackmann DE, Krause CJ (Eds). Advances in Otolaryngolgoy, vol. 12. St. Louis: Mosby, 1998: 61–80

192 Rudert HH. The CO_2laser in the management of hypopharyngeal cancer. Curr Opin Otolaryngol Head Neck Surg 2002; 10: 118–122

193 Czaja JM, Gluckman JL. Surgical management of early-stage hypopharyngeal carcinoma. Ann Otol Rhinol Laryngol 1997; 106: 909–913

194 Ogura JH, Jurema DA, Watson RK. Partial laryngopharyngectomy and neck dissection for pyriform sinus cancer. Laryngoscope 1960; 70: 1399–1417

195 Dumich PS, Pearson BW, Weiland LH. Suitability of near-total laryngo-pharyngectomy in piriform carcinoma. Arch Otolaryngol 1984; 110: 664–669

196 Glanz H. Pathomorphologische Aspekte zur transoralen Resektion von Hypopharynxkarzinomen mit Erhalt des Kehlkopfes. Laryngo-Rhino-Otol 1999; 78: 654–662

197 Zbären P, Egger C. Growth pattern of piriform sinus carcinomas. Laryngoscope 1997; 1107: 511–518

198 Ogura JH, Marks JE, Freeman RB. Results of conservation surgery for cancers of the supraglottis and pyriform sinus. Laryngoscope 1980; 90: 591–600

199 Laccourreye H, Lacau St Guily J, Brasnu D, Fabre A, Menard M. Supracricoid hemilaryngopharyngectomy. Analysis of 240 cases. Ann Otol Rhinol Laryngol 1987; 96: 217–221

200 Spector JG, Sessions DG, Emami B, Simpson J, Haughey B, Harvey J, Frederickson JM. Squamous cell carcinoma of the pyriform sinus: a nonrandomized comparison of therapeutic modalities and long-term results. Laryngoscope 1995; 105: 397–406

201 Chevalier D, Watelet JB, Darras JA, Piquet JJ. Supraglottic hemilaryngopharyngectomy plus radiation for the treatment of early lateral margin and pyriform sinus carcinoma. Head Neck 1997; 19: 1–5

202 Kraus DH, Zelefsky MJ, Brock HAJ, Huo J, Harrison LB, Shah JP. Combined surgery and radiation therapy for squamous cell carcinoma of the hypopharynx. Otolaryngol Head Neck Surg 1997; 116: 637–641

203 Laccourreye O, Merite-Drancy A, Brasnu D, Chabardes E, Cauchois R, Menard M, Laccourreye H. Supracricoid hemilaryngectomy in selected pyriform sinus carcinoma staged as T2. Laryngoscope 1993; 103: 1379

204 Bataini JP, Jaulerry C, Brunin F, Ponvert D, Ghossein NA. Significance and therapeutic implications of tumor regression following radiotherapy in patients treated for squamous cell carcinoma of the oropharynx and pharyngolarynx. Head Neck 1990; 12: 41–49

205 Jones AS. Tumours of the hypopharynx. In: Jones AS, Philipps DE, Hilgers FJ (Eds). Diseases of the Head and Neck, Nose and Throat. New York: Oxford University Press, Inc, 1998: 230–249

206 Million RR, Cassisi NJ. Radical irradiation for carcinoma of the pyriform sinus. Laryngoscope 1981; 91: 439–450

207 National Cancer Institut. PDQ® treatment health professionals. July 1999

208 Pameijer FA, Mancuso AA, Mendenhall WM, Parsons JT, Mukherji SK, Hermans R, Kubilis PS. Evaluation of pretreatment computed tomography as a predictor of local control in T1/T2 pyriform sinus carcinoma treated with definitive radiotherapy. Head Neck 1998; 20: 159–169

209 Amdur RJ, Mendenhall WM, Stringer SP, Villaret DB, Cassisi NJ. Organ preservation with radiotherapy for T1–T2 carcinoma of the pyriform sinus. Head Neck 2001; 23: 353–362

210 Garden AS, Morrison WH, Clayman GL, Ang KK, Peters LJ. Early squamous cell carcinoma of the hypopharynx: outcomes of treatment with radiation alone to the primary disease. Head Neck 1996; 18: 317–322

211 Wang CC. Carcinoma of the hypopharynx. In: Wang CC (Ed). Radiation Therapy for Head and Neck Neoplasms. New York, Chichester, Brisbane, Toronto, Singapore, Weinheim: John Wiley & Sons, Inc, 1998: 205–220

212 Mendenhall WM, Parsons JT, Stringer SP, Cassisi NJ, Million RR. Radiotherapy alone or combined with neck dissection for T1–T2 carcinoma of the pyriform sinus: an alternative to conservation surgery. Int J Radiat Oncol Biol Phys 1993; 27: 1017–1027

213 Rodriguez J, Point D, Brunin F, Jaulerry C, Brugere J. Surgery of the hypopharynx after radiotherapy. Bull Cancer Radiother 1996; 83: 17–23

214 Davidson J, Keane T, Brown D, Freeman J, Gullane P, Irish J, Rotstein L, Pintilie M, Cummings B. Surgical salvage after radiotherapy for advanced laryngopharyngeal carcinoma. Arch Otolaryngol Head Neck Surg 1997; 123: 420–424

215 Wahlberg PCG, Andersson KEH, Biörklund AT, Moller TR. Carcinoma of the hypopharynx: analysis of incidence and survival in Sweden over a 30-year period. Head Neck 1998; 20: 714–719

216 Khan A, Spiro JD, Dowsett R, Greenberg BR. Sequential chemotherapy and radiotherapy for organ preervation in advanced resectable nonlaryngeal head and neck cancer. Am J clin Oncol 1999; 22: 403–407

217 Pignon JP, Bourhis J, Domenge C, Designé L. Chemotherapy added to locoregional treatment for head and neck squamouscell carcinoma: three meta-anayses of updated individual data. Lancet 2000; 355: 949–955

218 Prades JM, Schmitt TM, Timoshenko AP, Simon PG, deCornulier J, Durand M, Guillot A, Martin C. Concomitant chemoradiotherapy in pyriform sinus carcinoma. Arch Otolaryngol Head Neck Surg 2002; 128: 384–388

219 Taylor Sg, Murthy AK, Griem, Recine DC, Kiel K, Belndowski C, Hurst PB, Showel JT, Hutchinson JC, Campanella RS, Chen S, Caldarelli DD. Concomitant cisplatin/5-FU infusion and radiotherapy in advanced head and neck cancer. 8-year analysis of results. Head Neck 1997; 19: 684–691

220 Samant S, Kumar P, Wan J, Hanchett C, Vieira F, Murry T, Wong FS, Robbins KT. Concomitant radiation therapy and targeted cisplatin chemotherapy for the treatment of advanced pyriform sinus carcinoma: disease control and preservation of organ function. Head Neck 1999; 21: 595–601

221 Kotz T, Abraham S, Beitler J, Wadler S, Smith RV. Pharyngeal transport dysfunction consequent to an organ-sparing protoco. Arch Otolaryngol Head Neck Surg 1999; 125: 410–413

222 Lazarus C, Logemann JA, Pauloski BR, Colangelo LA, Kahrilas PJ, Mittal BB, Pierce M. Swallowing disorders in head and neck

cancer patients treated with radiotherapy and adjuvant chemotherapy. Laryngoscope 1996; 106: 1157–1166

223 Lazarus C, Logemann JA, Shi G, Kahrilas P, Pelzer H, Kleinjan K. Does laryngectomy improve swallowing after chemoradiotherapy? A case study. Arch Otolaryngol Head Neck Surg 2002; 128: 54–57

224 Harari PM. Why has induction chemotherapy for advanced head and neck cancer become a united states community standard of practice? J Clin Oncol 1997; 15: 2050–2055

225 Lewin F, Damber L, Jonsson H, Andersson T, Berthelsen A, Biorklund A, Blomqvist E, Evensen JF, Hansen HS, Hansen O, Jetlund O, Mercke C, Modig H, Overgaard M, Rosengren B, Tausjo J, Ringsborg U. Neoadjuvant chemotherapy with cisplatin and 5-fluorouracil in advanced squamous cell carcinoma of the head and neck: a randomized phase III study. Radiother Oncol 1997; 43: 23–28

226 Lefebvre JL, Chevalier D, Luboinski B, Kirkpatrick A, Collette L, Sahmoud T. Larynx preservation in pyriform sinus cancer: preliminary results of a European Organization for Research and Treatment of Cancer Phase III Trial. J Natl Cancer Inst 1996; 88: 890–899

227 Urba SG, Wolf GT, Bradford CR, Thornton AF, Eisbruch A, Terrell JE, Carpenter V, Miller T, Tang G, Strawderman M. Neoadjuvant therapy for organ preservation in head and neck cancer. Laryngoscope 2000; 110: 2074–2080

228 Strong MS, Vaughan CW, Healy GB, Shapshay SM, Jako GJ. Transoral management of localized carcinoma of the oral cavity using the CO_2 laser. Laryngoscope 1979; 89: 897–905

229 Chies F, Tradati N, Sala L, Costa L, Podrecca S, Boracchi P, Bandieramonte G, Mauri M, Molinari R. Follo-up of oral leukoplakia after carbon dioxide laser surgery. Arch Otolaryngol Head Neck Surg 1990; 116: 177–180

230 Chu FWK, Silverman S, Dedo HH. CO_2 laser treatment of oral leukoplakia. Laryngoscope 1988; 98: 125

231 Frame JW, Morgan D, Rhys Evans PH. Tongue resection with the CO_2 laser: the effect of past radiotherapy on postoperative complications. Br J Oral Maxillofac Surg 1988; 26: 464–471

232 Davis RK. Laser surgery for oral cavity and oropharyngeal cancer. In: Davis RK (Ed). Lasers in otolaryngology – head and neck surgery. Philadelphia: Saunders, 1990

233 Guerry TL, Silverman S Jr. Dedo HH. Carbon dioxide laser resection of superficial oral carcinoma: indications, techniques, and results. Ann Otol Rhinol Laryngol 1986; 95: 547–555

234 Nagorsky NJ, Sessions DG. Laser resection for early oral cavity cancer. Results and complications. Ann Otol Rhinol Laryngol 1987; 96: 556–560

235 Wang CP, Chang SY, Wu JD, Tai SK. Carbon dioxide laser microsurgery for tongue cancer: surgical techniques and long-term results. J Otolaryngol 2001; 30: 19–23

236 Ben-Bassat M, Kaplan I, Shindel Y, Edlan A. The CO_2 laser in sergery of the tongue. Br J Plast Surg 1978; 31: 155–156

237 Carruth JA. Resection of the tongue with the carbon dioxide laser: 100 cases. J Laryngol Otol 1985; 99: 887–889

238 Hirano M, Ohkubo H, Kurita S, Maeda T, Kamimura M, Kawaguchi T, Watanabe Y. CO_2 laser in treating carcinoma of the tongue. Auris Nasus Larynx 1985; 12: 10–14

239 Williams SR, Carruth JA. The role of the carbon dioxide laser in treatment of carcinoma of the tongue. J Laryngol Otol 1988; 102: 1122–1123

240 Eckel HE, Volling P, Pototschnig C, Zorowka P, Thumfart W. Transoral laser resection with staged discontinuous neck dissection for oral cavitiy and oropharynx squamous cell carcinoma. Laryngoscope 1995; 105: 53–60

241 Bier-Laning C, Adams GL. Patterns of recurrence after carbon dioxide laser excision of intraoral squamous cell carcinoma. Arch Otolaryngol Head Neck Surg 1995; 121: 1239–1244

242 Alvi A, Myers EN, Johnson JT. Cancer of the oral cavity. In: Myers EN, Suen JY (Eds). Cancer of the Head and Neck. 3rd edition. Philadelphia: Mosby, 1996: 321–360

243 O'Brien CJ, Lahr CJ, Soong S. Surgical treatment of early stage carcinoma of the oral tongue. Head Neck Surg 1986; 8: 401–408

244 Sessions DG, Spector GJ, Lenox J, Haughey B, Chao C, Marks J. Analysis of treatment results for oral tongue cancer. Laryngoscope 2002; 112: 616–625

245 Spiro RH, Spiro JD, Strong EW. Surgical approach to squamous cell carcinoma cinfined to the tongue and the floor of the mouth. Head Neck Surg 1986; 9: 27–31

246 Shah JP, Lydiatt WM. Buccal mucosa, alveolus, retromolar trigone, floor of the mouth, hard palate, and tongue tumors. In: Thawley S, Panje WR, Batsakis J, Lindberg RD (Eds). Comprehensive Management of Head and Neck tumors. 2nd edition. Philadelphia: Saunders, 1999: 686–694

247 McConnel FM, Teichgraeber JF, Adler RK. A comparison of three methods of oral reconstruction. Arch Otolaryngol Head Neck Surg 1987; 113: 496–500

248 McConnel FMS, Pauloski BR, Logemann JA, Rademaker AW, Colangelo L, Shedd D, Carroll W, Lewin J, Johnson J. Functional results of primary closure vs flaps in oropharyngeal reconstruction. Arch Otolaryngol Head Neck Surg 1998; 124: 625–630

249 Konstantinovic VS, Dimic ND. Articulatory function and tongue mobility after surgery followed by radiotherapy for tongue and floor of the mouth cancer patients. Br J Plast Surg 1998; 51: 589–593

250 Konstantinovic VS. Quality of life after surgical excision followed by radiotherapy for cancer of the tongue and floor of the mouth: evaluation of 78 patients. J Craniomaxillofac Surg 1999; 27: 192–197

251 Schliephake H, Schmelzeisen R, Schonweiler R, Schneller T, Altenbernd C. Speech, deglutition and life quality after intraoral tumour resection. A prospective study. Int J Oral Maxillofac Surg 1998; 27: 99–105

252 Hicks WL, Loree TR, Garcia RI, Maamoun S, Marshall BS, Orner JB, Bakamjian VY, Shedd DP. Squamous cell carcinoma of the floor of mouth: a 20-years review. Head Neck 1997; 19: 400–405

253 Nason RW, Sako K, Beecroft WA, Razack MS, Bakamjian VY, Shedd DP. Surgical management of squamous cell carcinoma of the floor of the mouth. Am J Surg 1989; 158: 292–296

254 Sessions DG, Spector GJ, Lenox J, Parriott S, Haughey B, Chao C, Marks J, Perez C. Analysis of treatment results for floor of mouth cancer. Laryngoscope 2000; 100: 1764–1772

255 Ikeda H, Nishiyama K, Masaki N. Squamous cell carcinoma of the floor of mouth treated by radiotherapy. Nippon Acta Radiol 1985; 45: 877–893

256 Marsiglia H, Haie-Meder C, Sasso G, Mamelle G, Gerbaulet A. Brachytherapy for T1–T2 floor of the mouth cancer: the Gustave-Roussy Institute experience. Int J Radiat Oncol Biol Phys 2002; 52: 1257–1263

257 Foote RL, Schild SE, Thompson WM, Buskirk SJ, Olsen KD, Stanley RJ, Kunselmann SJ, Schaid DJ, Grill JP. Tonsil cancer. Patterns of failure after surgery alone and surgery combined with postoperative radiation therapy. Cancer 1994; 73: 2638–2647

258 Hicks WL, Kuriakose MA, Loree TR, Orner JB, Schwartz G, Mullins A, Donaldson C, Winston JM, Bakmjian VY. Surgery versus radiation therapy as single-modality treatment of tonsillar fossa carcinoma: the Rosewell Park Cancer Institute experience (1971–1991). Laryngoscope 1998; 108: 1014–1019

259 Leemans CR, Engelbrecht WJ, Tiwari R, Deville WL. Karim AB, van der Waal I, Snow GB. Carcinoma of the soft palate and anterior tonsillar pillar. Laryngoscope 1994; 104: 1477–1481

260 Perez CA, Patel MM, Chao KSC, Simpson JR, Spector GJ, Haughey B, Lockett MA. Carcinoma of the tonsillar fossa: prognostic factors and long-term therapy outcome. Int J Radiat Oncol Biol Phys 1998; 42: 1077–1084

261 Wang MB, Kuber N, Kerner MM, Lee SP, Juilliard GF, Abermayor E. Tonsillar carcinoma: analysis of treatment results. J Otolaryngol 1998; 27: 263–269

262 Zelefsky MJ, Harrison LB, Armstron JG. Long-term treatment results of postoperative radiation therapy for advanced stage oropharyngeal carcinoma. Cancer 1992; 70: 2388–2395

263 Jackson SM, Hay JH, Flores AD, Weir L, Wong FL, Schwindt C, Baerg B. Cancer of the tonsil: the results of ipsilateral radiation treatment. Radiother Oncol 1999; 51: 123–128

264 Mendenhall WM, Amdur RJ, Stringer SP, Villaret DB, Cassisi NJ. Radiation therapy for squamous cell carcinoma of the tonsillar region: a preferred alternative to surgery? J Clin Oncol 2000; 18: 2219–2225

265 Foote RL, Hilgenfeld RU, Kunselman SJ. Radiation therapy for squamous cell carcinoma of the tonsil. Mayo Clin Proc 1994; 69: 525–531

266 Parsons JT, Mendenhall WM, Stringer SP, Amdur RJ, Hinerman RW, Villaret DB, Moore-Higgs GJ, Green BD, Speer TW, Cassisi NJ, Million RR. Squamous cell carcinoma of the oropharynx. Surgery, radiation therapy, or both. Cancer 2002; 94: 2967–2980

267 DeNittis AS, Machtay M, Rosenthal DI, Sanfilippo NJ, Lee JH, goldfeder S, Chalian AA, Weinstein GS, Weber RS. Advanced oropharyngeal carcinoma treated with surgery and radiotherapy: Oncologic outcome and functional assessment. Am J Otolaryngol 2001: 22: 329–335

268 Steiner W, Fierek O, Ambrosch P, Hommerich CP, Kron M. Transoral laser microsurgery for squamous cell carcinoma of the base of tongue. Arch Otolaryngol Head Neck Surg 2003; 129: 36–43

269 Foote RL, Olsen KD, Davis DL, Buskirk SJ, Stanley RJ, Kunselman SJ, Schaid DJ, DeSanto LW. Base of tongue carcinoma: Patterns of failure and predictors of recurrence after surgery alone. Head Neck 1993; 15: 300–307

270 Nisi KW, Foote RL, Bonner JA, McCaffrey TV. Adjuvant radiotherapy for squamous cell carcinoma of the tongue base: Improved local regional disease control compared with surgery alone. Int J Radiat Oncol Biol Phys 1998; 41: 371–377

271 Weber RS, Gidley P, Morrison WH, Peters LJ, Hankins P, Wolf P, Guillamondegui O. Treatment selection for carcinoma of the base of the tongue. Am J Surg 1990; 160: 415–419

272 Gourin CG, Johnson JT. Surgical treatment of squamous cell carcinoma of the base of tongue. Head Neck 2001; 23: 653–660

273 Kraus DH, Vastola AP, Huvos AG, Spiro RH. Surgical management of squamous cell carcinoma of the base of the tongue. Am J Surg 1993; 166: 384–388

274 Nasri S, Oh Y, Calcaterra TC. Transpharyngeal approach to base of tongue tumors: a comparative study. Laryngoscope 1996; 106: 945–950

275 Brunin F, Mosseri V, Jaulerry C, Point D, Cosset JM, Rodriguez J. Cancer of the base of the tongue: Past and future. Head Neck 1999; 21: 751–759

276 Jaulerry C, Rodriguez J, Brunin F, Mosseri V, Pontvert D, Brugere J, Bataini JP. Results of radiation therapy in carcinoma of the base of the tongue. Cancer 1991; 67: 1532–1538

277 Mak AC, Morrison WH, Garden AS. Base of tongue carcinoma: Treatment results using concomitant boost radiotherapy. Int J Radiat Oncol Biol Phys 1995; 33: 289–296

278 Mendenhall WM, Stringer SP, Amdur RJ, Hinerman RW, Moore-Higgs G, Cassisi NJ. Is radiation therapy a preferred alternative to surgery for squamous cell carcinoma of the base of tongue? J Clin Oncol 2000; 18: 35–42

279 Harrison LB, Zelefsky MJ, Armstron JG, Carper E, Gaynor JJ, Sessions RB. Performance status after treatment for squamous cell cancer of the base of tongue – A comparison of primary radiation therapy versus primary surgery. Int J Radiat Oncol Biol Phys 1994; 30: 953–957

280 Moore GJ, Parsons JT, Mendenhall WM. Quality of life outcomes after primary radiotherapy for squamous cell carcinoma of the base of tongue. Int J Radiat Oncol Biol Phys 1996; 36: 351–354

281 Robertson ML, Gleich LL, Barrett WL, Gluckman JL. Base of tongue cancer: Survival, function, and quality of life after external beam irradiation and brachytherapy. Laryngoscope 2001; 111: 1362–1365

282 Horwitz EM, Frazier AJ, Martinez AA, Keidan RD, Clarke DH, Lacerna MD, Gustafson GS, Heil E, Dmuchowski CF, Vicini FA. Excellent functional outcome in patients with squamous cell carcinoma of the base of tongue treated with external irradiation and interstitial iodinge 125 boost. Cancer 1996; 78: 948–957

283 Harrison LB, Lee HJ, Pfister DG, Kraus DH, White C, Raben A, Zelefsky MJ, Strong EW, Shah JP. Long term results of rimary radiotherapy with/without neck dissection for squamous cell cancer of the base of tongue. Head Neck 1998; 20: 668–673

284 Vokes EE, Kies MS, Haraf DJ, Stenson K, List M, Humerickhouse R, Dolan ME, Pelzer H, Sulzen L, Witt ME, Hsieh YC, Mittal BB, Weichselbaum RR. Concomitant chemoradiotherapy as primary therapy for locoregionally advanced head and neck cancer. J Clin Oncol 2000; 18: 1652–1661

285 Vaughan CW, Strong MS, Jako GJ. Laryngeal carcinoma: transoral resection utilizing the CO_2 laser. Am J Surg 1978; 136: 490–493

286 Laccourreye O, Lawson G, Muscatello L, Biacabe B, Laccourreye L, Brasnu D. Carbon dioxide laser debulking for obstructing endolaryngeal carcinoma: a 10-year experience. Ann Otol Rhinol Laryngol 1999; 108: 490–494

287 Davis RK, Shapshay SM, Vaughan CW, Strong MS. Pretreatment airway management in obstructing carcinoma of the larynx. Otolaryngol Head Neck Surg 1981; 89: 209–214

288 McGuirt WF, Koufman JA. Endoscopic laser surgery. An alternative in laryngeal cancer treatment. Arch Otolaryngol Head Neck Surg 1987; 113: 501–505

289 Robson AK, Herrema I, Stafford FW. Laser debulking for obstructing laryngeal tumours. Clin Otolaryngol 1994; 430–432

290 Rudert H. Larynx- und Hypopharynxkarzinome – Endoskopische Chirurgie mit dem Laser: Möglichkeiten und Grenzen. Arch Oto-Rhino-Laryngol Suppl 1991; 1: 3–18

7 Lasers in Dermatology (Including Interstitial Therapy)

I. Hackert and C. Offergeld

■ Contents

◼ Abstract

Lasers are widely used in dermatology and surgical disciplines. The range of different laser devices enable the dermatologist to treat numerous skin diseases. For lasers to produce optimum results, they must be used for the correct indications by a surgeon who is knowledgeable in their broad range of therapeutic applications in dermatology and in neighboring specialties such as otolaryngology. In the interest of interdisciplinary cooperation, this chapter reviews and examines the current indications for traditional and innovative laser systems in dermatologic surgery.

◼ Introduction

Laser therapy is an established part of dermatologic treatment. For certain skin disorders laser therapy is the only effective treatment. This particularly applies to the port-wine stain (nevus flammeus), which is the most important vascular malformation in dermatology. The results of radium exposure, soft X-rays, thorium-X, cryosurgery, and sclerotherapy for this condition have been unsatisfactory. Plastic surgery has yielded excellent results in some cases but can also result in unsightly scars. The introduction of the argon laser expanded our treatment options for port-wine stains. The desired result was not achieved in many patients, however, and scarring was often unavoidable. The pulsed laser systems in use today permit the selective destruction of vascular lesions without collateral damage to surrounding cutaneous structures.

The new laser systems and innovative treatment strategies have resulted in significant advances in the treatment of vascular lesions and pigmentary changes as well as diseases of the hair and actinic skin damage.

◼ Laser Systems in Dermatology

A number of laser devices are used in the treatment of various skin diseases [1].

The lasers most commonly used in dermatologic surgery are:
- Lasers for selective photothermolysis:
  - Flashlamp-pumped pulsed lasers, dye lasers, Q-switched and long-pulse neodymium:yttrium aluminum garnet (Nd:YAG) lasers, alexandrite laser, ruby laser
- Lasers with a semiselective coagulating effect:
  - Argon, copper-vapor, krypton, frequency-doubled Nd:YAG laser (532 nm, called also the potassium-titanyl-phosphate (KTP)-532 laser)
- Lasers with a nonspecific coagulating effect:
  - continuous-wave (CW) Nd:YAG laser, diode laser
- Lasers for vaporization and ablation:
  - CW CO_2 laser, pulsed CO_2 laser, CW CO_2 laser with a scanner system, erbium:YAG laser

The biophysical principles of laser–tissue interactions are covered in Chapter 1.

Alexandrite Lasers

Q-switched Alexandrite Laser (755 nm, 50–100 ns)

Indications: removal of melanin-pigmented skin lesions and bluish-black, blue, green or yellow tattoo pigments.

Long-Pulse Alexandrite Laser (Pulse Length Up To 50 ms)

Indications: photoepilation, vascular lesions.

Side effects: see Ruby Lasers.

Argon Laser

The argon laser (wavelength 488/514 nm, continuous mode with pulse length of 0.1 s to seconds, maximum power 5–6 W, spot size 0.05–5 mm or scanner) has a penetration depth of 1 mm, which can be increased by cooling.

Indications: Since the advent of the dye laser, only tuberous port-wine stains are still treated with the argon laser. Other applications are telangiectasias, lip angiomas, senile and eruptive angiomas, angiofibromas, angiokeratomas, syringomas, xanthelasmas, soft epidermal nevi, sebaceous hyperplasia, and lentigines (see KTP Laser).

Concomitant reactions, side effects: Argon laser treatment may be followed by crusting and possible blistering of the skin. Other potential effects are irreversible hypopigmentation, transient hyperpigmentation, punctate atrophic and hypertrophic scars, and keloid formation.

CO_2 Laser

CW CO_2 Laser (Wavelength 10 600 nm)

CO_2 lasers for dermatologic surgery are used in the CW or pulsed (superpulse) mode with an initial power setting of 20–50 W.

Indications: Various exophytic skin lesions can be removed with the CO_2 laser, including papillomavirus lesions, epidermal or organoid nevi, lymphangiomas, neurofibromas, papillomatous dermal nevi, sebaceous adenomas, actinic premalignant lesions, actinic cheilitis, chondrodermatitis nodularis helicis, fibrous nasal papules, rhinophyma, trichoepitheliomas, and cysts.

Concomitant reactions, side effects: Healing time depends on the depth of laser ablation and ranges from 10 days to 12 weeks. Except with very superficial ablation, healing is accompanied by more or less pronounced scarring, and keloids may occur.

Pulsed CO$_2$ Laser or CW CO$_2$ Laser With a Scanner System

True pulsed (ultrapulsed) lasers and CW lasers used with a scanner system emit separate pulses of very short duration (<1 ms) with an extremely high energy density. There is very little collateral thermal damage to the surrounding tissues.

Indications: These laser systems are used chiefly in cosmetic medicine for the treatment of wrinkles and acne scars (skin resurfacing).

Concomitant reactions, side effects: Superficial tissue defects are reepithelialized in 10–12 days. Side effects may include prolonged erythema, postinflammatory hyperpigmentation, permanent hypopigmentation, scarring, bacterial or viral infection, as well as skin reactions due to contact allergy or toxic irritation.

Diode Lasers

Diode lasers emit at wavelengths of 800–980 nm in the CW or pulsed mode.

Indications: photodynamic therapy, photoepilation, treatment of vascular lesions (e.g., interstitial therapy, endoluminal therapy for saphenous or branch varicosity and reticular varices, and percutaneous treatment of spider veins.

Concomitant reactions, side effects: same as the CW Nd:YAG laser when operated in the continuous mode, and same as the long-pulse alexandrite and ruby lasers when operated in the pulsed mode.

Erbium:YAG Laser

This device is a flashlamp-pumped, pulsed solid-state laser (wavelength 2940 nm, pulse length 0.25–1 ms, pulse repetition rate 5–20 Hz, energy up to 2 J/pulse, spot size up to 7 mm, scanner).

One disadvantage of the almost athermal ablation produced by the erbium:YAG laser is its lack of efficacy in coagulating small blood vessels. As a result, systems are available that can be switched to a hemostatic mode or combine the erbium:YAG laser with a CO$_2$ laser for coagulation. Long-pulse erbium:YAG lasers (pulse length 10 ms) are increasingly used for their greater thermal component, which can produce hemostasis and collagen shrinkage.

Indications: removal of benign skin lesions, especially lesions in the eyelid region such as syringomas, xanthelasmas, fibromas, and seborrheic keratosis; also the treatment of acne scars and superficial wrinkles due to actinic elastosis.

Concomitant reactions, side effects: Postoperative swelling, weeping, and crusting should resolve in about 5 days. Erythema and transient hyperpigmentation are of shorter duration than with the CO$_2$ laser. Hypopigmentation and scarring are less common. The potential for infection and skin irritation is the same as with the CO$_2$ laser.

Dye Lasers

Flashlamp-pumped pulsed dye lasers are available in various wavelengths and pulse lengths (wavelengths 585, 590, 595, 600 nm). The classic flashlamp-pumped pulsed dye laser (FPDL, 585 nm, 450 µs) can selectively coagulate cutaneous vessels without affecting the surrounding tissue. The tunable flashlamp-pumped pulsed dye laser has a variable wavelength (585, 590, 595, or 600 nm) and long pulse length (1.5–40 ms, long-pulse tunable dye laser [LPTDL]). It can coagulate larger and more deeply situated vessels. Because of the high energy density, the skin surface must be cooled during laser use [2].

Indications: port-wine stains, congenital hemangiomas, spider nevi, telangiectasias, rubeosis, pyogenic granuloma, angiomas, and angiofibromas. Long-pulse dye lasers are useful particularly for large-caliber vessels such as telangiectasias in the nasal region, livid port-wine stains, and spider veins.

Concomitant reactions, side effects: Treatment with the FPDL is immediately followed by a bluish-gray to bluish-black discoloration that persists for 8–14 days. This is caused by intravascular coagulated blood and vessel wall damage. Swelling, blistering, and crusting may occur. Transient hypo- and hyperpigmentation, permanent pigmentary changes, atrophic and hypertrophic scars can occur after treatment. The purpuric changes are less pronounced with long-pulse lasers.

Pulsed Pigmented-Lesion Dye Laser (Wavelength 510 nm, Pulse Length 300 ns)

This laser is used to treat melanin-pigmented lesions as well as red, orange, and yellow tattoos.

Krypton Laser, Copper-Vapor Laser

The krypton laser (520/530 nm, 568 nm) and copper-vapor laser (510/578 nm) are pseudo-CW lasers. They are used in the treatment of pigmented and vascular lesions (see Argon Laser).

KTP Laser

The potassium-titanyl-phosphate (KTP) laser is a frequency-doubled Nd:YAG laser that emits at a wavelength of 532 nm. The relatively high power outputs allow the use of shorter pulse lengths with fewer side effects. The clinical applications and side effects are basically the same as with the argon laser.

Nd:YAG Laser

The Nd:YAG laser, which emits at a wavelength of 1064 or 532 nm, is the most versatile laser in dermatologic laser therapy.

CW Nd:YAG Laser (Wavelength 1064 nm)

The nonspecific coagulating effect of this laser is used in dermatology for percutaneous and interstitial therapy.

Indications: The main dermatologic indications are large, deeply situated hemangiomas, vascular malformations, and port-wine stains that have undergone massive nodular change.

Concomitant reactions, side effects: Postoperative swelling invariably occurs. Exudative reactions, scars, and permanent hypopigmentation may occur.

Long-Pulse Frequency-Doubled Nd:YAG Laser (532 nm)

The pulsed, frequency-doubled Nd:YAG laser is used to treat vascular lesions of varying depth and diameter.

Indications: telangiectasias, spider veins, angiomas [3].

Concomitant reactions, side effects: Treatment is followed by transient erythema and edema that persist for 2–4 days. Crusting and pigmentary changes can occur, especially on the lower leg.

Long-Pulse Nd:YAG Laser (1064 nm)

This laser penetrates deeply into the skin and is useful for treating darker skin types.

Indications: photoepilation [4], spider veins.

Q-Switched Nd:YAG Laser (1064/532 nm, 5–20 ns)

Indications: The Q-switched Nd:YAG laser, which emits at a wavelength of 1064 nm, is used for melanin-pigmented skin lesions and for black or blue tattoos. The frequency-doubled laser, which emits at 532 nm, is used to treat superficial melanin-pigmented lesions and red, orange, or yellow tattoos. It has the same mechanism of action as the Q-switched ruby laser.

Ruby Laser

Q-Switched Ruby Laser

The Q-switched ruby laser light (wavelength 694 nm, pulse length 20–40 ns, maximum energy density 40 J/cm^2, spot size up to 6 mm) is strongly absorbed by melanin and pig-

ments and has relatively deep penetration, enabling it to destroy pigmented keratinocytes, melanocytes, pigmented nevus cells, and exogenous color pigments without causing significant damage to surrounding cells. The absorbing target structure is rapidly heated (>1000 °C), and its integrity is disrupted by the resulting shock wave and thermal expansion. Pigment removal is accomplished through cellular mechanisms (macrophages) and by the lymphatic elimination of pigmentary particles released from the cells. Any pigment left at the target site is again phagocytized.

Indications: This laser can be used on black, blue and green tattoos, melanin-pigmented skin lesions, and Ota nevi.

Concomitant reactions, side effects: Treatment is followed by a whitish discoloration (intraepidermal and dermal vacuolation), punctate bleeding, blistering and crusting. Other possible effects are transient hypo- and hyperpigmentation for 3–6 months, scarring, irreversible color changes, and allergic reactions.

Long-Pulse or Normal-Mode Ruby Laser (Pulse Length 0.3–5 ms)

Indication: photoepilation.

Concomitant reactions, side effects: Erythema and edema lasting for hours or days, blistering and crusting, and transient hypo- and hyperpigmentation may occur. Folliculitis or herpes simplex can develop in rare cases.

■ Cutaneous Vascular Lesions (Including Interstitial Therapy)

Port-Wine Stains

The port-wine stain (nevus flammeus) is the most important extratruncal capillary malformation in dermatology (Fig. 7.1 a). Asymmetrical, lateral port-wine stains are present in approximately 2.8% of all newborns and, unlike median stains, do not regress. In adults they become darker and raised and undergo tuberous transformation. Port-wine stains are caused by a disturbance of vascular innervation with a decrease in vascular tone, usually due to the deficient development of α-adrenergic receptors and less commonly to a vasomotor defect. Since port-wine stains often cause psychosocial problems, treatment should be initiated early to avoid social isolation.

Flashlamp-Pumped Pulsed Dye Laser Therapy

Despite innovative laser systems, the FPDL (585 nm, 0.45 ms) is still considered the method of first choice for the treatment of port-wine stains. The results of treatment depend on the age of the patient and the location, color, size, and histologic structure of the lesions [5]. One or more test patches should be treated initially. Response is evident in 6–8 weeks (Fig. 7.1 b).

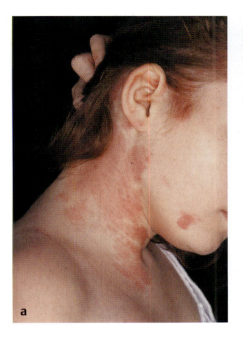 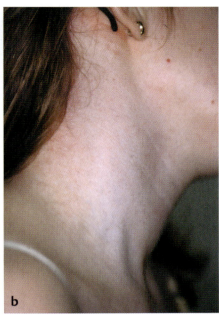

Fig. 7.**1** **a** Extensive port-wine stain. **b** Clearing produced by eight treatments with the flashlamp-pumped pulsed dye laser.

Timing: Treatment is begun in infancy owing to the low incidence of side effects. Excellent results are achieved in most cases (74% from birth to 2 years). Very good clearing is achieved in up to 50% of children and adolescents. This rate declines to 33% in adults over 35 years of age.

Location: Port-wine stains on the face, neck, and trunk respond better to treatment than those on the extremities. Particularly difficult areas are the distal portions of the arms and legs, the central facial region, and the region supplied by the second division of the trigeminal nerve.

Size: Unlike lesions smaller than 20 cm^2, uniform clearing is often not achieved in patients with extensive port-wine stains [2].

Color: The color of a port-wine stain depends on the size and depth of the vessels. Pale pink stains with deeply situated, very thin (16.5 µm) vessels and dark stains with deep, large-caliber vessels cannot be adequately lightened with the FPDL. The best results are obtained with red, purple, and pink stains. Complete coagulation is achieved only in vessels from 20 µm to 150 µm in diameter situated no deeper than 0.65 mm [5]. Since every port-wine stain contains vessels of varying sizes, complete removal is not possible in every case [1].

Multiple sessions are required to lighten or remove port-wine stains, with the greatest response achieved after the initial treatments. Patients from 0 to 2 years of age require the fewest number of sessions (5), while 11- to 20-year-olds require the most sessions (7.8) [5]. Port-wine stains may recur after the completion of treatment. This particularly applies to livid stains. Long-term follow-ups are currently underway for patients who have completed treatment and may show whether the low recurrence rates in young patients are maintained over the years [6]. Painfulness of the treatment varies from one individual to the next. Pain can be relieved by topical anesthesia with EMLA cream (lidocaine 2.5% and prilocaine 2.5%) or by cooling with cold air.

Side effects: bluish-black discoloration for 10–12 days, blistering, crusting, transient hypo- and hyperpigmentation (16.3% and 6.4%, respectively), and atrophic and hypertrophic scarring (4.6% and 3.2%, respectively) [5].

Alternatives To Dye Lasers

The long-pulse frequency-doubled Nd:YAG laser, long-pulse dye laser, or high-energy flashlamps can be used as alternatives and in difficult-to-treat cases [7]. Semiselective coagulating lasers (argon, copper-vapor lasers) should be used only for bright red or tuberous port-wine stains, while the CW CO_2 laser and CW Nd:YAG laser are used for livid tuberous stains and exophytic nodules.

Hemangiomas, Vascular Malformations

Hemangiomas and vascular malformations are the most common benign neoplasms of childhood, with more than 50% occurring in the head and neck region [8–11]. Classic hemangiomas are defined as benign tumors of the vascular epithelium that grow after birth and may undergo spontaneous involution [12, 13]. In contrast, vascular malformations are already present at birth and do not regress [13, 14].

Often it is not possible to wait for the spontaneous involution of hemangiomas due to functional, cosmetic, and/or health concerns (ocular or nasal region, orotracheal tract, internal organs) [9, 11, 12, 14–20]. Compared with treatment modalities described in the literature (e. g., surgery, cryosurgery, pharmacologic radiotherapy) [10, 12, 14, 21–25], laser use is a good therapeutic option offering good

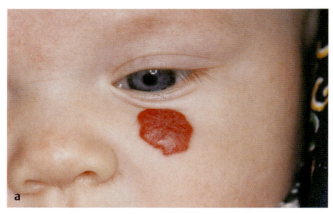
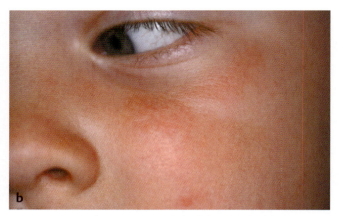

Fig. 7.**2**   **a** A fast-growing hemangioma in an 8-week-old infant. **b** Appearance at 1 year. Two laser treatments halted the growth of the lesion.

results. The Nd:YAG laser and FPDL are particularly effective for these lesions, depending on the indication and location [8, 9, 11, 15, 17, 18, 26–35] (Fig. 7.**2 a, b**).

The Nd:YAG laser has the largest range of indications for any currently available laser system. This is due to its low complication rate and favorable biophysical properties for treating hemangiomatous tissue (penetration depth, specific absorption properties, wavelength, coagulating effect) [8, 9, 11, 15, 17, 26, 28–30, 32–36]. This laser system has a

penetration depth of up to 1 cm, allowing the successful treatment of deep and extensive hemangiomas and even some vascular malformations [11, 26, 28, 30, 33] (Fig. 7.**3 a, b**). In contrast, the FPDL has a limited penetration depth of approximately 0.8 mm and produces a specific vascular effect (selective photothermolysis) [18]. As a result, this laser can be used easily and successfully (even in premature infants) for treating cutaneous and mixed cutaneous–subcutaneous hemangiomas with a maximum depth of 3 mm [14, 18, 32] (Fig. 7.**3 c, d**).

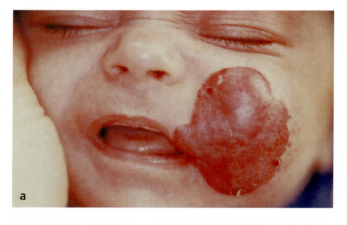
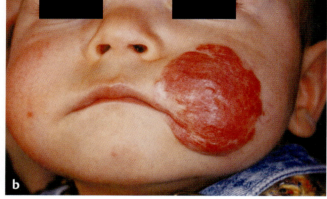
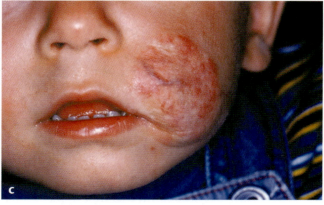
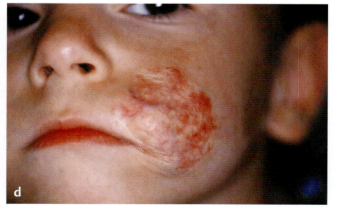

Fig. 7.**3**   **a** A cavernous hemangioma in an 8-week-old infant. **b** Appearance 6 months after interstitial Nd:YAG laser therapy. **c** Appearance at 2 years of age after supplementary treatment with the flashlamp-pumped pulsed dye laser. **d** Appearance at 3 years of age.

The current strategy for laser treatment of hemangiomas and vascular malformations involves the alternating use of both the Nd:YAG and FPDL systems combined with modern imaging procedures [33, 34]. In this approach, color duplex sonography (CDS) is used to assess and classify the vascular lesions as a basis for selecting further diagnostic and therapeutic measures (e. g., magnetic resonance imaging [MRI], angiography, embolization, laser therapy). This information is necessary because, for example, the Nd:YAG laser may be unable to coagulate arterial vessels that are larger than 3 mm or perfused by high-velocity flow [29, 33, 34, 38, 39]. While primary percutaneous treatment with the FPDL is generally satisfactory for superficial vascular lesions of limited extent, deeper and more extensive lesions require primary interstitial (or combined interstitial–percutaneous) Nd:YAG laser therapy supplemented by secondary cutaneous treatments with the FPDL. When the Nd:YAG laser is used percutaneously, it is important to maintain constant cooling and compression of the treated area, preferably using ice cubes free of air bubbles or an ice-cooled glass slide [8, 9, 11, 15, 17, 26, 33].

In interstitial Nd:YAG laser therapy (Fig. 7.**4**), the laser treatment fiber is positioned at the exact center of the lesion under real-time color duplex ultrasound guidance, and the laser energy is applied intralesionally or used for selective vascular coagulation [9, 11, 17, 33–35] (Fig. 7.**5**). Vascular lesions of the mucosae and upper aerodigestive tract can be successfully treated under vision with the Nd:YAG laser while the site is constantly cooled with ice-chilled Ringer solution (using endoscopic or endosonographic guidance as needed) [15, 40]. The laser fibers for this application measure 400–600 µm in diameter and have variable tip geometry (ITT, bare fiber) for producing specific effects on the treatment volume [15, 21]. As the Nd:YAG laser light is transformed into heat, it initiates involution of the lesion through a process of intravascular hemoglobin coagulation, thrombosis, and endothelial fusion; this culminates in postoperative fibrosis of the treated area [9, 11, 15–17, 33, 34, 40]. At the time the laser energy is applied, ultrasound demonstrates changes in tissue echogenicity caused by gas generation about the fiber tip (Fig. 7.**6**; CO_2 and water vapor, depending on the temperature), providing indirect confirmation that adequate therapeutic temperatures have been reached [11, 15, 26, 33, 34]. Due to the large penetration depth of the Nd:YAG laser, anatomic structures at risk (eye, facial nerve, skin) should be protected by measures such as neuromonitoring, maintaining adequate safety clearance, constant cooling, and individual dosing of the applied energy to avoid thermal injuries [9, 11, 33].

The diverse characteristics of vascular lesions in terms of color, consistency, location, and extent account for the varying energy and application-time parameters found in the literature for Nd:YAG laser use, ranging from 2 W to 25 W (0.2–5 s) for percutaneous therapy and from 4 W to 10 W (10–120 s) for interstitial therapy [9, 11, 15, 17, 29, 30, 32, 40]. When the interstitial therapy has been completed and the lesion has been substantially reduced in size, secondary treatment with the FPDL is applied with the goal of clearing and leveling the remaining cutaneous components. Interstitial Nd:YAG laser therapy generally requires an average

Principle of color duplex-guided interstitial laser therapy

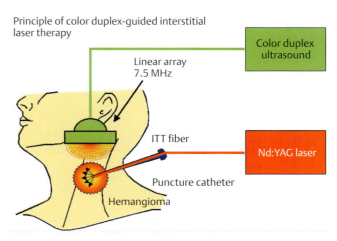

Fig. 7.**4** Principle of color duplex ultrasound-guided interstitial laser therapy with the Nd:YAG laser.

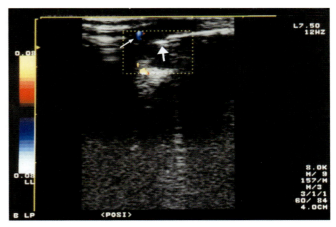

Fig. 7.**5** Placement of the interstitial laser fiber under color duplex ultrasound guidance. One remaining vessel (blue; thin white arrow) is targeted with the fiber tip (broad white arrow).

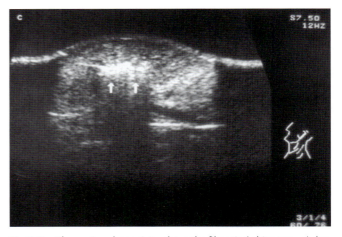

Fig. 7.**6** Change in echogenicity about the fiber tip (white arrows) during direct Nd:YAG laser light application under B-mode ultrasound guidance.

of two sessions under general endotracheal anesthesia during a two-day hospital stay. Cutaneous FPDL therapy requires an average of five sessions and can be performed on an ambulatory basis.

Alternative laser systems for the treatment of vascular lesions include the copper-vapor laser for superficial lesions and the diode laser for deep, extensive tumors [11, 15, 41, 42]. Various authors have described the possible use of argon and KTP laser systems, but their indications are usually limited to small, circumscribed, superficial vascular lesions. The low penetration depth (1–3.6 mm) and relatively high risk of scarring limit the therapeutic results that can be achieved with these systems [10, 32, 43–45].

The CO_2 laser is used almost exclusively for the ablation of subglottic, symptomatic vascular lesions [10, 46]. One drawback of this system is the risk of circumferential subglottic scarring, prompting some authors to recommend the systemic administration of interferon alpha or corticosteroids as an alternative therapy [10, 46]. Excision or vaporization of (sub)cutaneous vascular lesions with the CO_2 laser has not been described as advantageous over conventional surgical methods [15, 27, 32]. This laser has a limited penetration depth, depending on the applied energy density (0.3–6 mm), and can cause thermal skin injuries [32].

Lymphangiomas

Lymphangiomas are classified as a vascular malformation. They frequently coexist with hemangiomas and are treatable with the CO_2 laser [27, 32]. The laser can be used to vaporize lymphangiomas and their mixed forms and can also seal their lymphatic channels. Nd:YAG and argon lasers are also available for the treatment of lymphangiomas [27, 47, 48]. As a rule, however, lymphangiomas are considerably less responsive to laser therapy than hemangiomas.

Lip Angiomas

Lip angiomas can be treated with semiselective coagulating lasers or with the long-pulse frequency-doubled Nd:YAG laser. Nodules larger than 5 mm require multiple treatments. Swelling and crusting may occur. Scarring is rare.

Osler Disease

The argon, diode or CW Nd:YAG laser can be used to treat angiomatous nodules on the mucosa, depending on the size of the lesions. Cutaneous angiomas can be treated with the argon laser, pulsed dye laser, or long-pulse frequency-doubled Nd:YAG laser. The lesions may be incompletely removed despite repeated treatments, and recurrences are possible.

Telangiectasias

All lasers with a semiselective action can be used in the treatment of primary and secondary telangiectasias. Scars

should not be a problem if the treatment is carefully administered. The pulsed dye laser is an excellent tool for progressive, disseminated telangiectasias and for vascular dilatations in connective tissue diseases. In most cases this laser is not tolerated in the facial region, however, where post-therapeutic purpuric macules can develop (see Dye Laser). The long-pulse frequency-doubled Nd:YAG laser is a very good alternative. Swelling may persist for up to 3 days after treatment. Excessive light exposure should be avoided before and after each treatment session.

■ Benign Tumors and Epidermal or Organoid Nevi

Neurofibromas

The CO_2 laser can be used in the CW mode for the excision or vaporization of multiple neurofibromas. Recurrence can be prevented by opening the epidermis, expressing the neurofibroma in a "buttonhole" fashion, and completely removing it or vaporizing its deepest portion. The lesion will heal with scarring, depending on the size of the defect. The erbium:YAG laser can also be used for facial lesions.

Rhinophyma

Large exophytic nodules are removed with the CO_2 laser applied in the CW mode using a focused beam. The general shape of the nose in rhinophyma can be sculpted with a defocused beam, and a pulsed beam can be used in peripheral areas. The laser treatment of rhinophyma is more time-consuming than dermaplaning with a scalpel.

Xanthelasmas, Syringomas, Seborrheic Keratosis

These lesions can be removed with ablating lasers (pulsed CO_2 laser and erbium:YAG laser) or with an argon laser in one or more sittings. The pulsed dye laser can be used on shallow xanthelasmas. Transient or occasionally permanent hypopigmentation can occur, especially when the area around the eyes is pigmented.

Cysts

Cysts in steatocystoma multiplex, mucous cysts, and mucoid dorsal cysts can be opened at their center with a focused CO_2 laser beam, the cyst contents expressed, and the cyst wall ablated with a defocused beam. The erbium:YAG laser can also be used.

Epidermal and Organoid Nevi

Verrucous epidermal nevi are the most common type. Besides cosmetic problems, these lesions cause itching as well as fetor and infections involving the body folds. Soft nevi can be removed with semiselective coagulating lasers (e.g., argon laser), and prominent verrucous nevi can be removed with the CO_2 laser (CW or pulsed mode) [49]. The erbium:YAG laser is particularly useful in sensitive regions such as the upper chest and the area around the eyes. Because epidermal proliferation and differentiation are controlled by the dermis, an insufficient depth of ablation can lead to a recurrence, and transgressing the papillary layer of the dermis can lead to scarring.

Sebaceous nevi occur predominantly in the head and neck region. Various tumors can arise from these lesions with aging (approximately 30%), mostly trichoblastomas and less commonly basal cell carcinomas. Because the hyperplastic sebaceous glands lie deep in the corium, lasers are unable to remove the nevus completely for prevention of basal cell carcinoma. Semiselective coagulating and ablating lasers can do no more than plane away the exophytic elements. Follow-up is recommended. Operative removal is advised for circumscribed nevi.

Scars, Keloids

Various laser systems can produce cosmetic improvement, depending on the nature of the scar. The FPDL can be used to lighten erythematous scars and striae atrophicae, flatten hypertrophic scars, and reduce keloid-associated pain. Keloids can be planed with an ablating laser beam and subsequently treated with cryosurgery, intralesional corticosteroid injection, and compression.

■ Benign Pigmented Cutaneous Lesions

For psychological and cosmetic reasons, it is particularly desirable to remove pigmented skin lesions without scarring. An essential prelude to laser therapy for these cases is a definitive diagnosis based on light microscopic and/or histologic examination in order to exclude premalignant and malignant lesions. In principle, laser therapy is feasible for benign lesions. The laser systems of choice for this application are Q-switched systems such as ruby, alexandrite and Nd:YAG lasers. However, experience about the long-term development of melanocytes that have sustained sublethal damage is still lacking. For this reason, pigmented acquired and congenital nevus cell nevi should not be treated with laser; other melanocytic lesions require long-term follow-up after treatment.

Benign Lentigines

Lentigines can occur on the skin and mucous membranes or as solar lentigines. Their superficial location makes them easily accessible to laser therapy. Q-switched devices as well as ablative and semiselective coagulating lasers can be used.

Café-Au-Lait Spots

Lasers are less successful in the removal of café-au-lait spots. Ablative lasers are not recommended due to the po-

tential for scarring. Treatment with Q-switched lasers may be followed by irregular lightening, pigmentary changes, and recurrence. Better results are usually obtained in adolescent patients. Several test patches should be treated before the definitive treatment of a larger area.

Ota Nevus, Ito Nevus

These nevi occur predominantly in people of Asian descent. Histologic examination shows increased numbers of spindle-shaped and stellate melanocytes and melanophages in the mid-corium. Since an acceptable operative treatment is not available, treatment with Q-switched lasers may be tried. Partial to complete clearing can be achieved with this therapy [50]. Long-term follow-up is recommended.

Nevus Cell Nevi

The results of selective photothermolysis lasers or with ablative laser systems are not satisfactory. In most cases a pseudomelanoma-like recurrence develops from residual nevus cells. Given the moderate success rates, the lack of histologic information about remaining nevus cells, and the uncertain long-term results, laser therapy should be used only in very selected cases. It is suitable for congenital nevi, especially on the eyelids, ears, lips, and hands; these lesions can be lightened by dermabrasion with the erbium:YAG laser, following the principle of early dermabrasion in infancy. Extensive, superficial forms of congenital nevi located in cosmetically sensitive areas can be lightened or removed in multiple sittings with a Q-switched laser or a normal-mode ruby laser [1].

Skin-colored papillomatous dermal nevi can be removed with ablating lasers but may recur after treatment.

Chloasma, Postinflammatory Hyperpigmentation

Pigment-selective lasers do not afford improvement in most patients. Treatment is often followed by increased pigmentation, which may persist. Hyperpigmented burn scars often respond well to treatment with the Q-switched ruby laser.

Decorative Tattoos

Decorative tattoos done by amateurs are usually applied with needles using India ink, ordinary ink, or soot. Professional tattoos are applied with tattooing machines, which use high-density pigments. Metal salt-based pigments were once commonly used. Modern tattooists use industry manufactured organic pigments, and iron-containing pigments are used for cosmetic tattooing. Professional tattoos are more difficult and time-consuming to remove than amateur tattoos. A Q-switched ruby laser, alexandrite laser, Nd:YAG laser, or pigment dye laser may be effective, depending on the color of the tattoo (see under Laser Types).

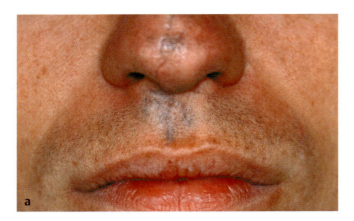

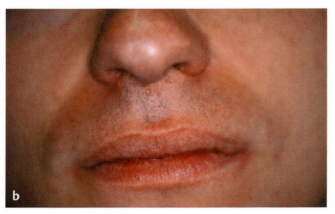

Fig. 7.**7** **a** Traumatic tattooing of the nose and upper lip. **b** Appearance after four treatments with the Q-switched ruby laser.

A test patch should be tried for cosmetic tattoos, since irreversible color changes may occur.

Traumatic Tattoos

Dirt, paint, or other particle driven into the skin by a traumatizing force can be removed with a Q-switched laser with varying degrees of efficacy, depending on the location of the pigment (Fig. 7.7 **a, b**). A test patch should be treated first, especially on skin that has been tattooed by a pyrotechnic injury.

Dyschromias

Pigmented areas caused by an amalgam, amiodarone, iron, or minocycline can be lightened with the Q-switched ruby laser or Nd:YAG laser.

■ Premalignant Lesions, Semimalignant and Malignant Tumors

Laser therapy for malignant tumors is not an established part of dermatologic treatment. Operative surgery is always the treatment of first choice. "Blind" methods that do not allow for precise histologic control of margins should be used only in exceptional situations. These include palliative indications, inoperability, and multiple tumors.

Premalignant Lesions

Actinic Cheilitis

Actinic cheilitis is an obligate premalignant lesion encountered in older individuals. Early lesions can be removed with the CO_2 laser (CW, pulsed) or erbium:YAG laser following histologic confirmation [51]. It takes 2–3 weeks for the treated area to reepithelialize. The reported recurrence rate is 2%. More pronounced lesions should be referred for operative treatment.

Actinic Keratosis

This premalignant lesion is caused by the proliferation of atypical keratinocytes. Malignant transformation to squamous cell carcinoma occurs in 10–20% of cases after a course of years or decades. A number of conservative and operative treatment options are available. The keratotic lesions can be removed with the erbium:YAG laser or pulsed CO_2 laser. As with other treatment methods, recurrence is possible and regular follow-ups should be scheduled.

Lentigo Maligna

See the following section.

Basal Cell Carcinoma, Spindle Cell Carcinoma, Malignant Melanoma

Reports on the laser treatment of these entities have been published [2]. However, we do not feel that laser therapy is justified. Laser use may be considered in selected cases strictly for the palliative treatment of multiple cutaneous metastases from melanoma.

■ Esthetic Uses of Lasers

Photoepilation

Long-term epilation is usually desired for cosmetic and cultural reasons. Medical causes of hypertrichosis include polycystic ovaries, adrenocortical hyperplasia, and side effects of drug (e.g., minoxidil, cyclosporin A). Long-term epilation is also desirable in transsexual patients, hair-bearing skin grafts, and for ingrowing hairs. A number of light and laser systems are currently available for photoepilation, including the long-pulse alexandrite laser, ruby laser, Nd:YAG laser, diode laser, and high-energy flashlamps (Ellipse, EpiLight, Photoderm) [2].

The efficacy of treatment depends on physical factors (wavelength, pulse duration, energy density) and biological factors (hair growth cycle, hair color, target structure). Wavelengths in the range of 700–1000 nm are ideal. Light at this wavelength has a high penetration depth and is preferentially absorbed by melanin (eumelanin). The pulse duration is geared toward the size of the hair follicle, which releases the absorbed energy to its surroundings less efficiently than the small epidermal cells and therefore is preferentially damaged. Because of the high energy density, continuous skin cooling is necessary to protect the epidermis. Energy density appears to be important for good long-term response.

The depth of the follicle varies with the body region and the phase of the hair cycle. Only the actively growing and pigmented hair follicle in the early anagen phase is responsive to laser therapy. Response consists of miniaturization of the follicles, with a corresponding decrease of hair density and pigmentation.

The advantage of laser therapy is that it can be applied easily over a large area. Dark, thick hairs are easy to remove, unlike light, thin hairs. The incidence of side effects is considerably lower in light-skinned patients [52]. Three to eight sessions scheduled at approximately 4–6-week intervals are usually necessary to achieve significant hair reduction (Fig. 7.**8 a, b**). This is followed by two or three maintenance treatments per year. Currently, permanent, complete epilation cannot be achieved.

Photoepilation is not a painless procedure. Effective surface cooling should be provided to reduce pain. EMLA cream can be applied for topical anesthesia. To avoid pigmentary changes, the skin should not be tanned. Excessive light exposure should be avoided for up to 8 weeks after treatment (see Ruby Laser).

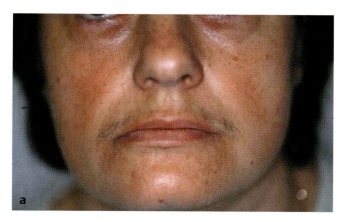

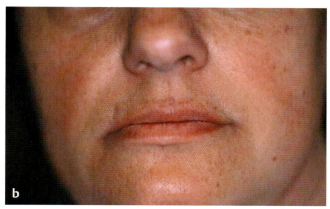

Fig. 7.**8** **a** Hypertrichosis of the upper lip. **b** Appearance after four treatments with the long-pulse ruby laser.

Ablative Skin Resurfacing

The pulsed CO_2 and erbium:YAG lasers are established tools for this indication. Usually they are used with special scanner applicators for large-area skin resurfacing in older patients with elastotic or actinic skin damage and wrinkles and for the smoothing of acne scars [53]. The laser beam vaporizes the aged, sun-damaged epidermal layer while tightening the underlying corium. The thermal damage to the corium is desired to induce superficial fibrosis. Besides an immediately visible shrinkage effect on collagen fibers, new collagen formation occurs at the histologic level [54]. The result is a cosmetically desirable skin-smoothing effect. The less damaging erbium:YAG laser is used to treat problem areas like the periorbital, perioral, and cervical regions and the dorsum of the hand.

Patient selection is essential for a good response. Laser therapy is appropriate for superficial actinic facial wrinkles, radial lip lines, infraorbital wrinkles, crow's feet, and sleep lines. Caution is advised in patients with a dark skin type (Fitzpatrick type III or IV) or suntanned skin due to the risk of hyper- and hypopigmentation. Ablative skin resurfacing is contraindicated in patients who have received systemic isotretinoin therapy during the past 6 months and in patients who have plastic or Gortex implants. The complication rate is increased in patients who have had prior facial cosmetic surgery (facelift, blepharoplasty, chemical peel) and in cases prone to postinflammatory hyperpigmentation and keloid formation.

Concomitant reactions, side effects: Treatment is followed by significant exudation, swelling, crusting, and an unpleasant burning sensation.

The most common side effect is prolonged erythema lasting up to 8 months or longer. Other side effects are itching for up to 3 weeks; infections, especially with herpes virus (7.4%); irritative dermatitis (5–10%); postinflammatory hyperpigmentation (CO_2 laser: 2.8–83%, erbium:YAG laser: 3.4–24%); hypopigmentation (CO_2 laser: 1–19.2%, erbium:YAG laser: 4%); irreversible loss of melanocytes (5–16%); and scarring (>1–3.8%) [1, 2, 53].

Acne Scars

Deep acne scars can be corrected with the CO_2 laser, shallow scars with the erbium:YAG laser. Acne scars generally require two or three treatments spaced 6 months apart. The smoothing effect will increase somewhat over the next 12 months.

Nonablative Skin Resurfacing

Skin rejuvenation by tightening the skin without damaging the epidermis ("subsurfacing") has been a subject of intense research for several years [55]. Various flashlamp and laser systems have been used such as the pulsed dye laser (585 nm), Q-switched Nd:YAG laser (1064/532 nm), long-pulse Nd:YAG laser (1320 nm), diode laser (1450 nm), erbuim:glass laser (1540 nm), and high-energy flashlamp (IPL technology, 500–1200 nm).

Histologic studies have demonstrated new collagen formation and fibroblast proliferation. To date, however, reported results of nonablative skin resurfacing have not been encouraging enough to justify the use of this cost-intensive procedure. Ablative skin resurfacing is still considered the gold standard for the treatment of age-related skin changes.

■ Photodynamic Therapy

Photodynamic therapy (PDT) is used in dermatology to induce immune-modulating effects in inflammatory and malignant skin lesions. It is still classified as an experimental therapy.

Systemic PDT is used to treat large or multiple basal cell carcinomas or early spindle-cell carcinomas in cases where the tumors are deemed to be inoperable. The photosensitizing agent (Photofrin, 2 mg/kg bodyweight i.v.) is administered 24–48 hours before the lesion is exposed to red light. The same regimen is used for Kaposi sarcomas of the skin. Good results can be achieved with indocyanine green followed by irradiation with the diode laser (805 nm) [56].

Topical PDT with 5-aminolevulinic acid (ALA) and exposure to a noncoherent light source is suitable for superficial lesions such as actinic keratosis, Bowen disease, and superficial basal cell carcinoma. The demonstration of immune-modulating effects is opening up new applications for topical PDT such as the treatment of warts, alopecia, and other dermatoses. Studies are currently under way on the efficacy of systemic PDT in the treatment of psoriasis. We should know in the next few years whether systemic PDT will become an effective alternative to PUVA therapy.

■ References

1 Landthaler M, Hohenleutner U. Lasertherapie in der Dermatologie. Berlin, Heidelberg: Springer 1999: 15–21
2 Raulin Ch, Greve B. Laser- und IPL-Technologie in der Dermatologie und Ästhetischen Medizi., Stuttgart, New York: Schattauer, 2001: 23, 113
3 Gambilchler T, Avermaete A, Wilmert M, Altmeyer P, Hoffmann K. Generalized essential teleangiectasia successfully treated with high-energy, long-pulse, frequency-doubled Nd:YAG laser. Dermatol Surg 2001; 27: 355–357
4 Alster Ts, Bryan H, Williams CM. Long-pulsed Nd:YAG laser-assisted hair removal in pigmented skin: a clinical and histological evaluation. Arch Dermatol 2001; 137: 885–889
5 Wimmershoff MB, Wenig M, Hohenleutner U, Landthaler M. Die Behandlung von Feuermalen mit dem blitzlampengepumpten gepulsten Farbstofflaser. Hautarzt 2001; 52: 1011–1015
6 Michel S, Landthaler M, Hohenleutner U. Recurrence of portwine stains after treatment with the flashlamp-pumped dye laser. Br J Dermatol 2000; 143: 1230–1234
7 Strempel H, Klein G. Behandlung von therapieresistenten Feuermalen mit einem Langpuls-Farbstofflaser. Z Hautkr 2000; 75: 129–131
8 Böhm M, Berlien H-P, Müller G, Philip C, Scholz C, Waldschmidt J. Technik und Klinik der Therapie oberflächlicher und tiefer Hämangiome mit verschiedenen Lasersystemen im Kindesalter. Lasermedizin 1990; 5: 45–51
9 Gosepath K, Pfeiffer N, Mann WJ. Die Behandlung kavernöser Hämangiome mit dem Neodymium:YAG-Laser. Laryngo-Rhino-Otol 1997; 76: 284–288
10 Drolet BA, Esterly NB, Frieden IJ. Hemangiomas in children. NEJMAG 1999; 341: 173–181
11 Werner Ja, Lippert BM, Gottschlich S, Folz BJ, Fleiner B, Hoeft S, Rudert H. Ultrasound-guided interstitial Nd:YAG laser treatment of voluminous hemangiomas and vascular malformations in 92 patients. Laryngoscope 1998; 108: 463–470
12 Cremer HJ. Gefäßanomalien im Bereich der Haut. Monatsschr Kinderheilkd 1998; 146: 622–638
13 Mulliken JB, Glowacki J. Hemangiomas and vascular malformations in infants and children: a classification based on endothelial chrraracteristics. Plast Reconstr Surg 1982; 69: 412–422
14 Siegert E, Hackert I, Offergeld Ch. Hämangiome und vaskuläre Fehlbildungen – eine interdisziplinäre Aufgabe. Ärzteblatt Sachsen 2000; 11: 510–512
15 Hoffmann P, Offergeld Ch, Hüttenbrink K-B, Hackert I, Scholz A. Ultrasound-guided interstitial Nd:YAQG laser therapy of cavernous hemangiomas. In: Anderson RR (ed). Proceedings of Lasers in Surgery: Advanced characterization. Therapeutics and Systems V. Proc. SPIE 2395, 1995: 160–169
16 Joppich I, Schiele U. Die Indikation zur operativen Behandlung von Hämangiomen im frühen Säuglingsalter. Kinderarzt 1988; 19: 619–625
17 Werner JA, Lippert BM, Godbersen G, Rudert H. Die Hämangiombehandlung mit dem Heodym:Yttrium-Aluminium-Granat-Laser (Nd:YAG-Laser). Laryngo-Rhino-Otol 1992; 71: 388–395
18 Poetke M, Philipp C, Berlien H-P. Die Behandlung von Hämangiomen im Säuglings- und Kindesalter mit dem blitzlampengepumpten Farbstofflaser. Hautarzt 2001; 52: 120–127
19 Robertson JS; Wiegand DA, Schaitkin BM. Life-threatening hemangioma arising from the parotid gland. Otolaryngol Head Neck Surg 1991; 104: 858–862
20 Hellmann JR, Myer IIICM, Prenger EC. Therapeutic alternatives in the treatment of life-threatening vasoformative tumors. Am J Otolaryngol 1992; 13: 48–53
21 Apfelberg D, Lane B, Marx M. Combined (Team) Approach to Hemangioma Management: Arteriography with Superselective Embolization plus YAG Laser/Sapphire-Tip Resection. Plast Reconstr Surg 1991; 88: 71–82
22 Azzolini A, Bertani A, Riberti C. Superselective embolization and immediate surgical treatment: our present approach to treatment of large vascular hemangiomas of the face. Ann Plast Surg 1982; 9: 42–60
23 Bartohesky LE, Bull M, Feingold M. Corticosteroid treatment of cutaneous hemangiomas: How effective? Clin Pediatr 1978; 17: 625
24 Greinwald Jr JH, Burke DK, Bonthius DJ, Baumann NM, Smith RJ. An update on the treatment of hemangiomas in children with interferone alfa-2a. Arch Otolaryngol Head Neck Surg 1999; 125: 21–27
25 Schild SE, Buskirk SJ, Frick LM, Cupps RE. Radiotherapy of large symptomatic hemangiomas. Int J Radiat Oncol Biol Phys 1991; 21: 729–735
26 Berlien H-P, Waldschmidt J, Müller G. Laser treatment of cutan and deep vessel anomalies. In: Waidelich W, Waidelich R (eds). Laser 87 – Optoelectronics in Medicine. Berlin: Springer 1987: 526–528
27 Landthaler M, Hohenleutner U. Laser treatment of congenital vascular malformations. Int Angiol 1990; 9: 208–213
28 Rudert H, Werner JA. Lasertherapie von Hämangiomen und vaskulären Malformationen im Kopf-Hals-Bereich. In: Ganz H, Schätzle W (Hrsg). HNO Praxis Heute 16. Berlin, Heidelberg, New York, Tokio: Springer, 1996: 206–211

29 Shapshay SM, David L, Zeitels S. Neodymium-YAG laser photocoagulation of hemangiomas of the head and neck. Laryngoscope 1987; 97: 323–330

30 Werner JA, Lippert BM, Hoffmann P, Rudert H. Nd:YAG-laser therapy of voluminous hemangiomas and vascular malformations. In: Rudert H, Werner JA (eds). Lasers in Otorhinolaryngology and in Head and Neck Surgery. Basel: Adv. Otorhinolaryngol Karger, 1995; 49: 75–80

31 Gosepath K, Mann W. Der gepulste Farbstofflaser zur Behandlung gutartiger, oberflächenartiger, oberflächennaher Gefäßmißbildungen. Laryngo-Rhino-Otol 1995; 74: 500–503

32 Landthaler M, Hohenleutner U, El Raheem TA. Therapy of vascular lesions in the head and neck area by means of Argon, Nd:YAG, CO_2 and Flashlampf-pumped pulsed Dye lasers. In: Rudert H, Werner JA (eds). Lasers in Otorhinolaryngology and in Head and Neck Surgery. Basel: Adv Otorhinolaryngol Karger, 1995; 49: 81–86

33 Offergeld Ch, Schellong S, Hackert I, Schmidt A, Hüttenbrink K-B. Die farbduplexsonographisch-gesteuerte interstitielle Nd:YAG-Lasertherapie von Hämangiomen und vaskulären Malformationen. HNO 2003; 51: im Druck

34 Offergeld Ch, Schellong S, Hackert I, Hüttenbrink K-B. Color-Doppler imaging-guided laser therapy of hemangiomas in children. In: Ruben RJ, Karma P (eds). Advances in Pediatric Otorhinolaryngology. Amsterdam: Elsevier Science, 1999; Article No. 116 (CD-ROM)

35 Hoffmann P, Werner JA, Rudert H. Die sonographisch gesteuerte interstitielle Nd:YAG-Lasertherapie cavernöser Hämangiome. Ultraschall 1993; 8: 170

36 Enjoiras O, Mulliken JB. The current management of vascular birthmarks. Pediatric Dermatol 1993; 10: 311–333

37 Waldschmidt J, Schier F, Bein U, Soerensen M. The use of the laser in the treatment of arterio-venous malformations and vascular tumors of the liver. Eur J Pediatr Surg 1993; 3: 217–223

38 Offergeld Ch, Schellong S, Hackert I, Hüttenbrink K-B. Wertigkeit der farbcodierten Duplexsonographie bei der interstitiellen Lasertherapie cutaner Hämangiome und vaskulärer Malformationen. Laryngo-Rhino-Otol 1998; 77: 342–346

39 Issing PR. Möglichkeiten und Grenzen der Dopplersonographie im Kopf-Hals-Bereich. HNO 1999; 47: 6–13

40 Waner M, Suen J, Dinehart S. Treatment of hemangiomas of the head and neck. Laryngoscope 1992; 102: 1123–1132

41 Höhmann D, Waner M, Schwager K. Gelblichtlaserphotokoagulation vaskulärer Malformationen im Kopf- und Halsbereich. HNO 1993; 41: 173–178

42 Höhmann D, Waner M, Schwager K. Therapiekonzept bei Hämangiomen – Photokoagulation mit dem Kupferdampflaser. Laryngo-Rhino-Otol 1995; 74: 238–241

43 Apfelberg DB. Intralesional laser photocoagulation – steroids as an adjunct to surgery for massive hemangiomas and vascular malformations. Ann Plast Surg 1995; 35: 144–149

44 Achauer BM, Chang CJ, Vander Kam VM. Management of hemangiomas of infancy: review of 245 patients. Plast Reconstr Surg 1997; 99: 1301–1308

45 Achauer BM, Celikoz B, Vander Kam VM. Intralesional bare fiber laser treatment of hemangioma of infancy. Plast Reconstr Surg 1998; 101: 1212–1217

46 Sie KC, McGill T, Healy GB. Subglottic hemangioma: ten years' experience with the carbon dioxide laser. Ann Otol Rhinol Laryngol 1994; 103: 167–172

47 Bailin PL, Kantor GR, Wheeland RG. Carbon dioxide laser vaporization of lymphangioma circumscriptum. J Am Acad Dermatol 1986; 14: 257–262

48 Landthaler M, Haina D, Waidelich W, Braun-Falco O. Behandlung zirkumskripter Lymphangiome mit dem Argonlaser. Hautarzt 1982; 33: 266–270

49 Murad A, Kenneth A. A method for carbon dioxide laser treatment of epidermal nevi. J Am Acad Dermatol 2002; 46: 554–556

50 Park SH, Koo SH, Choi EO. Combined laser therapy for difficult dermal pigmentation: resurfacing and selective photothermolysis. Ann Plast Surg 2001; 47: 31–36

51 Hohenleutner S, Landthaler M, Hohenleutner U. CO_2-Laservaporisation der Cheilitis actinica. Hautarzt 1999; 50: 562–565

52 Raulin C, Greve B. Aktueller Stand der Photoepilation. Hautarzt 2000; 51: 809–817

53 Kaufmann R. Die Rolle des Erbium:YAG-Laser zur Behandlung der alternden Haut. Z Hautkr 2001; 76: 671–676

54 Pozzner JM, Goldberg DJ. Histologic effects of a variable pulsed Er:YAG laser. Dermatol Surg 2000; 26: 733–736

55 Grema H, Raulin C, Greve B. „Skin rejuvation" durch nichtablative Laser- und Lichtsysteme. Hautarzt 2002; 53: 385–392

56 Szeimies RM, Lorenzen T, Karrer S, Abels C, Plettenberg A. Photochemotherapie Aids-assoziierter Kaposi-Sarkome mit Indocyaningrün und Laserlicht. Hautarzt 2001; 52: 322–326

8 Lasers in Otologic Research

T. Zahnert

■ Contents

■ Abstract

By virtue of its physical nature, laser light application in otolaryngology has gone far beyond the "laser scalpel." The laser is also an optical measuring instrument that has become an indispensable tool in modern middle ear and inner ear research. The laser beam is unique in its ability to measure vibrational displacements as small as a few nanometers in the middle ear and cochlea without touching the object being measured.

This chapter reviews the principal laser measurement technologies that have been used in modern otologic research. It includes detailed applications and new experimental results of laser interferometry in the middle and inner ear. Taking the middle ear as an example, it shows how laser measurements can provide an image of the vibrational pattern of the healthy tympanic membrane–ossicular chain complex in various frequency ranges. Experiments in temporal bone specimens demonstrate how lasers are used to perfect the design of middle ear implants. Initial clinical studies describe the use of laser interferometry for measuring the vibrational properties of the ossicular chain in patients. One day this method will be a useful adjunct to audiologic testing and supply additional information on the function of the middle ear behind an intact tympanic membrane. Laser interferometry can be used in inner ear research to analyze basilar membrane vibrations and study the micromechanics of the organ of Corti. As an example, it is shown how this method can measure vibrations of the basilar membrane down to the cellular level. The results can advance the design of existing cochlear models and improve our understanding of the cochlear amplifier.

■ Introduction

The otolaryngologist is familiar with the laser as a precision surgical instrument that divides tissue structures without contact. But lasers can do more than cut. The physical properties of laser light offer additional advantages. This chapter deals with the capabilities of the laser as a noncontact measuring instrument. It reviews common applications that have helped improve our understanding of middle and inner ear functions in recent years. Particular attention is given to middle ear mechanics, for which the author presents original experimental results. Laser scanning microscopy, a method with new capabilities for tissue structural analysis, comes under microscopy and is beyond the scope of the present chapter.

For a better understanding of laser measurement technology, the chapter begins with a review of the physical properties of laser light that form the basis for its use as an optimal measuring instrument.

Interesting Physical Properties of Laser Light

Laser light is produced by the artificial amplification of light by stimulated emission. The physical properties of la-

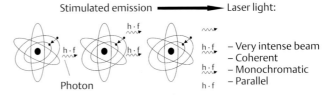

Fig. 8.**1** Production of laser light by stimulated emission. The stimulated atoms have identical structures and constitute the laser medium (e.g., CO_2 gas) (after Spengler, 2002 [2]).

ser light are derived from the nature of light. Light has properties of both a wave and a particle (wave–particle duality). While the wave theory describes all phenomena related to the propagation of light, the quantum theory explains the energy transformation occurring in the production and extinction of light at the atomic level [1]. Atoms have the unique ability to absorb, store, and release energy in discrete quantities. When an atom absorbs energy, an electron is raised to an orbit that is more distant from the nucleus (quantum leap). When the atom releases energy, the electron returns to a lower level while a discrete amount of energy is released. Energy is absorbed and released in the form of quanta (photons), and this process can occur spontaneously.

Energy release can also be induced by an extrinsic force (stimulated emission). This principle is applied in the production of laser light. A photon generated by spontaneous emission encounters other atoms, where it triggers the emission of more photons. This is the basic process by which electromagnetic radiation is produced. In contrast to the visible light from an incandescent bulb, the propagation of this radiation is controlled by a resonator in such a way that the light rays travel in a single direction (Fig. 8.1, resonator not shown).

A special feature of lasers is that all emitted laser light has the same frequency and wavelength (monochromatism). While ordinary light propagates in all spatial directions, the laser light rays are "bundled" into an approximately parallel path (collimation). And finally, all the wave trains in laser light have a definite phase relationship to one an-

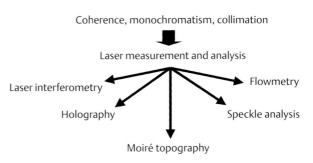

Fig. 8.**2** Techniques of laser measurement and analysis in otologic research based on the physical properties of laser light.

other in both time and space (coherence). These essential properties of laser light are used for optical methods of analysis in otologic research (Fig. 8.2).

Principles of Optical Methods in Otologic Research

Since the early days of middle and inner ear research, efforts have been made to measure vibrational processes and document them in the form of images. Optical methods are ideal for detecting these vibrational amplitudes, which measure only a few nanometers, because generally they are noncontact techniques, i. e., they work without placing any mechanical stresses on the structures being examined.

Laser Interferometry

The principle of laser interferometry is based on the Doppler effect. When coherent laser light strikes a moving object (e. g., a vibrating tympanic membrane) and is reflected back, the frequency of the reflected beam is shifted relative to the frequency of the incident beam (the Doppler shift, Fig. 8.3). This frequency shift (fd) is proportional to the velocity v of the moving object, as defined by the equation:

$$fd = 2v/\lambda$$

where λ is the wavelength of the laser light and v is the velocity of the moving object.

Thus the frequency shift is a measurable quantity corresponding to the vibrational speed (velocity) of the object, and the amplitude of the vibration can be calculated from the integral of the velocity. Due to the high frequency of laser light (4.7×10^{14} Hz), it is not possible to measure the frequency shift directly. Instead, the reflected beam is combined with a superimposed reference beam. A photodetector then measures the differences that occur in the laser light intensity when the object and reference beams are combined (interference).

To achieve high sensitivity, the measuring instrument, called an interferometer, must satisfy two conditions:
- the structure being examined must have high reflectivity so that sufficient light is reflected back to the photodetector, and
- the system must be mechanically stable enough to provide an undistorted interference pattern.

These conditions are difficult to fulfill in measurements of biological structures. The pulse and respiration transmit synchronous movements to the ear which are several orders of magnitude greater than the vibrational amplitudes to be measured. Generally the reflectivity (e. g., of the tympanic membrane) is extremely poor when compared with smooth artificial surfaces. Most of the laser light passes through the tympanic membrane and is not reflected [3]. Additional losses result from diffuse reflection due to surface roughness. An obliquely incident laser beam further reduces the intensity of the light returning to the detector (Fig. 8.4).

One way to minimize reflection problems is by using reflectors. In the earliest laser measurements in otology, small reflective targets were glued to the tympanic membrane to increase its reflectivity (Fig. 8.5) [4]. In experiments on temporal bone specimens, this resulted in relatively high sensitivity for displacements up to 100 pm, so that vibrations could be measured using acoustic stimuli of only 60 dB SPL (sound pressure level) at low frequencies. In live animals, the sensitivity was considerably lower (1 nm corresponding to 80 dB SPL) despite the use of reflectors due to greater mechanical artifacts, caused mainly by respiration. To reduce these artifacts, the animal's head had to be immobilized with cortical bone screws. The high laboratory costs of this procedure, plus the susceptibility of the Michelson interferometer to mechanical artifacts, limited the use of the instrument to a few experimental animals.

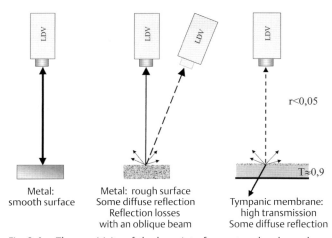

Metal: smooth surface

Metal: rough surface Some diffuse reflection Reflection losses with an oblique beam

r<0,05

T≈0,9

Tympanic membrane: high transmission Some diffuse reflection

Fig. 8.**4**   The sensitivity of the laser interferometer also depends on the reflectivity (f) of the object under study. With an object like the tympanic membrane, which reflects diffusely and has high through-transmission (T), the sensitivity is poor and varies with the angle of the laser beam.

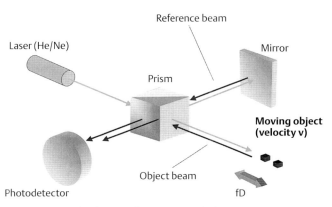

Reference beam

Laser (He/Ne)

Mirror

Prism

Moving object (velocity v)

Object beam

Photodetector

fD

Fig. 8.**3**   Principle of an interferometer (Michelson type). The laser light reflected from a moving object is combined with a reference beam.

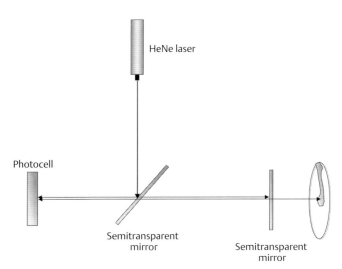

Fig. 8.**5** Modified Michelson interferometer for measuring tympanic membrane vibrations (after Tonndorf and Khanna, 1968 [4]).

Another way to improve the sensitivity of interferometers is by modifying the measurement principle. "Heterodyne interferometers" were introduced into otologic research during the 1970s. These instruments could make measurements in vivo with a high degree of sensitivity. In contrast with the Michelson interferometer, the reference beam is modulated in its frequency or phase. Modulating the reference beam with a high frequency (in the MHz range), which is done using a Bragg cell, Kerr cell, or a rotary grating disk, results in an improved signal-to-noise ratio. Low-frequency mechanical artifacts, such as pulse or respiratory movements, cause less distortion of the high-frequency measurement signal and are easier to filter out [5].

The design of a heterodyne interferometer is illustrated in Fig. 8.6, showing that modern vibrometers can measure both the velocity and displacement of vibrating structures.

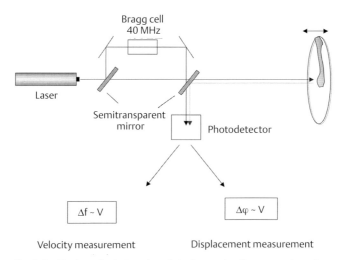

Fig. 8.**6** Design of a heterodyne interferometer for measuring vibrations and distance changes.

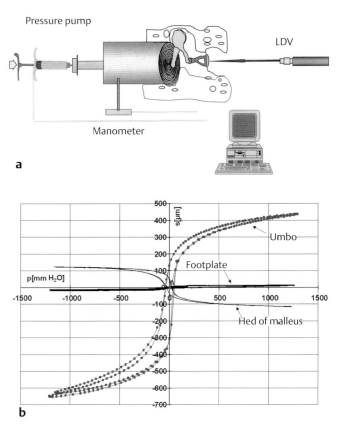

Fig. 8.**7** **a** Setup for measuring quasistatic displacement of the footplate and umbo in response to pressure changes in the auditory canal using a laser Doppler vibrometer. **b** Corresponding pressure–displacement diagram for the footplate and umbo. LDV, laser interferometer.

The phase information is used for measuring displacement. The distance change $\lambda/2$ (where $\lambda = 316$ nm for a helium neon [HeNe] laser) corresponds to one phase shift of 360°. Absolute displacement is measured by electronically counting the number of 360° phase cycles. This method is useful, for example, for measuring the quasistatic displacements of the tympanic membrane or ossicular chain in response to atmospheric pressure changes (Fig. 8.7).

Heterodyne interferometers are now considered the standard tool for vibration analysis in biological structures. The high linearity of these instruments is cited as a particular advantage over other optical methods [6–9].

Various types of heterodyne interferometer are available for investigations of the middle and inner ear. For simplicity, they can be broadly classified as single-point or multipoint vibrometers (Fig. 8.**8**). In a single-point system, only the vibrations at a single point on the object are measured in the direction of the beam. These instruments can be used to determine the "transfer functions" (transmission characteristics) of the middle and inner ear. Generally this is done by relating the applied sound pressure to the vibration amplitude measured at a particular point by the equation:

$$TF = n/p$$

where TF is the transfer function, n is the vibration amplitude and velocity (measured with a laser interferometer), and p is the sound pressure (e. g., in front of the tympanic membrane).

The advantage of this method is that the specific micromechanical function between the two sampled points need not be known—only the transmission of the middle or inner ear as a whole. The transfer function of the middle ear can be used, for example, to investigate implant materials or reconstructive techniques in temporal bone specimens. Usually this is done by relating the vibration amplitude of the stapes and perhaps the umbo to the sound pressure at the tympanic membrane. This transfer function displays a characteristic shape (Fig. 8.**9**). The first resonance frequency of the middle ear occurs at 800 Hz, and a second resonance frequency occurs at 1400 Hz. Both curves are roughly horizontal up to the first resonance frequency and then slope downward at approximately 12 dB/octave. A number of authors have documented this pattern in temporal bone specimens by means of laser interferometry, including Vlaming, Vlaming et al., Nishihara et al., Goode et al., Kurakowa and Goode, Rodriguez et al., Eiber et al., Murakami et al., Schön and Müller, Decreamer and Khanna, Voss et al., and Stenfelt et al. [8, 10–20].

Scanning vibrometry (see Fig. 8.**8**, center) is also based on single-point measurements. The sensor head is scanned point-by-point over the entire object surface in a predetermined pattern. The measurements taken at the various points are then assembled into a composite image of the object surface, and the vibration patterns can be displayed on a computer monitor. Unlike holography, this method also yields phase information and makes it possible to display time-changing vibration patterns by computer animation. One disadvantage of scanning vibrometry is that, like holography, it requires broad optical access to the structure being examined. In the case of the tympanic membrane, for example, this means that the entire surface of the membrane cannot be scanned in the living patient. The method has broad industrial applications, where it is used to analyze vibrating parts in machinery and musical instruments.

Recently, laser interferometers that can analyze vibrational patterns in three dimensions have been developed (see Fig. 8.**8**, bottom). In this process, three laser beams are emitted from a sensor head at various angles and converge at a single spot. The three-dimensional vibration pattern at that site can be computed from the direction of the sampling beam and the measured displacement. If the sensor head is scanned over the body surface similar to the scanning vibrometer described above, the measurements can be assembled to create a three-dimensional image of the surface vibrations. To date, this type of interferometer has not yet been used in otologic research.

The sensitivity of the devices depends on the reflectivity of the structure examined, the frequency of the acoustic stimulus, and mechanical artifacts. Sensitivity is also controlled by the manufacturer. Under ideal conditions (high reflectivity, no mechanical artifacts), a typical system (Polytec Hearing Vibrometer, Waldbronn) has a rated sensitivity of

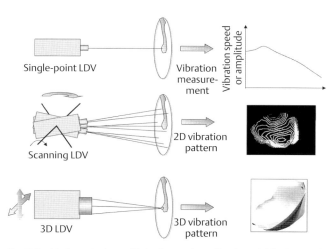

Fig. 8.**8**   Various designs of interferometers. Single-point instruments (top) are mainly used to measure the acoustic transfer functions of the middle or inner ear, while scanning and 3D devices are used to analyze vibration patterns. LDV, laser interferometer.

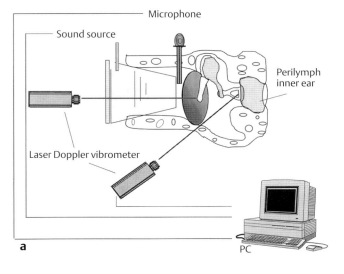

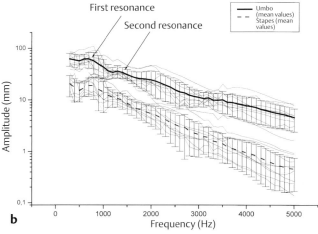

Fig. 8.**9**   **a** Measuring setup for determining transfer functions in a temporal bone specimen. **b** Amplitude curves for umbo and stapes vibrations, stimulated at 94 dB SPL (sound pressure level).

16 pm at a frequency of 1 kHz. This corresponds roughly to the vibration amplitude of the umbo of the human tympanic membrane when stimulated at a level of 25 dB SPL. To help understand the magnitude of this displacement, it is equal to about one-sixth the diameter of a hydrogen atom. Unfortunately, this high sensitivity has not yet been achieved with measurements in vivo.

Holography, Holographic Interferometry

The principle of holographic measurement utilizes the interference properties of monochromatic laser light. In this process, a laser beam is passed through a shutter and is separated by a beam splitter into an object beam and a reference beam. While the reference beam is trained directly on a photographic plate, the object beam is diffusely reflected from the object surface before it strikes the plate. This creates an interference pattern that is recorded on the photographic plate. When this plate (holographic plate) is again illuminated with a laser beam, it creates a virtual three-dimensional image of the object in space through wavefront reconstruction.

Besides generating three-dimensional displays for artistic purposes, holography can also demonstrate movements and deformations (vibrations) of an object surface. For this purpose the object under study is illuminated twice (before and after deformation), and the resulting holograms are superimposed on the photographic plate. The resulting interference rings provide a measure of the surface deformation. "Time-average" holography can be used to record periodic oscillating processes (e.g., tympanic membrane vibration in response to a sine-wave tone). In this technique the laser shutter remains open for several vibration periods so that several successive vibration maxima are recorded in the hologram. Reconstructing the time-average hologram creates interference lines that represent the amplitude lines of the vibration pattern of the object under study (Fig. 8.10) [21].

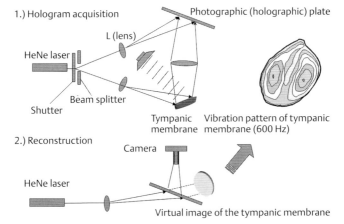

Fig. 8.**10** Experimental setup for time-average holography of the tympanic membrane (image acquisition and reconstruction) following stimulation with a 600-Hz sine-wave tone.

Powel and Stetson introduced time-average holography into medicine in 1965 [22]. The first holographic studies of vibrational patterns in the ear were done on the tympanic membrane of the locust and on the round window membrane of the cat [23, 24]. Holography was the first method that could measure vibration patterns over the entire surface of the tympanic membrane without having to reconstruct the patterns from data acquired at various points (as in the capacitive probe method of von Bekesy [25]). Holography was used in cat temporal bone specimens to provide experimental confirmation of the theory, postulated by Helmholtz, of an inherent amplification factor in the tympanic membrane [25]. This study also slightly revised the eardrum vibration characteristics described earlier by von Bekesy. The lines of equal deflection that Tonndorf and Khanna determined holographically were not circumferential and parallel to the limbus of the tympanic membrane, as described by von Bekesy but ran parallel to the malleus handle (see Fig. 8.5, vibration pattern of the tympanic membrane at 600 Hz). This results in two vibration maxima at low frequencies, located in front of and behind the malleus handle showing the same pattern of movement. The malleus follows this movement of the tympanic membrane, but at a smaller amplitude.

Von Bally performed holographic studies of the tympanic membrane to diagnose impaired sound conduction in temporal bone specimens. When the incus was removed, the vibration amplitudes in the anterior quadrant of the tympanic membrane increased [26]. Dancer et al. studied the deformation of the guinea pig tympanic membrane stimulated by acoustic impulses. Based on the maximum deflection, they were able to predict injury patterns in response to explosion trauma [27].

Hogmoen and Gundersen used time-average holography to determine the pattern of stapes footplate vibrations in human temporal bone specimens. When an acoustic stimulus was applied at 600 Hz, they observed a predominantly piston-like movement of the footplate accompanied by a rocking movement about its longitudinal axis [28].

Although the holographic technique has the advantage of being able to measure vibration patterns over a large area, the method also has several disadvantages. It requires broad optical access, i.e., the external ear canal must be removed in order to examine the tympanic membrane. Generally the reflectivity of the structure under study must be artificially enhanced (e.g., with aluminum powder) [29]. The sensitivity of the technique is predetermined by the wavelength of the applied laser light and is in the order of 1 μm. As a result, unphysiologically high sound pressures of 120 dB or more must be applied to investigate the many smaller vibrational amplitudes occurring in the ossicular chain [30]. According to Michelsen, this method is useful only for studying linear vibration processes, whereas phase information is difficult to obtain. Moreover, holograms cannot be unambiguously interpreted when higher frequencies are applied due to the complex vibration patterns that arise [7]. Because of these disadvantages, in addition to high equipment costs, the holographic technique is seldom used today to investigate vibrational processes in the middle ear.

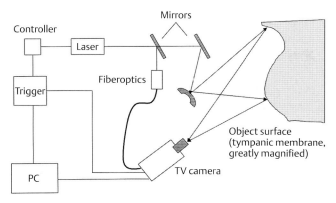

Fig. 8.**11** Experimental setup for recording a speckle pattern, e. g., of the tympanic membrane (after Höfling, 1992 [31]).

Fig. 8.**12** Principle of moiré topography of the tympanic membrane. A grating projected onto the object surface is superimposed over a reference grating (after Heymann and Lingner, 1986 [34]).

Speckle Analysis

Speckle analysis is based on a peripheral phenomenon that occurs in laser examinations of reflective surfaces, first referred to as "noise in coherent images." When a laser beam strikes the rough surface of an object, the diffusely reflected light is diffracted at every point on the surface. These diffractions produce a typical surface pattern called speckle, which changes when the surface is deformed (e. g., by vibration). The speckle patterns are recorded with a television camera before and after the deformation and are superimposed by digital image processing. The result is a pattern of lines that reflects the surface deformation of the object [31]. This technique is more sensitive than holography and also permits phase analysis (Fig. 8.**11**).

While speckle analysis is widely used in material testing, so far it has found very limited application in otologic research. Wada et al. used this technique to investigate the vibration patterns of the guinea pig tympanic membrane, which they were able to do even with a relatively low-level stimulus of only 70 dB (SPL) at 4 kHz with good resolution [32]. The speckle technique can also be used for flow measurements. For example, speckle flowmetry has been used to measure blood flow in the human tympanic membrane [33].

Moiré Effect

The French word *moiré* originally referred to certain silk fabrics producing fleeting wavy patterns when illuminated at different angles. Today it refers to a principle of optical analysis based on the use of superimposed optical gratings [34]. A grating projected onto the surface of the object (object grating) is superimposed with a known reference grating. When the surface of the object is deformed, the fringe pattern produced by the superimposed gratings will also be deformed. This geometric change can be recorded (e. g., with a camera) and measured. The shadow cast by reflected surface light can also be used instead of an object grating (shadow moiré technique). The method can thus be used to measure quasistatic deformations of surfaces, such as deformations of the tympanic membrane in response to atmospheric pressure changes.

The moiré technique is used in otologic research to define the geometry of the tympanic membrane and measure its deformation in response to stresses, from which the elasticity properties of the membrane can be determined (Fig. 8.**12**). The shape of the tympanic membrane is relatively complex, especially when displaced by external forces. The moiré technique is a noncontact method providing a topographic image of the tympanic membrane surface displaying lines of equal slopes and surface displacement, analogous to the contour lines on a map (moiré topography) [35].

This method can be used, for example, to investigate the displacement of the tympanic membrane in response to atmospheric pressure loads [36]. The traditionally poor depth resolution of moiré has been significantly improved by the introduction of phase-shift moiré technology [37], which can measure even the displacement of the relatively small pars flaccida of the human tympanic membrane under static pressure loads with high resolution (25 μm) [38]. In the classic shadow moiré technique, the reference grating must be mounted close to the tympanic membrane to obtain acceptable contrast. This requires removal of the external ear canal, limiting the in-vivo application of this technique. One solution to this problem is optoelectronic moiré topography, in which a projector is used to superimpose the object grating on the tympanic membrane. The shadow image of black and white lines appearing on the object is altered by the shape and deformation of the tympanic membrane (bowing of the contour lines). This image is recorded with a video camera. The actual topogram is produced by digitizing the image and superimposing it electronically in a computer [39, 40]. While the resolution in initial studies was low (80 μm), the sensitivity of the video moiré technique was subsequently improved to 10–15 μm by analysis of the phase shift (high-resolution phase-shift projection moiré interferometer) [41].

An important application of the moiré technique is in obtaining the geometric and material parameters of the tympanic membrane for use in computer models (finite-element models) of the middle ear [41, 42]. For example, this technique can be used to analyze the stiffness of the pars flaccida relative to the pars tensa in response to various pressures in the middle ear [40]. It can also be used to conduct mechanical investigations of the tympanic membrane under varying stresses. Experimental studies in the gerbil have shown that cutting the tensor tendon and removing the cochlea and stapes had no effect on the deformation of the tympanic membrane in response to pressure changes in the ear canal. The elastic resilience of the tympanic membrane limits its outward movement in response to negative pressure in the ear canal, while its inward movement is further constrained by the malleus and incus [41].

Laser Doppler Flowmetry

Laser Doppler flowmetry is an optical method for the noninvasive assessment of blood circulation. Its principle is based on the interaction of the laser with the perfused tissue. Monochromatic laser light is delivered to the tissue through a probe and is reflected from stationary tissues as well as moving red blood cells. While the frequency of light reflected from stationary tissue is unchanged, that of light reflected from moving particles undergoes a frequency shift (Doppler effect). The probe has a built-in photocell that detects these frequency changes.

Laser Doppler flowmetry is useful for investigating capillary blood flow and was used as early as 1972 for the assessment of retinal perfusion [43]. It is logical to assume that its use would also be rewarding in inner ear research. It has been shown that the function of the cochlea depends partly on a stable oxygen supply, which is controlled by the blood supply to the lateral cochlear wall [44]. Since the wavelength of the laser light enables it to pass through the intact bone of the cochlear wall, laser Doppler flowmetry has been used to perform functional blood flow measurements in animal models (Fig. 8.**13**). Experiments have demonstrated the dependence of cochlear blood flow, measured at the promontory, on various factors such as cardiovascular drugs, nicotine, oxygen saturation, anemia, and body temperature [45–47]. Other experiments in

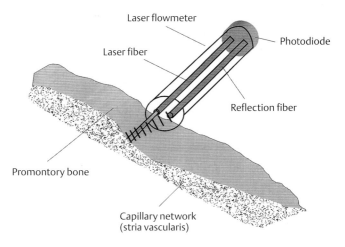

Fig. 8.**13** Laser flowmetry of the inner ear, measured at the promontory.

noise-exposed animals showed that short-term exposure to noise levels of 100–120 dB for 6 minutes had no effect on cochlear blood flow [48].

Although the human promontory bone is relatively thick (1–1.6 mm), this method can also be applied in humans [50–53]. Initial measurements in patients diagnosed with sudden hearing loss were performed through an exploratory tympanotomy and showed no significant change in cochlear blood flow [52]. In more recent studies using a smaller probe, measurement were performed via paracentesis in a larger group of patients (n = 115) [54]. The authors doubted that Ménière disease and sudden hearing loss had a predominantly vascular etiology, but they discovered a statistically significant correlation between hearing level and cochlear blood flow in patients with progressive sensorineural hearing loss.

■ Laser Interferometric Studies of Middle Ear Mechanics

Vibration Patterns of the Tympanic Membrane

Laser interferometry is a powerful tool for investigating the vibration characteristics of the tympanic membrane and ossicular chain. The technical costs incurred by the use of industrial scanning or three-dimensional vibrometers are low compared with holographic techniques. Also, these devices make it possible to display the time-varying amplitude and phase of vibration processes by computer animation, making it easier to understand the complex vibration patterns developing at high frequencies. The vibration patterns determined by interferometry are useful for analyzing middle ear mechanics and creating more precise computer models (finite-element models).

Like all techniques of optical analysis in otology, laser scanning interferometry of the tympanic membrane requires broad optical access, which is obtained either by removing the external bony ear canal or by removing the tegmen tympani and portions of the medial wall of the tympanic cavity. Thus, except for the studies by Huber et al. [55], all previous laser scanning studies of the tympanic membrane were done strictly in animal models or in human temporal bone specimens [56, 57].

Figure 8.**14** shows the experimental setup we used to measure the vibration patterns of the tympanic membrane and ossicular chain. According to the results of laser scanning vibrometry, the vibration pattern of the tympanic membrane up to the first resonance frequency (approximately 1 kHz) is a predominantly in-phase movement of the entire membrane surface, as previous holographic and microstroboscopic measurements have shown [32, 55, 56, 58, 59]. Laser measurements, which are superior to holographic studies by permitting the analysis of phase distribution, showed that the tympanic membrane had another vibration mode between 1 kHz and 3 kHz, in which the anterior and posterior surfaces of the membrane move out of phase (Fig. 8.**15**) [32, 60]. This movement necessarily caus-

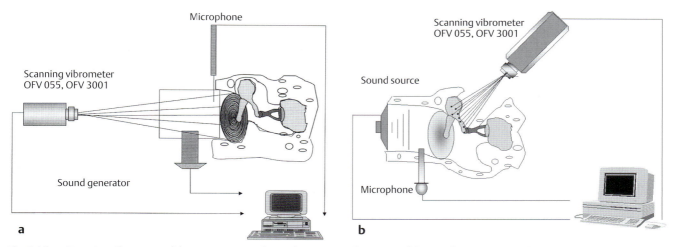

Fig. 8.**14**   **a** Scanning vibrometry of the tympanic membrane. **b** Scanning vibrometry of the ossicles in a temporal bone specimen.

es the malleus handle to rotate about its longitudinal axis during one phase cycle, and so it also affects the vibration pattern of the ossicular chain. Our laser scanning measurements suggest that the tympanic membrane has a third vibration mode between 3 kHz and 4 kHz. This mode is characterized by the appearance of four vibration peaks on the surface of the tympanic membrane (Fig. 8.15). These peaks move out of phase in relation to one another, depending on the frequency of the acoustic stimulus.

Frequencies above 4 kHz do not give rise to additional, typical vibration modes. Instead, they produce a number of vi-

bration peaks like those previously observed by Tonndorf and Khanna [4]. The different areas vibrate independently of one another, showing no definite phase relationship, giving rise to a complex vibrational pattern.

Vibration Patterns of the Ossicular Chain

Laser interferometry also has advantages over holography in investigating the vibration patterns of the ossicular chain. Holographic studies of the malleus-incus-stapes complex require acoustic stimulus levels up to 140 dB SPL

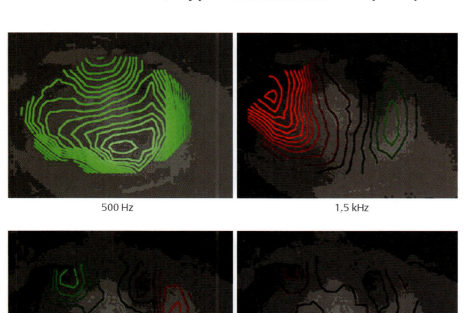

Fig. 8.**15**   Vibration patterns of the tympanic membrane measured at various frequencies by scanning vibrometry.

500 Hz

1,5 kHz

3.5 kHz

4.5 kHz

to measure the vibration amplitudes, which are much smaller than those of the tympanic membrane [30]. At these sound pressure levels, however, the middle ear is already functioning in a nonlinear range, i. e., the physiologic vibration mode is distorted by concomitant movements in the ossicular joints or by rocking movements of the ossicles. Since the vibration amplitudes fall off at higher frequencies, holographic measurements of the malleus and incus can be performed only up to 1.5 kHz, and measurements of the footplate up to 1 kHz [28, 30]. Laser interferometric measurements, on the other hand, can be performed at frequencies as high as 10 kHz [18].

The first laser interferometric studies of ossicular chain vibration patterns were done on the stapes footplate in human temporal bone preparations using a single-point technique [10]. On the assumption that the bone of the footplate vibrates without bending, the vibration pattern can be calculated by taking measurements from at least three points on the footplate. Vlaming and Feenstra took measurements at four points, directing the laser beam onto the footplate through a posterior tympanotomy. The maximum differences between the sampled points were less than a factor of 1.25 (2 dB) [10]. Since this difference was within the accuracy range of the method, they concluded that the footplate underwent a purely piston-like movement, as other methods had previously shown [28, 30, 61, 62]. However, more recent laser interferometric studies in temporal bone specimens and in vivo have shown that the stapes footplate actually undergoes both longitudinal and transverse rocking movements that are in this order of magnitude (Fig. 8.16). Heiland et al. made measurements in human temporal bone specimens showing that the footplate undergoes an anterior–posterior rocking motion beginning above 2 kHz, increases with frequency, and equals the displacement of the piston-like movement at 4 kHz. Based on correlation equations, it is assumed that the rocking motion continues to increase up to 5 kHz [63]. In laser studies on temporal bone specimens, Voss et al. measured rocking movements of the footplate above 2 kHz in two of five specimens and concluded that the footplate had a complex motion pattern above that frequency [19]. Huber et al. even measured rocking movements of the human footplate in vivo by performing scanning vibrometry through a posterior tympanotomy [64]. Although the facial nerve prominence markedly obscures the view of the footplate in the live subject compared with a temporal bone specimen, these studies and subsequent animated vibration displays also demonstrated complex movements of the footplate above 1 kHz.

The characteristics of the vibration of the stapes at frequencies above 4 kHz are still controversial. While Decreamer et al. describe a predominantly piston-like movement at 7 kHz, the "rocking ratio" measured by Heiland indicates a linear increase (measured up to 5 kHz) [63, 65].

For many years it was believed that the malleus and incus rotated like a hinge on a fixed axis passing through the short process of the incus and the anterior process of the malleus (the "axial ligament," see Fig. 8.17) [66–70]. Later studies using stroboscopy and holography showed that at frequencies above 1 kHz, the axis of rotation was shifted or translated in the caudal direction [30, 61, 71]. These results are called into question, however, by the high level of the acoustic stimulus (120–140 dB SPL). Measurements with laser interferometry, which permit the reconstruction (by single-point measurements) or direct animation of vibration patterns (scanning vibrometry), were able to correct the vibration pattern of the malleus and incus at intermediate frequencies using considerably lower stimulus levels. While the malleus and incus basically undergo a hinge-like movement about the axial ligament up to the first resonance frequency, at frequencies above 800 Hz the malleus also rotates about its longitudinal axis and translates in the plane of the tympanic membrane over one phase cycle. These additional movements are transmitted to the incus, resulting in a see-saw–like movement of the malleus–incus complex (Fig. 8.17 b) that does not have a fixed axis of rotation [18, 72]. While Decreamer observed this pattern only in an animal model (cat), we were able to confirm this

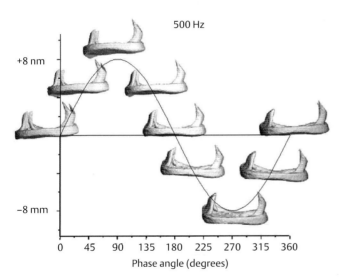

500 Hz

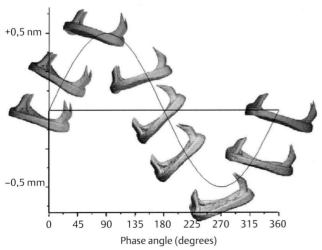

Fig. 8.**16** Relative displacement of the stapes footplate over one phase cycle at 500 kHz and 4000 Hz, reproduced from laser scanning measurements (by the author). For purposes of illustration, the footplate is shown much smaller than scale.

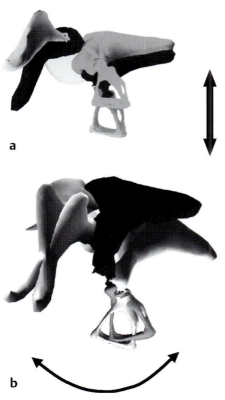

a

b

Fig. 8.**17** **a** Diagram of the vibration patterns of the ossicular chain, which basically undergoes a hinge-like movement up to the resonance frequency at 1 kHz. **b** The entire complex also undergoes see-saw movements at higher frequencies.

complex vibration pattern in a human temporal bone specimen (Fig. 8.**17**).

These see-saw movements are transmitted to the incudomalleolar joint, producing relative movements in the joint space once thought to occur only in response to unphysiologically high acoustic pressures. Recent studies using laser interferometry indicate relative motion in the incudomalleolar joint based on reconstructed vibration modes or relative phase information between the umbo and lenticular process [65, 71, 73, 74]. As our own laser scanning studies demonstrate, the isoamplitude lines measured at 2.5 kHz run parallel to the joint space, showing a maximum on the malleus head and a concomitant minimum on the body of the incus as well as rotation of the malleus handle about its longitudinal axis (Fig. 8.**18**). This line pattern shows that a slight gliding movement occurs in the incudomalleolar joint, even at physiologic sound pressure levels. On the other hand, our measurements to date have not shown any gliding movements in the incudostapedial joint. Single-point laser measurements from various angles have not shown any amplitude or phase differences between the lenticular process and stapes head, suggesting that this joint allows rotational movements that are transmitted toward the stapes footplate with very little loss [8, 61].

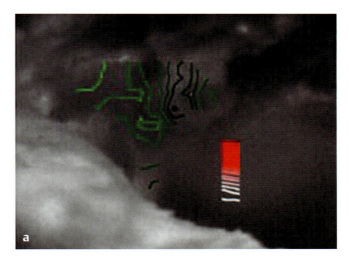

a

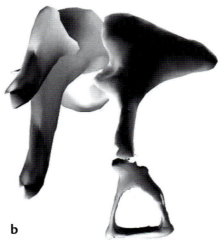

b

Fig. 8.**18** **a** Isoamplitude lines measured by laser scanning interferometry at 2.5 kHz (90°) indicate relative motion in the incudomalleolar joint caused by rotation of the malleus about the long axis of the malleus handle. **b** Diagram of the gliding motion in the joint revealed by computer animation.

Middle Ear Transfer Functions

Analysis of Middle Ear Joints

While older methods of measurement (e. g., SQUID magnetography) could determine middle ear transfer functions in temporal bone specimens with high sensitivity, laser interferometry is an optical method offering new capabilities at relatively low cost. By coupling an ordinary interferometer to a dissecting or operating microscope, it is possible to manipulate the ossicular chain and tympanic membrane without altering the measurement conditions or having to exchange the specimen during the manipulation. This increases not only the reproducibility of the measurement but also its sensitivity. Even miniscule changes in middle ear impedance can be detected by keeping the laser beam in a constant position during the manipulations.

This application is illustrated by studies of altered articular function in the middle ear. It is of interest to surgeons to

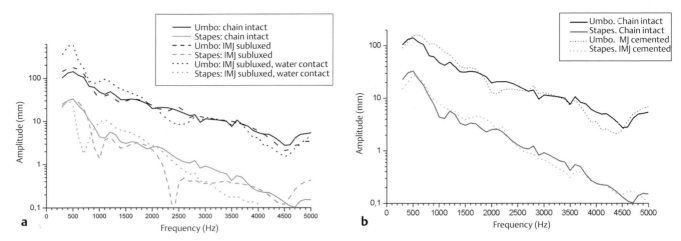

Fig. 8.**19** **a** Vibration amplitudes of the middle ear, measured at the umbo and stapes after separation of the incudomalleolar joint (IMJ). **b** Amplitudes measured after cementing the joint.

know how the dislocation or fixation of ossicular joints affects the acoustic transmission properties of the middle ear. While removing large cholesteatomas or glomus tumors, it can be helpful to interrupt the ossicular chain temporarily by removing the incus. This step would be easier if it were certain that it would not cause irreparable damage from an acoustic standpoint. In earlier experimental studies, very little work was done on the effects of joint subluxations. It was found that cementing the malleus to the incus at the incudomalleolar joint had no discernible effect on transmission properties or vibration patterns [71, 75]. Hudde and Engel determined the change in middle ear input impedance after joint fixation with cement and found that the difference was negligibly small (5 dB between 0.3 kHz and 2 kHz) [76].

With laser interferometry, the effects of subluxation and cement fixation of the incudomalleolar joint in temporal bone specimens can be investigated with a laser beam kept stationary during the manipulations. The transfer functions obtained by this method demonstrate that the fre-

quency response at the umbo changes very little after subluxation of the incudomalleolar joint, while the frequency response at the stapes shows frequency-dependent discontinuities of up to 20 dB (Fig. 8.19 a).

A subluxed incudomalleolar joint can be reapposed with a dissecting needle, and the articular surfaces will remain apposed through adhesion. A joint reapposed in this way will transmit vibrations without the unwanted resonances in the mid-frequency range that occur with a subluxed joint, but the first resonance frequency will be increased. Losses due to damping occur at high frequencies up to a level of 10 dB. When the joint surfaces are cemented together, the transfer function is approximately equal to that of a healthy middle ear. The only appreciable effect is an increase in the stiffness of the ossicular chain up to the first resonance frequency, with an approximately 5-dB decrease in the vibration amplitudes of the footplate (see Fig. 8.**19 b**).

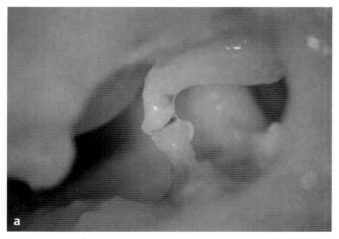

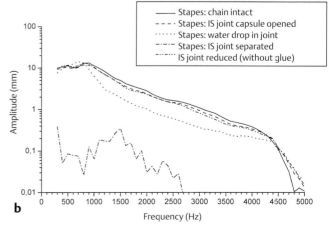

Fig. 8.**20** **a** A separated incudostapedial (IS) joint with only a drop of water bridging the gap. **b** Footplate vibration with an intact, separated, and reapposed joint. A drop of water in the joint space causes relatively small transmission losses (10 dB) above 1 kHz. Stimulus 94 dB SPL.

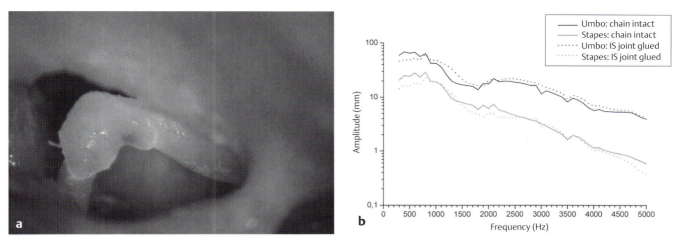

Fig. 8.**21**   **a** Incudostapedial (IS) joint cemented with acrylate glue. **b** Footplate and umbo vibration after cement application, showing only minor losses at low frequencies (6 dB). Stimulus 94 dB SPL.

Similar laser interferometric studies can be performed on the incudostapedial joint. After separation of the incudostapedial joint, the transmission properties of the healthy middle ear have been restored simply by reducing the joint with a dissecting needle. Surprisingly, placing a drop of water in the open joint space provided relatively good acoustic transmission up to the first resonance frequency (Fig. 8.**20**). Above that point, transmission fell by only 10 dB due to damping.

We found that cementing the joint space between the stapes head and incus caused transmission losses of approximately 6 dB up to the first resonance frequency, and that these losses could even be measured at the umbo (Fig. 8.**21**). Apparently the cemented joint space restricts the mobility of the entire chain at lower frequencies. Reapposing the joint surfaces without cement appears to be more favorable for acoustic transmission than creating a rigid connection, as the study by Maassen and Zenner also suggests [77].

Analysis of Middle Ear Muscles

Laser interferometry can also be used for functional evaluation of middle ear muscles. Tensile stresses on the middle ear muscles lead to characteristic changes in the transfer functions of the ear, which can be detected by single-point measurements on the footplate. Traction on the tensor tendon leads to a decrease in malleus and stapes vibrations at low frequencies and to an increase at high frequencies. The first resonance frequency at the umbo is shifted from 1 kHz to 1.5 kHz as a sign of increased chain stiffness (Fig. 8.**22 a**).

On the other hand, traction on the stapedius tendon leads to stiffening of the annular ligament with a decline at low frequencies and to a dampening of footplate vibrations between 2 kHz and 4 kHz. Even at physiologic forces estimated at 50 mN [78], the transfer function at the footplate is decreased by 6 dB at low frequencies (Fig. 8.**22 b**). These typical frequency changes are comparable to the effects of a high-pass filter [78–80]. We cannot deduce the physio-

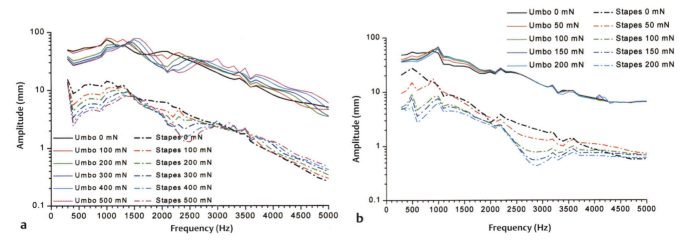

Fig. 8.**22**   **a** Vibration of the umbo and stapes with tension on the tensor tympani muscle. **b** Vibration of the umbo and stapes with tension on the stapedius muscle. Stimulus 94 dB SPL.

logic significance of the stapedius reflex based on these laser measurements in temporal bone specimens, but the slight damping of the transfer function does not support the theory that middle ear muscles protect the ear from unphysiologic acoustic events. It is more plausible that the muscles protect the joints from degenerative changes by keeping them in motion. "Disuse osteoarthritis" would lead to joint fixation, compromising the ability of the joints to transmit sound and protect against atmospheric pressure changes [78].

Analysis of Middle Ear Implants

In the past, experimental studies were rarely done on the function of the reconstructed middle ear and had very little impact on the development of middle ear implants, which were usually designed empirically. Transfer functions were measured with a microphone in the round window niche [81–83], electrocochleography [84], stroboscopic studies [85], and dynamic measurements of intracochlear pressure [86]. It is only in recent years that progress has been made toward optimizing the mechanical properties of middle ear implants and operating techniques based on model calculations and experiments [12, 87–90].

Laser interferometry has greatly simplified the technique for measuring the vibration amplitudes of the stapes footplate or round window in temporal bone specimens [16, 57, 91–95]. Unfortunately, these experiments have been compromised by a number of methodologic problems. Besides the known problems associated with the drying of temporal bone specimens, methodologic errors result from a change in laser position; a change in measuring angle; a change of implant position on the tympanic membrane,

malleus handle, or footplate; a change in coupling strength to the stapes head; or changes in the primary tension of the reconstruction. Also, little information is gained by comparing implants from different manufacturers with different material properties, as many authors have done [12, 77, 94, 96]. It is more rewarding to conduct a separate analysis of the specific material properties of implants. The effect of stiffness, for example, can be measured in isolation by minimizing the effects of other parameters (design, coupling, position, mass) by producing implant blanks of identical shapes (Fig. 8.**23 b**) placed perpendicular on the stapes head without primary tension and braced against a designated site.

As our own laser interferometric studies on the effect of stiffness on sound transmission have shown, only the implant made of soft silicone leads to transmission losses of 20 dB over the entire frequency range due to the strong damping properties of the silicone (Fig. 8.**23 a**). All other materials differ only at frequencies above 3 kHz (up to a maximum of 12 dB). The favorable transmission properties of the bone implant suggest an optimum solution of the mass and stiffness problem by nature. It is not surprising that many surgeons swear by autologous ossicles for reconstructions in the uninflamed middle ear. The general principle of preferring autologous material continues to justify this policy.

Besides stiffness, laser interferometry can also be used to investigate the effect of implant mass on sound transmission. Small weights can be attached to an implant already in place without altering the position of the laser spot on the footplate [94]. According to studies by Nishihara and Goode, adding just 5 mg of mass to a partial ossicular replacement prosthesis (PORP) (4 mg) leads to transmission

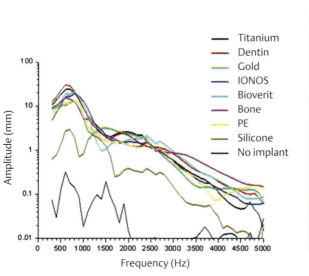

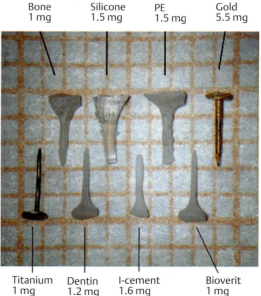

Fig. 8.**23** **a** Vibration of the stapes after ossicular chain reconstruction with partial ossicular replacement prosthesis (PORP) implants made of various materials. Coupled to the tympanic membrane, stimulus 94 dB SPL. **b** Implants of the same design (PE, polyethylene; I-cement, ionomer cement; Bioverit, glass ceramic).

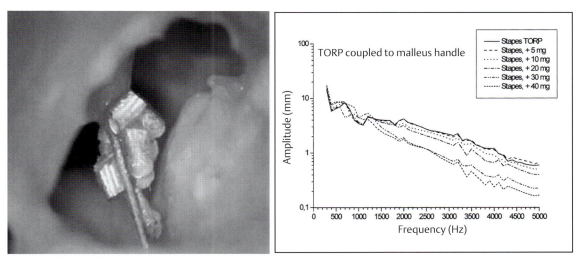

Fig. 8.**24 a** Titanium implant mass increased by progressively adding 5-mg weights. **b** Footplate vibration after reconstruction as a function of mass. Stimulus 94 dB SPL.

losses of 10 dB in the range from 3 kHz to 5 kHz (6 dB) [94]. Our own measurements in temporal bone specimens showed that the effect of mass varied with the position of the prosthesis.

The critical mass that should not be exceeded with middle ear implants to avoid transmission losses of 5 dB or more is estimated at 10 mg (coupled to the tympanic membrane) or 15 mg (coupled to the malleus handle) for PORP implants. It is estimated at 5 mg (tympanic membrane) or 15 mg (malleus handle) for total ossicular replacement prosthesis (TORP) implants (see the example of a TORP coupled to the malleus handle in Fig. 8.**24**).

Another key factor affecting sound transmission is implant design. The shape of the implant can affect the coupling conditions. Lately there has been growing experience with metallic implants, which are distinguished by their slender shape and their potential for plastic deformation in the middle ear [97–100]. There have been few reports to date on the contact area between the prosthesis and bone.

Laser interferometric experiments with identically shaped PORP implants demonstrate the effect of prosthesis coupling to the stapes head on acoustic transmission (Fig. 8.**25**). While the soft tabs of the gold bell could be accurately form-fitted to the stapes head, this condition could not be consistently achieved with the titanium bell due to the greater resilience and "memory" of the material. When the tabs are crimped together, the material tends to spring back to its original shape. This results in transmission losses up to 12 dB at low frequencies and approximately 6 dB at high frequencies. These losses disappear at once when the titanium bell is cemented to the head of the stapes with a drop of acrylate glue. Since gluing the implant or crimping the relatively stiff titanium entails certain risks under clinical conditions (foreign-body reaction or stapes dislocation), one possible solution is to redesign the titanium bell with thin, springy tabs that press against the bone when the implant is pushed into place (Dresden Clip Prosthesis, Fig. 8.**26**).

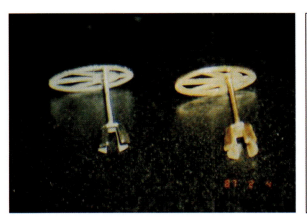
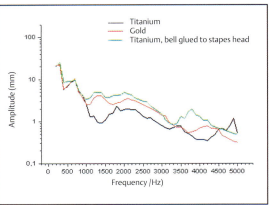

Fig. 8.**25 a** Identically shaped PORP implants made of gold and titanium. **b** Footplate vibration as a function of the bell/stapes head attachment. Stimulus 94 dB SPL.

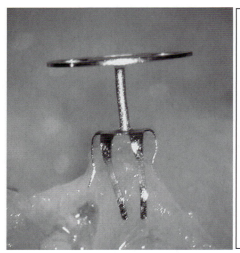

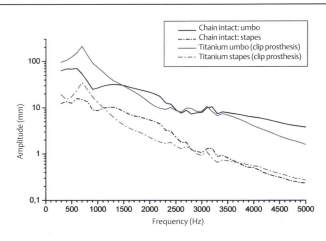

Fig. 8.**26** **a** Dresden clip prosthesis on the stapes head, consisting of a thin titanium bell with springy tabs providing a secure hold on the stapes head with good contact. **b** Footplate vibration before and after reconstruction with the implant. Stimulus 94 dB SPL.

Laser Audiometry

Temporal bone specimens are not the only setting for analyzing the transfer functions of the middle ear. Today the sensitivity of commercially available interferometers is high enough to permit the measurement of umbo vibrations in live subjects [14, 55, 101, 105]. It is hoped that studies of this kind will provide information on the function of the middle ear or even the inner ear. This means that laser interferometry could provide an objective method of middle and inner ear investigation as an adjunct to subjective pure-tone audiometry. This has given rise to the interesting concept of "laser audiometry." As we shall see below, however, interferometry is still a long way from becoming a standard technique for everyday clinical use.

The setup for measuring umbo vibrations in vivo is very similar to the setup for experimental studies in temporal bone specimens. Certain distinctions, however, could lead to serious errors or misinterpretations if ignored. The sound generator and microphone are introduced into the subject's ear canal, taking care to position the microphone no more than 2–3 mm from the umbo. Placing the microphone too far from the eardrum leads to measurement errors at high frequencies. Most authors prefer a closed sound delivery system, using a glass coverslip to produce an airtight seal and ensure a sufficiently high sound pressure at low frequencies [14, 15, 101–104]. The acoustic stimulus may consist of single- or multisine tones. The single-sine stimulus allows for better sound-pressure regulation in front of the tympanic membrane but prolongs the examination time, which is why a multisine or sweep stimulus is better for clinical use. For the measurement, the laser beam is passed through the glass coverslip of the closed meatal sound chamber and focused onto the umbo. While reflectors had to be affixed to the umbo in the early days of laser interferometry [102, 103, 105], modern heterodyne interferometers are sensitive enough to record useful signals, eliminating the need for reflective material [14, 55, 104]. Omitting the reflectors, which generally were placed on the umbo with an instrument following local anesthesia of the tympanic membrane, simplifies the measurement protocol and lowers the risk of the examination. It also eliminates potential artifacts caused by the reflector mass or relative motion between the umbo and reflector [3]. Errors can still arise from mechanical vibrations or drifting of the laser beam during the examination due to movements of the head during breathing. To minimize this error, the head of the subject should be stabilized during the examination, e. g., by placing it in a vacuum pillow [55]. At present there is no standard technical protocol for delivering the acoustic stimulus or positioning the microphone. Most studies to date have employed homemade sound generators (Fig. 8.**27**).

While ossicular chain lesions such as malleus head fixation, ossicular chain disruption, and stapes fixation can be experimentally produced and differentiated in temporal bone specimens under laboratory conditions [10, 105], previous studies in vivo have yielded only illustrative case results in clinical use, usually involving small numbers of patients. In studies with larger case numbers, interindividual amplitude differences in the transfer function of 15–20 dB [103, 104] and 10–15 dB [55] have been reported even in normal-hearing subjects. It is still uncertain how

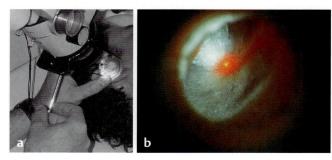

Fig. 8.**27** **a** Laser interferometry in a patient. **b** Laser spot on the tympanic membrane.

these large discrepancies arise. Hypothetically, they may relate to qualitative differences in the mechanical properties of the middle ear that are not detected with pure-tone audiometry; this means simply that some middle ears transmit better than others [106]. It is also possible, however, that the examination technique itself is the cause of the large interindividual differences in the location of the resonance frequencies and in the amplitude curve (Fig. 8.**28 a**). This large variability makes it difficult to distinguish true abnormalities in the ossicular chain. As temporal bone experiments have shown, fixation of the malleus head reduces the amplitude of umbo vibrations by a maximum of 30 dB, while disrupting the ossicular chain leads to an amplitude increase of approximately 15 dB, and otosclerosis reduces umbo vibrations by only 6 dB (Fig. 8.**28 b**). It is clear, then, that amplitude analysis alone is not sufficient for the clinical differentiation of ossicular chain abnormalities.

When the shift of the first resonance frequency is included in the analysis, it appears that a statistically reliable differentiation can be made even with otosclerotic fixation of the footplate, although so far this has been demonstrated only in anecdotal case reports [55]. For the future, there appears to be a good chance that changes in the malleus and incus (fixation or disruption) will be diagnosed by laser interferometry, whereas changes involving the stapes, such as otosclerosis, are more difficult to detect due to the multiple degrees of freedom of the incudostapedial joint [104]. It appears that laser interferometry of the umbo is not useful for the diagnosis of cochlear hearing loss. For example, testing the function of the cochlear amplifier, and thus of the outer hair cells, would require the use of stimulus levels far below 60 dB SPL. But there are physical limits to the sensitivity of the laser interferometer, making it likely that stimulus levels of 60 dB or more will have to be used for in vivo examinations, both now and in the future. Thus, hair cell damage or damage to the basilar membrane was diagnosed only outside the working range of the outer hair cells (above 60 dB) and would be reflected more clearly in impedance changes in the basilar membrane [14]. Because the impedance of the cochlea is small in relation to middle ear impedance and above 1 kHz is determined chiefly by the mass of the cochlear fluid, even the complete loss of cochlear impedance (e. g., by drainage of the inner ear) has only a minor effect on tympanic membrane impedance, consisting of a slight increase in the first resonance frequency [76]. This means that the prospects for inner ear investigation by laser interferometry are extremely poor, and the term "laser audiometry" appears too optimistic.

■ Laser Interferometric Studies of Inner Ear Mechanics

Studies of the Basilar Membrane

Since von Bekesy performed stroboscopic studies of the basilar membrane, efforts have been made to gain a deeper understanding of the mechanical processes in the cochlea [69]. Few measuring techniques are sensitive enough to resolve the extremely small amplitudes of the vibrations. Before laser interferometry was introduced into inner ear research, the frequency characteristics of the basilar membrane were investigated using optical levers, capacitive probes, laser speckle analysis, and the Mössbauer technique [107]. Of these methods, the Mössbauer technique was found to have the highest resolution, but it still has considerably less sensitivity and dynamic range than laser interferometry (Mössbauer technique 30–1000 μm/s, laser interferometry 0.5–10 000 μm/s) [108].

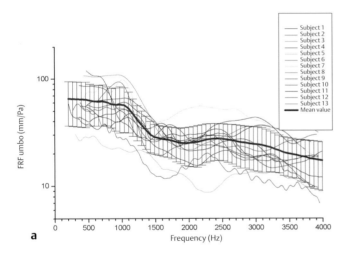

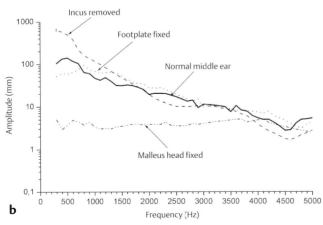

Fig. 8.**28** **a** Laser interferometry of umbo vibrations in 13 subjects, showing large interindividual variations. **b** Measurement of umbo vibrations in temporal bone specimens with various ossicular chain lesions. Stimulus 94 dB SPL.

Laser interferometry offers key advantages over traditional methods. As an optical method of analysis, it can examine the basilar membrane without touching it, i.e., without adding to the mass of the membrane or destroying its cells. The small diameter of the laser beam (3–7 μm) makes it possible to take point vibration measurements at various selected sites on the basilar membrane and from various angles. These data can be used to reconstruct the vibration patterns of the membrane. Laser interferometry also has a much larger dynamic range than traditional methods and can detect even nonlinear vibration processes, which are characteristic of the cochlea [109].

These advantages notwithstanding, laser interferometry is not free of methodologic problems. As studies in animal models have shown, the frequency response of the basilar membrane depends on the vitality of its very delicate cellular structures. For this reason, vibrations should be measured as atraumatically as possible and under "in vivo" conditions. The mere act of opening the bony shell can damage the outer hair cells at high frequencies due to mechanical alterations or a change in nutritive conditions [110]. Making an opening in the cochlea also changes the cochlear impedance, with an associated effect on traveling wave propagation, especially at low frequencies [111]. This effect can be prevented by covering the bony cochlear window with a glass coverslip [112]. When measurements are taken in the isolated cochlear preparation, the stiffness and resonance properties of the basilar membrane are altered due to cell death within a few hours. Consequently, the investigation of cochlear mechanics requires a largely noninvasive examination technique [110]. The round window membrane provides a natural access route for directing the laser beam through the fluid-filled scala tympani and onto the basilar membrane "from below" (Fig. 8.29). Unfortunately, the reflectivity of the round window membrane is high relative to the basilar membrane because of its curved surface, thickness, and vascularity, so that a large portion of the laser light intensity is lost, resulting in decreased sensitivity [113].

Khanna and Leonard developed their own high-sensitivity laser interferometer and integrated it into the optical path of a confocal microscope, enabling them to perform the first laser measurements through the intact round window membrane of the live cat [114]. Other in vivo studies of the basilar membrane in the area of the basal turn were subsequently undertaken in other species such as the guinea pig, chinchilla, and gerbil, in some cases after the creation of a small bone window [115–118]. Unfortunately, these measurements reflect only the frequency response of the

basilar membrane at high frequencies (7–40 kHz). Studies of cochlear mechanics at the low frequencies important for speech comprehension, i. e., in the apical turn, require meticulous dissection in live animals due to the confined anatomy and have only a relatively narrow route for optical access. Because of this limitation, an in vitro dissection technique was developed for studying low and middle frequencies, permitting measurements of the isolated cochlea in the basal, third, and fourth turns. The disadvantage is a rapid decline of hair cell function over a period of minutes to hours [119]. In this method the apical turns are not scanned via the scala tympani but via the scala vestibuli through the optically transparent Reissner membrane [120]. Due to the weak reflection of the basilar membrane, reflectors are commonly used in this approach, and the Reissner membrane must be opened to place the reflectors [121].

These problems aside, laser interferometry has become the current method of choice for investigating the mechanics of the basilar membrane. It has been used to confirm experimentally the active amplification of the traveling wave, discovered by the Mössbauer technique [108, 114, 115, 122–124]. Laser interferometric measurements in vivo show 100 times greater displacement of the basilar mem-

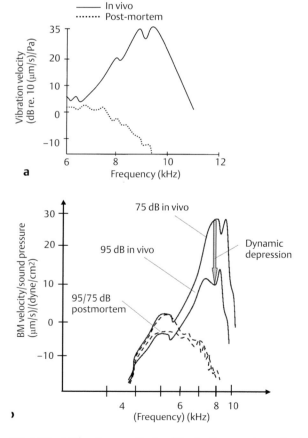

a

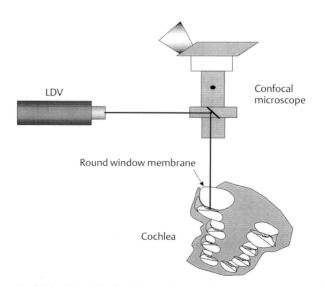

Fig. 8.**29**   Principle of basilar membrane vibration measurement in the guinea pig with a laser interferometer coupled to the microscope. The laser beam passes through the round window membrane and traverses the fluid-filled scala tympani. LDV, laser interferometer.

Fig. 8.**30**   **a** Vibration amplitude of the basilar membrane in vivo and post-mortem. **b** Effect of dynamic depression at high stimulus levels about the characteristic frequency (CF = 8 kHz) (after Ruggero and Rich, 1991 [108]).

brane than in the temporal bone specimen, proving that active mechanisms amplify the vibrations in vivo (Fig. 8.**30 a**). The amplification factor in this process is not constant, however, but changes as a function of the intensity of the sound stimulus and its frequency. With a sine-wave stimulus at a low sound pressure, the traveling wave initially undergoes constant amplification by a factor of 100 near the characteristic frequency (site of maximum basilar membrane displacement). The amplification factor declines at moderate sound pressures (40–80 dB SPL), and it plateaus at high sound pressures [112]. This dynamic depression of the live cochlea, known also as compressive nonlinearity, can be considered the mechanical cause of the recruitment phenomenon. To perceive a change of loudness at moderate sound levels above the hearing threshold, a very much greater increase in the sound level is required with a healthy inner ear than when hearing function is impaired [125].

The nonlinearity of the cochlea is not reflected merely in a declining amplification factor. Laser interferometry can measure sharply defined vibration maxima near the characteristic frequency at low and moderate sound pressures, and the curves of these maxima are identical to neuronal tuning curves [123]. Contrary to earlier beliefs, the sharp frequency tuning of the ear is not based on a neural effect but on an active mechanical process in the area of the basilar membrane, as point laser interferometric measurements have demonstrated. There is considerable evidence that the outer hair cells, considered the generators of otoacoustic emissions, are mechanical amplifiers that interact with the supporting cells, basilar membrane, and tectorial membrane in a complex way, amplifying the mechanical input signal for the inner hair cells within a sharply localized area [125]. When the outer hair cells are lost, the inner ear becomes less sensitive and also less discriminating. The basilar membrane undergoes a linear type of displacement.

Previously, basilar membrane vibrations in vivo have been measured strictly in animals and usually in the area of the easily accessible basal turn (Fig. 8.**31**). Recent studies have shown that the apical basilar membrane also shows nonlinearities, expressed not in the fundamental frequency but in the appearance of harmonic waves and distortions [120]. The basilar membrane behaves differently in the apical turn than in the basal turn. While the contraction of the outer hair cells in the basal turn leads to the amplification of basilar membrane vibrations (positive feedback between the organ of Corti and basilar membrane), a negative feedback mechanism is believed to exist in the apical turn, i.e., active mechanisms reduce the vibration of the basilar membrane. Since this has the effect of smoothing the amplitude of the fundamental frequency, the behavior of the apical basilar membrane has long been regarded as linear (see Fig. 8.**31**).

While home-made devices were used initially for the investigation of cochlear mechanics by laser interferometry, today a range of commercially available laser interferometers are available for vibration measurements [127]. Laser feedback interferometry is a potential new method for examining the weakly reflective basilar membrane. This technique uses diffusely returned laser light for analysis,

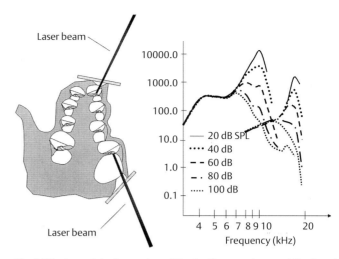

Fig. 8.**31**   Laser interferometry of the basilar membrane at the basal and apical turns of the cochlea. The displacement amplitudes were divided by the stimulus sound pressure. The vibration amplitude declined at different stimulus levels as a sign of nonlinearity (after Robles and Ruggero, 2001; Cooper, 1999 [112, 126]).

making it possible to measure with greater sensitivity [128]. Further details on the frequency characteristics of the basilar membrane can be found in survey works by Ulfendahl and Robles and Ruggero [107, 112] and other authors.

Studies of the Organ of Corti

With its extremely narrow measuring beam (approximately 3–7 µm), laser interferometry can also perform direct vibration measurements of the organ of Corti at the cellular level, including the hair cells, Hensen cells, and tectorial membrane [129–132]. The data from these single-point measurements can be analyzed to reconstruct the vibration patterns of the organ of Corti, which are essential for understanding the electromechanical transduction process in the inner ear. According to traditional concepts, the traveling wave of the basilar membrane induces a concomitant movement of the organ of Corti in the transverse direction. Due in part to the geometry and mechanical properties (mass, stiffness, friction) of the cellular structures of the organ of Corti, this up-and-down motion generates a shearing motion between the plane of the stereocilia (reticular membrane) and the tectorial membrane. This shearing motion is considered the cause of the bowing (deflection) of the stereocilia and thus of the depolarization of the outer hair cells. The outer hair cells can also amplify and sharpen the traveling wave through their active motor properties (rapid length change in the axial direction), while their slow motility helps control the position of the basilar membrane and stereocilia. This latter process is believed to be a protective mechanism against high noise levels and mechanical acoustic trauma [133].

Laser interferometry can measure relative movements within the organ of Corti if the measuring beam can be focused at different levels. Unfortunately, the cellular struc-

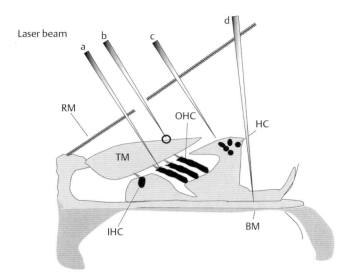

Fig. 8.**32** Schematic diagram of laser measurement of the organ of Corti at the cellular level in the apical cochlea through the scala vestibuli. RM, Reissner membrane; TM, tectorial membrane; OHC, outer hair cells; HC, Hensen cells; IHC, inner hair cells; BM, basilar membrane. The laser beam can be directed through the intact Reissner membrane onto the outer hair cells, Hensen cells, or basilar membrane (a, c, d), or the Reissner membrane can be opened for placing a reflective bead to measure the vibration of the optically transparent tectorial membrane (b) (after Ulfendahl, 1997; Robles and Ruggero, 2001 [107, 112]).

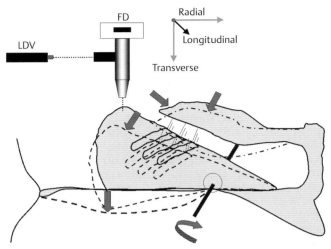

Fig. 8.**33** Three-dimensional vibration measurement of the organ of Corti using a laser interferometer (LDV) and photodiode (FD). Up to the characteristic frequency (CF), the organ of Corti rotates like a rigid body around a point close to the inner limbus (see rotational axis). Near the CF, the tectorial membrane vibrates parallel to the lamina reticularis in a radial direction (after Hemmert et al., 2000 [111]).

tures of the organ of Corti reflect light waves extremely poorly (0.002–0.009 %) [134]. This makes it difficult not only to identify the cellular structures but also to focus the laser beam. Indeed, the reflectivity of the cell under study may be so low that the laser beam does not measure the vibrations in the focal plane but the vibrations of an underlying cell that is a better reflector. This problem can be reduced by integrating the interferometer into a confocal microscope [135]. The microscope can filter out any reflected light that does not come from the focal plane. Although the sensitivity of the interferometer is not sufficient to measure the vibration of the hair cells via the round window and scala tympani through the intact basilar membrane, this technique is sensitive enough to examine the organ of Corti through the scala vestibuli and the intact Reissner membrane (Fig. 8.**32**). Particularly good study objects are the third and fourth turns of the guinea pig cochlea, fenestrated with a small bone window so that the laser beam can be directed onto the organ of Corti "from above."

Cooper developed an improved interferometer sensitive enough to make cellular measurements in the organ of Corti [126]. Commercially available interferometers can also be used for these measurements, but often the reflectivity of the cell under study must be increased by adding reflectors [136]. Usually these consist of glass or polystyrene microspheres 5–30 μm in diameter. The advantages of these reflectors lie in their omnidirectional reflection, de-emphasizing the importance of the incidence angle of the laser beam [115]. There is a danger, however, that the mass of the microspheres (5 μm = 0.18 ng) could affect the vibration mode of the cells or distort the measurement due to relative motion between the structure of interest and

the reflective sphere [115, 137]. When reflectors are used for measurements of the organ of Corti, the Reissner membrane must be opened to insert the spheres, allowing the mixing of perilymph and endolymph and thereby altering the endocochlear potential. This artifact can be reduced by introducing artificial endolymph [111]. To avoid adding reflectors, in theory the sensitivity of the interferometer can be increased by boosting the intensity of the laser light. It is still uncertain, however, whether this can damage the hair cells. No reliable data are available to answer this question for the inner ear, but an intensity threshold of 0.5 W/cm² has been determined for the retina of the eye. It is reasonable to assume that this value is a good approximation for the hair cells as well [9].

Previously, individual cells of the organ of Corti were measured through the scala vestibuli perpendicular to the basilar membrane and showed vibrations with only small phase and amplitude differences between the Hensen cells, the three rows of outer hair cells, and the inner hair cells and basilar membrane [111, 130, 136]. We may conclude from this that the organ of Corti vibrates like a rigid body up to the characteristic frequency, driven by the motion of the basilar membrane [111]. Recent three-dimensional vibration studies, performed in guinea pig temporal bone specimens using an interferometer for the transverse direction and a photodiode for motion in the cellular plane (radial direction), have revealed two different modes of vibration. Up to the characteristic frequency, the organ of Corti rotates like a rigid body about a point near the edge of the inner limbus. A second vibration mode occurs close to the characteristic frequency. There the tectorial membrane vibrates parallel to the lamina reticularis in the radial direction (Fig. 8.**33**) [111]. The authors believe that this motion reflects a control mechanism for the deflection of the outer hair cell bundle. Further details on the micromechanics of the organ of Corti and outer hair cells can be found in survey works by authors such as Rhode, Ruggero, Zenner, Ulfendahl, and Robles and Ruggero [107, 112, 133, 138, 139].

We can analyze the micromechanics of the organ of Corti in greater detail only by making the interferometer more sensitive to weakly reflecting structures and improving its focusing. One approach to this problem is the development of interferometers that detect displacement rather than velocity [126]. In the future, we may also expect that signal analysis will improve by digital processing. Further advances in laser measurements of the inner ear will involve extending the scope of investigations to the subcellular and molecular levels. Even today, it is possible to measure stereociliary stiffness and cell membrane stiffness in the isolated hair cell [140, 141]. As studies in renal cell cultures have shown, the viscoelastic properties of the cytoplasm can be determined by laser tracking microrheology [142]. The mechanical parameters obtained with this technology can be used to perfect existing hair-cell models and thus advance our understanding of their active contractile properties.

■ References

1 Westphal WH. Physik. Berlin, Heidelberg: Springer-Verlag, 1947; Bd. 12.
2 Spengler B. Grundlagen der Lasertechnik. www.uni-duesseldorf.de/www/MedFak/LaserMedizin/Laserkurs_skript/Laserkurs_Skript.PDF, 2002
3 Vogel U, Zahnert T, Hofmann G, Offergeld C, Hüttenbrink K-B. Laser vibrometry of the middle ear: opportunities and limitations. In: Hüttenbrink KB (ed). Middle Ear Mechanics in Research and Otosurgery. Dresden: Dept. of Oto-Rhino-Laryngology, Univ. Hospital, Univ. of Technology, 1997: 128–133
4 Tonndorf J, Khanna SM. Submicroscopic displacement amplitudes of the tympanic membrane (cat) measured by a laser interferometer. J Acoust Soc Amer 1968; 44: 1546–1554
5 Dragsten PR, Webb WW, Paton JA, Cabranica RR. Light scattering heterodyne interferometer for vibration measurements in auditory organs. J Acoust Soc Am 1976; 60: 665–671
6 Eberhadt FJ, Anrews FA. Laser heterodyne system for measurement of and analysis of vibration. J Acoust Soc Am 1970; 48: 603–609
7 Michelsen A. Laser Techniques in Studies of Hearing. In: Sattelle DB, Lee WI, Ware BR (eds). Biomedical Applications of Laser Light Scattering. Elsevier Biomedical Press, 1982: 357–370
8 Vlaming MS. Middle ear mechanics studied by laser Doppler interferometry. TU Delft/NL: Dissertation, 1987
9 Willemin JF, Dandliker R, Khanna SM. Heterodyne interferometer for submicroscopic vibration measurements in the inner ear. J Acoust Soc Am 1988; 83: 787–795
10 Vlaming MS, Feenstra L. Studies on the mechanics of the normal human middle ear. Clin Otolaryngol 1986; 11: 353–363
11 Nishihara S, Aritomo H, Goode RL. Effect of changes in mass on middle ear function. Otolaryngol Head Neck Surg 1993; 109: 899–910
12 Goode RL, Killion M, Nakamura K, Nishihara S. New knowledge about the function of the human middle ear: development of an improved analog model. Am J Otol 1994; 15: 145–154
13 Kurokawa H, Goode RL. Sound pressure gain produced by the human middle ear. Otolaryngol Head Neck Surg 1995; 113: 349–355
14 Rodriguez JJ, Zenner HP, Hemmert W, Burkhardt C, Gummer AW. Laservibrometrie. HNO 1997; 45: 997–1007
15 Murakami S, Gyo K, Goode RL. Effect of increased inner ear pressure on middle ear mechanics. Otolaryngol Head Neck Surg 1998; 118: 703–708
16 Eiber A, Freitag H-G, Burkhardt C, Hemmert W, Maassen MM, Jorge JR, Zenner HP. Dynamics of middle ear prostheses – simulations and measurements. Audiol Neuro-Otol 1999; 4: 178–184
17 Schön F, Müller J. Measurements of ossicular vibrations in the middle ear. Audiol Neuro-Otol 1999; 4: 142–149
18 Decraemer WF, Khanna SM. New insights into vibration of the middle ear. In: Rosowski JJ, Merchant SN (eds). Second International Symposium on Middle-Ear Mechanics in Research and Otosurgery, Boston, MA, USA, 1999. The Hague, The Netherlands: Kugler Publications, 2000: 23–38
19 Voss SE, Rosowski JJ, Merchant SN, Peake WT. Acoustic responses of the human middle ear. Hearing Research 2000; 150: 43–69
20 Stenfelt S, Hato N, Goode RL. Factors contributing to bone conduction: The middle ear. J Acoust Soc Am 2002; 111: 947–959
21 Brünings S. Zeitmittelungsverfahren zur Schwingungsanalyse. GMA-Bericht. Verfahren AO, 1991
22 Powell RL, Stetson KS. Interferometric vibration analysis by wavefront reconstruction. J Opt Soc Amer 1965; 55: 1593–1598
23 Michelsen A. The physiology of the locust ear. Zeitschr vergl Physiol 1971; 71: 49–128
24 Khanna SM, Tonndorf J. The vibration pattern of the round window in cats. J Acoust Soc Am 1971; 50: 1475–1483
25 Khanna SM, Tonndorf J. Tympanic membrane vibrations in cats studied by time-averaged holography. J Acoust Soc Amer 1972; 51: 1904–1920
26 von Bally G. Holografische Schwingungsanalyse des Trommelfelles. Laryng Rhinol 1978; 57: 444–450
27 Dancer AL, Franke AB, Smigielski P, Albe F, Fogot H. Holographic interferometry applied to the investigation of tympanic-membrane dispacements in guinea-pig ears subjected to acoustic impulses. J Acoust Soc Am 1975; 58: 223–228
28 Hogmoen K, Gundersen T. Holographic investigation of stapes footplate movements. Acoustica 1977; 37: 198–202
29 Tonndorf J, Khanna SM. The role of the tympanic membrane in middle ear transformation. Ann Otol 1970; 79: 743–753
30 Gundersen T, Hogmoen K. Holograpic vibration analysis of the ossicular chain. Acta Otolaryngol 1976; 82: 16–25
31 Höfling R. Specklemesstechnik. Technische Mitteilungen 1992; 1: 29–33
32 Wada H, Takeuchi M, Hozawa K, Gemma T, Nara M. Vibration measurement of the tympanic membrane usint the time-averaged speckle pattern interferometry. Abstract of the Assoc Res Otolaryngol, 1998; 27
33 Yamaguchi M, Agawa K, Kanetake H, Koike Y, Kashima K. Measurement of blood flow in human tympanic membrane with spectrophotometry and laser speckle flow meter. Nippon Jibiinkoka Gakkai Kaiho 1990; 93: 1354–1362
34 Heymann J, Lingner A. Moiréverfahren. Leipzig: VEB Fachbuchverlag, 1986; Bd 1
35 Khanna SM, Tonndorf J. Tympanic membrane shape determined by moiré topography. J Acoust Soc Am 1975: 1: 72
36 Suehiro M. Effects of an increase or decrease in the middle ear pressure on tympanic membrane vibrations (experimental study by holographic interferometry). Nippon Jibiinkoka Gakkai Kaiho 1990; 93: 398–406
37 Decraemer WF, Dirckx JJ, Funnell WR. Shape and derived geometrical parameters of the adult, human tympanic membrane measured with a phase-shift moire interferometer. Hear Res 1991; 51: 107–121
38 Dirckx JJ, Decraemer WF. Area change and volume displacement of the human tympanic membrane under static pressure. Hear Res 1992; 62: 99–104
39 von Unge M, Decraemer WF, Dirckx JJ, Bagger-Sjoback D. Tympanic membrane displacement patterns in experimental cholesteatoma. Hear Res 1999; 128: 1–15
40 Dirckx JJ, Decraemer WF, von Unge M, Larsson C. Measurement and modeling of boundary shape and surface deformation of the Mongolian gerbil pars flaccida. Hear Res 1997; 111: 153–164
41 Dirckx JJ, Decraemer WF. Effect of middle ear components on eardrum quasi-static deformation. Hear Res 2001; 157: 124–137

42 Funnell WR, Decraemer WF. On the incorporation of moire shape measurements in finite-element models of the cat eardrum. J Acoust Soc Am 1996; 100: 925–932

43 Riva C, Ross B, Benedek GB. Laser Doppler measurements of blood flow in capillary tubes and retinal arteries. Invest Ophthalmol 1972; 11: 936–944

44 Nilsson GE, Tenland T, Oberg PA. Evaluation of a laser Doppler flowmeter for measurement of tissue blood flow. IEEE Trans Biomed Eng 1980; 27: 597–604

45 Miller JM, Marks NJ, Goodwin PC. Laser Doppler measurements of cochlear blood flow. Hear Res 1983; 11: 385–394

46 Miller JM, Goodwin PC, Marks NJ. Inner ear blood flow measured with a laser Doppler system. Arch Otolaryngol 1984; 110: 305–308

47 Wright JW, Dengerink HA, Miller JM, Goodwin PC. Potential role of angiotensin 2 in noise-induced increases in inner ear blood flow. Hear Res 1985; 17: 41–46

48 Hultcrantz E, Angelborg C, Beausang-Linder M. Noise and cochlear blood flow. Arch Otol Rhinol Laryngol 1979; 224: 103–106

49 Laurikainen E, Kanninen P, Aho H, Saukko P. The anatomy of the human promotory for laser Doppler flowmetrie. Eur Arch Otolaryngol 1997; 254: 264–268

50 Miller FM, Bredberg G, Grénman R, Suonpää J, Lindström B, Didier A. Measurement of human blood flow. Ann Otol Rhinol Laryngol 1991; 100: 44–53

51 Scheibe F, Haupt H, Berndt H, Magnus S, Waymar P. Laser light transmission and laser Doppler blood flow measurements on the human, rat and guinea pig cochlea. Eur Arch Otolaryngol 1990; 247: 20–23

52 Nakashima T, Suzuki T, Morisaki H, Yanagita N. Measurement of cochlear blood flow in sudden deafness. Laryngoscope 1992; 102: 1308–1310

53 Haapaniemi J, Schrey A, Laurikainen E. The effect of promotorial bone on laser light transmission in measuring capillary blood flow in vivo. Eur Arch Otolaryngol 2001; 258: 209–212

54 Selmani Z, Pyykkö I, Ishizaki H, Martilla TI. Cochlear blood flow measurement in patients with Meniere's disease and other inner ear disorders. Acta Otolaryngol 2001; 545: 10–13

55 Huber A, Schwab C, Linder T, Stoeckli S, Ferrazzini M, Dillier N, Fisch U. Evaluation of eardrum laser Doppler interferometry as a diagnostic tool. Laryngoscope 2001; 111: 501–507

56 Konradsson K, Ivarsson A, Bank G. Computerized laser Doppler interferometric scanning of the vibrating tympanic membrane. Scand Audiol 1987; 16: 159–166

57 Huber A, Ball G, Asai M, Goode R. The vibration pattern of the tympanic membrane after placement of a total ossicular replacement prosthesis (TORP). Hüttenbrink K-B (ed). Middle ear mechanicks in research and otosurgery. Dresden: Dept of Oto-Rhino-Laryngology, Univ. Hospital, Univ. of Technology, 1997: 219–223

58 Tonndorf J, Khanna SM. Tympanic-membrane vibrations in human cadaver ears studied by time-averaged holography. J Acoust Soc Amer 1972; 52: 1221–1233

59 Helms J. Experimentelle und klinische Untersuchungen zur Funktion des normalen, erkrankten und operierten Trommelfells. Acta Otolaryngol 1977; 350: 1–59

60 Lokberg OJ, Hogmoen K, Gundersen T. Vibration measurement of the human tympanic membrane – in vivo. Acta Otolaryngol 1980; 89: 37–42

61 Guinan JJ, Peake WT. Middle-ear characteristics of anaesthetized cats. J Acoust Soc Am 1967; 41: 1237–1261

62 Cancura W, Stark H. Über die Schwingungsform des Steigbügels in Abhängigkeit von der Lautstärke. Experimentelle Untersuchungen am menschlichen Schläfenbeinpräparat. Arch Oto-Rhino-Laryng 1977; 215: 121–128

63 Heiland KE, Goode RL, Asai M, Huber AM. A human temporal bone study of stapes footplate movement. Am J Otol 1999; 20: 81–86

64 Huber A, Linder T, Ferrazzini M, Schmid S, Dillier N, Stoeckli S, Fisch U. Intraoperative assessment of stapes movement. Ann Otol Rhinol Laryngol 2001; 110: 31–35

65 Decraemer WF, Khanna SM, Funnell WR. Measurement and modelling of three-dimensional vibration of the stapes in cat. In: Wada H, Takasaka T, Ikeda K, Ohyama K, Koike T(eds). Recent developments in auditory mechanics. Sendai: World Scientific, 1999: 36–44

66 Dahmann D. Zur Physiologie des Hörens; experimentelle Untersuchungen über die Mechanik der Gehörknöchelkette sowie über deren Verhalten auf Ton und Luftdruck. Z f Hals-Nasen-Ohrenheilk 1930; 27: 329–368, 462–488

67 Barany E. A contribution to the physiology of bone conduction. Acta Otol Laryngol 1938; 26

68 Helmholtz H. Die Mechanik der Gehörknöchelchen und des Trommelfells. Pflügers Archiv Ges Physiol 1868; 1: 1–60

69 von Bekesy G. Experiments in hearing (Reprint). Huntington / NY: Robert E. Krieger Publ. Comp., 1960/1980

70 Wever Eg, Lawrence M. Physiological Acoustics. Princeton: Princeton University Press, 1954

71 Gyo K, Aritomo H, Goode RL. Measurement of the ossicular vibration ration in human temporal bones by use of a video measuring system. Acta Otolaryngol Stockh 1987; 103: 87–95

72 Decraemer WF, Khanna SM. Vibrations on the malleus measured through the ear canal. In: Hüttenbrink K-B (ed). Middle Ear Mechanichs in Research and Otosurgery. Dresden: Dept. of Oto-Rhino-Laryngology: Univ. Hospital, Univ of Technology, 1997: 32–39

73 Ball GR, Huber A, Goode RL. Scanning laser Doppler vibrometry of the middle ear ossicles. Ear Nose Throat J 1997; 76: 213–222

74 Huber A et al. Analysis of ossicular vibration in three dimensions. In: Hüttenbrink K-B (ed). Middle ear mechanics in research and otosurgery. Dresden: Dept. of Oto-Rhino-Laryngology: Univ. Hospital, Univ. of Technology, 1997: 82–87

75 Elpern BS, Greisen O, Andersen HC. Experimental studies on sound transmission in the human ear. VI: Clinical and experimental observations on non-otosclerotic ossicle fixation. Acta Otolaryngol 1965; 60: 223–230

76 Hudde H, Engel A. Measuring and modeling basic properties of the human middle ear and ear canal. Part III: Eardrum impedances, transfer functions and model calculations. Acustica & acta acustica 1998; 84: 1091–1109

77 Maassen MM, Zenner HP. Tympanoplasty typ 2 with ionomeric cement and titanium-gold-angle prostheses. Amer J Otol 1998; 19: 693–699

78 Hüttenbrink KB. Die Mechanik und Funktion des Mittelohres: Teil 1: Die Ossikelkette und die Mittelohrmuskeln. Laryngo-Rhino-Otol 1992; 71: 545–551

79 Fletcher JL, Riopelle AJ. Protective effect of the acoustic reflex for impulsive noises. J Acoust Soc Am 1960; 32: 401–404

80 Dallso P. The Auditory Periphery. Biophysics and Physiology. New York, London: Academic Press Inc., 1973

81 Elbrond O, Elpern BS. Reconstruction of ossicular chain in incus defects. Arch Otolaryngol 1965; 82: 603–608

82 Elbrond O, Elpern BS: Reconstruction of the ossicular chain. Arch Otolaryngol 1966; 84: 490–494

83 Elbrond O, Elpern BS. Rekonstruktion der Gehörknöchelchenkette. Experimentelle Untersuchungen. Mschr Ohrenheilkunde 1968; 102: 102–105

84 Cottle RD, Tonndorf J. Mechanical aspects of stapedial substitution. An experimental study. Arch Otolaryngol 1966; 83: 547–553

85 Kreutzer UA. Experimentelle Untersuchungen über die Mechanik der Gehörknöchelchenkette nach Tympanoplastik unter Berücksichtigung der Stapesfußplatte. Tübingen: Inaug. Diss., 1978

86 Hüttenbrink KB, Hudde H. Untersuchungen zur Schalleitung durch das rekonstruierte Mittelohr mit einem Hydrophon; erste Ergebnisse. HNO 1994; 42: 49–57

87 Rosowski JJ, Merchant SN. Mechanical and acoustic analysis of middle ear reconstruction. Am J Otol 1995; 16: 486–497

88 Williams KR, Blayney AW, Lesser THJ. A 3-D finite element analysis of the natural frequencies of vibration of a stapes prosthesis replacement reconstruction of the middle ear. Clin Otolaryngol 1995; 20: 36–44

89 Hüttenbrink K-B. Mechanical aspects of middle ear reconstruction. In: Hüttenbrink K-B (ed). Middle Ear Mechanics in Research and Otosurgery. Dresden: Dept. of Oto-Rhino-Laryngology: Univ. Hospital, Univ. of Technology, 1997: 165–169

90 Zahnert T, Schmidt R, Hüttenbrink K-B, Hardtke H-J. FE-Simulation of vibrations of the Dresden middle ear prosthesis. Hüttenbrink K-B (ed). Middle Ear Mechanics in Research and

Otosurgery. Dresden: Dept. of Oto-Rhino-Laryngology: Univ. Hospital, Univ. of Technology, 1997: 200–206

91 Asai M, Heiland KE, Huber AM, Goode RL. Evaluation of a cement incus replacement prosthesis in a temporal bone model. Acta Otolaryngol 1999; 119: 573–576

92 Asai M, Huber A, Goode RL. Analysis of the best site on the stapes footplate for ossicular chain reconstruction. Acta Otolaryngol 1999; 119: 356–361

93 Feenstra L, Vlaming MS. Laser interferometry with human temporal bones. Adv Oto-Rhino-Laryng 1987; 37: 36–38

94 Nishihara S, Goode R. Experimental study of the acoustic properties of incus replacement prostheses in a human temporal bone model. Am J Otol 1994; 15: 485–494

95 Gasn RZ, Wood MW, Dyer RK, Dormer KJ. Mass loading on the ossicles and middle ear function. Ann Otol Rhinol Laryngol 2001; 110: 478–485

96 Meister H, Walger M, Mickenhagen A, Stennert E. Messung der Schwingungschaften von Mittelohrimplantaten mit einem mechanischen Mittelohrmodell. HNO 1998; 46: 241–245

97 Tange RA, Brujin AJG, Grolman W. Experience with a new pure gold piston in stapedotomy for cases of otosclerosis. Auris Nasus Larynx 1998; 25: 249–253

98 Gjuric M, Schagerl S. Gold prostheses for ossiculoplasty. Am J Otol 1998; 19: 273–276

99 Stupp GH, Dalchow C, Grün D, Stupp HF, Wustrow J. Titan-Prothesen im Mottelohr. 3-Jahres-Erfahrungsbericht. Laryngo-Rhino-Otol 1999; 78: 299–303

100 Fisch U. Total reconstruction of the ossicular chain. Otolaryngol Clin N Amer 1994; 27: 785–797

101 Dyer Jr RK, Dormer KJ, Pineda M, Conley K, Saunders J, Dennis M. The hearing laser vibrometer. Initial clinical results. In: Rosowski JJ, Merchant SN (eds). Second International Symposium on Middle-Ear Mechanics in Research and Otosurgery. Boston, MA, USA. The Hague, The Netherlands: Kugler Publications, 2000: 383–397

102 Goode RL, Ball G, Nishihara S. Measurement of umbo vibration in human subjects – method and possible clinical applications. Am J Otol 1993; 14: 247–251

103 Goode RL, Ball G, Nishihara S, Nakamura K. Laser Doppler Vibrometer (LDV) – A new clinical tool for the otologist. Amer J Otol 1996; 17: 813–822

104 Merchant SN, Whittemore KR, Poon B, Lee C-Y, Rosowski JJ. Clinical measurements of tympanic membrane velocity using laser Doppler vibrometry. Preliminary results, methodological issues and potential applications. In: Rosowski JJ, Merchant SN (eds). Second International Symposium on Middle-Ear Mechanics in Research and Otosurgery. Boston, MA, USA. The Hague, The Netherlands: Kugler Publications, 2000; 367–381

105 Stasche N, Foth H-J, Hörmann K, Baker A, Huthoff C. Middle ear transmission disorders – tympanic membrane vibration analysis by laser-Doppler-vibrometry. Acta Otolaryngol (Stockh) 1994; 114: 59–63

106 Goode RL. Middle Ear Function, Biologic Variation, and Otosurgical Alchemy. Can we turn tin ears into gold? Arch Otolaryngol 1986; 112: 923–924

107 Ulfendahl M. Mechanical response of the mammalian cochlea. Progress Neurobiol 1997; 53: 331–380

108 Ruggero MA, Rich NC. Application of a commercially-manufactured Doppler-shift laser velocimeter to the measurement of basilar-membrane vibration. Hear Res 1991; 51: 215–230

109 Lynch TJ, Nedzelnitsky V, Peake WT. Input impedance of the cochlea in cat. J Acoust Soc Am 1982; 72: 108–131

110 Khanna SM, Figueroa LY. Need for noninvasive technique to measure cochlear responses. Acta Otolaryngol (Stockh) 1989; 467: 19–26

111 Hemmert W, Zenner HP, Gummer AW. Three-dimensional motion of the organ of Corti. Biophys J 2000; 78: 2285–2297

112 Robles L, Rugerro MA. Mechanics of Mammalian Cochlea. Physiological Reviews 2001; 81: 1305–1351

113 Khanna SM, Koester CJ, Willemin JF, Dändliker R, Rosskothen H. A noninvasive optical system for the study of the function of inner ear in living animals. Selected papers on coherence domain methods in biomedical optics. SPIE 2732.Tuchin V, 1996: 64–81

114 Khanna SM, Leonard DG. Basilar membrane tuning in the cat cochlea. Science 1982; 215: 305–306

115 Nuttal AL, Dolan DF, Avinash G. Laser Doppler velocimetry of basilar membrane vibration. Hear Res 1991; 51: 203–213

116 Cooper NP, Rhode WS. Basilar membrane mechanics in the hook region of the cat and guinea-pig cochleae: Sharp tuning and nonlinearity in the absence of baseline position shifts. Hear Res 1992; 63: 163–190

117 Rugerro MA, Robles L, Rich NC. Basilar membrane mechanics at the base of the chinchilla cochlea. 2. Response to low-frequency tones and relationship to microphonics and spike initiation in the 8. nerve. J Acoust Soc Am 1986; 80: 1375–1383

118 Xue S, Mountain DC, Hubbard AE. Direct measurement of electrically-evoked basilar membrane motion. In: Duifhuis H, Horst JW, van Dijk P, van Netten SM (ed). Biophysics of hair cell sensory system. Singapore: World Scientific Publishing Co., 1993: 361–369

119 ITER. Cellular vibration and motility in the organ of corti. Acta Otol Laryngol (Stockh) 1989; 467: 1–279

120 Khanna SM, Hao LF. Nonlinearity in the apical turn of living guinea pig cochlea. Hear Res 1999; 153: 89–104

121 Gummer AW, Hemmert W, Zenner HP. Resonant tectorial membrane motion in the inner ear: Its crucial role in frequency tuning. Proc Natl Acad Sci USA 1996; 93: 8727–8732

122 Rhode WS. Observations of the vibration of the basilar membrane in squirrel monkeys using the Mössbauer technique. J Acoust Soc Am 1971; 49: 1218–1231

123 Rhode WS. Some observations on cochlear mechanics. J Acoust Soc Am 1978; 67: 158–176

124 Sellick PM, Patuzzi R, Johnstone BM. Comparison between the tuning properties of inner hair cells and basilar membrane motion. Hear Res 1983; 10: 93–100

125 Janssen T. Schwellennahe und überschwellige Schallverarbeitung des Innenohres, Teil 1: Physiologie und Pathophysiologie. Z Audiol 2000; 39: 100–117

126 Cooper NP. An improved heterodyne laser interferometer for use in studies of cochlear mechanics. J Neurosci Meth 1999; 88: 93–102

127 Nuttall AL, Ren T, de Boer E, Zheng J, Parthasarathi A, Grosh K, Guo M, Dolan D. In vivo micromechanical measurements of the organ of Corti in the basal cochlear turn. Audiol Neurootol 2002; 7: 21–26

128 O'Neill MP, Bearden A. Laser-feedback measurements of turtle basilar membrane motion using direct reflection. Hear Res 1995; 84: 125–138

129 Rhode WS, Cooper NP. Two-tone suppression and distortion production on the basilar membrane in the hook region of cat and guinea pig cochleae. Hear Res 1993; 66: 31–45

130 Cooper NP, Rhode WS. Nonlinear mechanics at the apex of the guinea-pig cochlea. Hear Res 1995; 82: 225–243

131 Ulfendahl M, Khanna SM, Fridberger A, Flock A, Flock B, Jager W. Mechanical response characteristics of the hearing organ in the low-frquency regions of the cochlea. J Neurophysiol 1996; 76: 3850–3862

132 Zinn C, Maier H, Zenner HP, Gummer AW. Evidence for active, nonlivear, negative feedback in the vibration response of the apical region of the in-vivo guinea-pig cochlea. Hear Res 2000; 142: 159–183

133 Zenner HP. Hören: Physiologie, Biochemie, Zell- und Neurobiologie. Stuttgart, New York: Thieme, 1994

134 Khanna SM, Willemin JF, Ulfendahl M. Measurement of optical reflectivity in cells of the inner ear. Acta Otolaryngol Suppl 1989; 467: 69–75

135 Koester CJ, Khanna SM, Rosskohten HD, Takaberry RB. Incident light optional sectioning microscope for visualisation of cellular structures in the inner ear. Acta Otolaryngol Suppl 1989; 476: 27–33

136 Gummer AW, Hemmert W, Morioka I, Reis P, Reuter G, Henner HP. Cellular motility measured in guinea-pig cochlea. In: Duifhuis H, Horst JW, van Dijk P, van Netten SM (eds). Biophysics of Hair Cell Sensory Systems. Singapore: World Scientific Publishing Co., 1993: 229–239

137 Khanna SM, Ulfendahl M, Steele CR. Vibration of reflective beads on the basilar membrane. Hear Res 1998; 116: 71–85

138 Rhode WS. Cochlear mechanics. A Rev. Physiol 1984; 46: 231–246

139 Rugerro MA. Responses to sound of the basilar membrane of the mammalian cochlea. Curr Opin Neurobiol 1992; 2: 449–456

140 Barrett MD, Peterson EH, Grant JW. Extrinsic Fabry-Perot Interferometer for measuring the stiffness of ciliary bundles on hair cells. IEEE Trans Biomed Eng 1999; 46: 331–339

141 Li Z, Anvari B, Takashima M, Brecht P, Torres JH, Brownell WE. Membrane tether formation from outer hair cells with optical tweezers. Biophys J 2002; 82: 1386–1395

142 Yamada S, Wirtz D, Kuo SC. Mechanics of living cells measured by laser tracking microrheology. Biophys J 2000; 78: 1736–1747

Index